RECOVERY ROOM PRACTICE

Editor
ELIZABETH A.M. FROST, M.D.
Department of Anesthesiology
Albert Einstein College of Medicine

BLACKWELL SCIENTIFIC PUBLICATIONS, INC.
Boston Oxford London Edinburgh Melbourne Palo Alto

Blackwell Scientific Publications, Inc.
© 1985, by Blackwell Scientific Publications, Inc.
Printed in the United States of America
88 87 86 85 5 4 3 2 1

All rights reserved. No part of this book may be reproduced in any form or by any electronic or mechanical means, including information storage and retrieval systems, without permission in writing from the publisher, except by a reviewer who may quote brief passages in a review.

Library of Congress Cataloging in Publication Data

Main entry under title:
Recovery room practice.

Includes index.
1. Postoperative care.   2. Recovery room (Surgery)
I. Frost, Elizabeth A.M. [DNLM: 1. Postoperative Care—
nurses' instruction.   2. Recovery Room—nurses'
instruction.   3. Surgical Nursing. WY 154 R3116]
RD51.R283 1985   617'.919   84-14447
ISBN 0-86542-017-3

Blackwell Scientific Publications

Editorial Offices:
52 Beacon Street, Boston, Massachusetts 02108, USA
Osney Mead, Oxford OX2 0EL, England
8 John Street, London, WC1N 2ES, England
23 Ainslie Place, Edinburgh, EH3 6AJ, Scotland
107 Barry Street, Carlton, Victoria 3053, Australia
744 Cowper Street, Palo Alto, California 94301, USA

Distributors:
USA
  Blackwell Mosby Book Distributors
  11830 Westline Industrial Drive
  St. Louis, Missouri 63146

Canada
  Blackwell Mosby Book Distributors
  120 Melford Drive
  Scarborough, Ontario, M1B 2X4

Australia
  Blackwell Scientific Book Distributors, Pty., Ltd.
  31 Advantage Road
  Highett, Victoria 3190

Outside North America and Australia
  Blackwell Scientific Publications Ltd.
  Osney Mead
  Oxford OX2 0EL
  England

To my mother and father

Contents

Preface		xiii
Contributors		xv
Part I.	General Care	1
Chapter 1.	Admitting Assessment and Monitoring *Elizabeth A.M. Frost*	3
	Admission Assessment	4
	Monitoring	6
	Conclusion	10
	Suggestions for Further Reading	11
Chapter 2.	Treatment of Postoperative Pain *Cedric Prys-Roberts*	13
	Origin and Transmission of Pain Impulses	14
	Endogenous Opioids and Their Receptors	14
	Pharmacology of Opioids	16
	Pharmacology of Local Anesthetics	18
	Practical Aspects of Postoperative Pain Relief	19
	Treatment of Opioid Side Effects	23
	Regional and Local Anesthetics	25
	Suggestions for Further Reading	27
Chapter 3.	Respiration: Mechanical Ventilation and Oxygen Therapy *Elizabeth A.M. Frost*	29
	O_2 Failure	29
	CO_2 Failure	30
	Causes of Respiratory Dysfunction	32

vi CONTENTS

	Oxygen Therapy	36
	Respiratory Assistance	46
	Conclusion	50
	Suggestions for Further Reading	50
Chapter 4.	Cardiovascular Action: Too Much, Too Little, or Irregular *Cedric Prys-Roberts*	53
	Monitoring	53
	Cardiovascular Disturbances and Their Management	59
	Suggestions for Further Reading	69
Chapter 5.	Postanesthetic Fluid Management *Walter Backus and Jeffrey Askanazi*	71
	Normal Body Composition	71
	Normal Daily Balance	72
	Serum Electrolyte Concentrations	73
	Gastrointestinal Tract Losses	74
	Fluid and Electrolyte Changes in Injury	76
	Use of Colloid in Fluid Resuscitation	80
	Fluid and Electrolyte Requirements in Convalescence	80
	Clinical Evaluation of the Patient	81
	Suggestions for Further Reading	83
Chapter 6.	Why Is the Patient Not Awake Yet? *Elizabeth A.M. Frost*	87
	Prolonged Anesthetic Effect	87
	Drug Interaction	90
	Respiratory Insufficiency	92
	Cardiovascular Instability	95
	Thermoregulatory Dysfunction	96
	Fluid and Electrolyte Imbalance	96
	Allergic and Atypical Drug Reaction	98
	Intraoperative Catastrophe	98
	Suggestions for Further Reading	101
Chapter 7.	Criteria for Discharge *Marilyn Schneider*	103
	JCAH	103
	ASA	104
	ASPAN	104
	Numerical Scoring Systems	105

	Discharge by Anesthesiologist	109
	Discharge Criteria	111
	Discharge (Transfer) of Patients from PACU	115
	Summary	117
	Suggestions for Further Reading	117
Part II.	Patients Who Require Special Consideration	119
Chapter 8.	Children in the Recovery Room *Nirmala Balan*	121
	Differences between Children and Adults	121
	Transfer from the Operating Room to the Recovery Room	125
	Monitoring	126
	Respiratory Complications	126
	Special Circumstances	131
	Respiratory Support	132
	Pain and Agitation	133
	Temperature Regulation	135
	Fluid Replacement	137
	Drug Dosages	140
	Special Situations	142
	Suggestions for Further Reading	147
Chapter 9.	Postoperative Care of Neurosurgical Patients *Somasundaram Thiagarajah*	149
	Pathophysiology	151
	Monitoring	152
	Intracranial Pressure	152
	Respiratory System	160
	Cardiovascular System	161
	Temperature	164
	Fluid and Electrolytes	164
	Seizures	164
	Restlessness and Pain	164
	Spinal Column Surgery	165
	Suggestions for Further Reading	167
Chapter 10.	Recovery from Regional Anesthetic Techniques *Richard B. Lilly, Jr.*	169
	General Considerations after Regional Anesthesia	169
	Local Anesthetic Toxicity	170
	Pneumothorax	173
	Sympathetic Nervous System Blockade	174

	Spinal and Epidural Anesthesia	176
	Suggestions for Further Reading	182

Chapter 11. **Recovery Room Care of the Patient with Renal Disease** — 183
Rhoda D. Levine

- Chronic Renal Disease — 183
- Renal Failure in the Patient with Previously Normal Renal Function — 191
- Renal Transplants — 196
- Suggestions for Further Reading — 196

Chapter 12. **Recovery Room Care after Intrathoracic Surgery** — 199
Patricia Hartwell

- Lobectomy — 201
- Pneumonectomy — 205
- Pericardial Window — 206
- Mediastinoscopy and Bronchoscopy — 207
- Thymectomy — 207
- Cardiac Surgery — 208
- Summary — 208
- Suggestions for Further Reading — 208

Chapter 13. **The Recovery Room as an Ambulatory and Special Procedures Unit** — 211
Elizabeth A.M. Frost

- Ambulatory Surgery — 212
- Special Procedures — 213
- Legal Issues — 223
- Suggestions for Further Reading — 224

Chapter 14. **Cardiopulmonary Arrest** — 225
Marcelle M. Willock

- Airway — 225
- Breathing — 226
- Circulation — 227
- Intravenous Fluids — 229
- Drug Therapy — 229
- Dysrhythmia — 231
- Defibrillators — 234
- Postresuscitation Management — 237
- Equipment — 238
- Summary — 239
- Suggestions for Further Reading — 239

Chapter 15.	Criteria for Establishment of Brain Death *Ashok Kumar*	241
	Brain Stem Death	242
	Protocols	244
	Legal and International Status of Brain Death	247
	Suggestions for Further Reading	247
Part III.	Administration	249
Chapter 16.	Planning the Physical Structure of the Recovery Room *Margaret DeFranco*	251
	General Physical Considerations	252
	Location of Equipment and Supplies	256
	Sensory Deprivation	262
	Sensory Bombardment	262
	Individual Patient Care Units	263
	Proximity of Support Services and Facilities	264
	Infection Control	266
	Fire Regulations and Codes	267
	Conclusion	269
	Suggestions for Further Reading	269
Chapter 17.	Nursing Requirements in the Recovery Room *Karen D. Spadaccia*	271
	Position Requirements	271
	Staffing Patterns	274
	Documentation	274
	Nursing Standards of Care	278
	Quality Assurance Programs	281
	Summary	281
	Suggestions for Further Reading	282
Chapter 18.	Educational Program for Recovery Room Personnel *Dorothy M. Williams*	285
	Role and Responsibilities of the Clinical Instructor	285
	Preceptor Selection and Training	286
	Weekly Orientation Outline for Preceptor Program	287
	Suggestions for Further Reading	291
Chapter 19.	A Role for the Recovery Room Nurse in the Wards *Ann Marie Terra*	293

CONTENTS

	Holistic Nursing	293
	Pediatric Patients	300
	Ambulatory Patients	301
	Summary	301
	Suggestions for Further Reading	302
Chapter 20.	Liabilities of the Recovery Room Team *Stephanie Putkowski*	303
	Malpractice	303
	Nursing Liability	305
	Suggestions for Further Reading	309

Part IV. Appendices — 311

Appendix 1. Guidelines for Blood Component Therapy — 313

Appendix 2. Postanesthetic Recovery Score — 317
J.A. Aldrete

Appendix 3. Nursing Care Standard: Care of the Patient in the Recovery Room — 319

Appendix 4. Orientation Checklist — 323

Appendix 5. Abbreviations, Normal Values, Conversion Factors, and Blood Gas and Acid-Base Analyses — 331

Appendix 6. American Heart Association Advanced Cardiac Life Support—Algorithms for Cardiac Dysrhythmias—Adult — 339

Appendix 7. American Heart Association Cardiopulmonary Resuscitation and Emergency Cardiac Care Rationale for One Rescuer CPR (Heartsaver) — 350

Appendix 8. American Heart Association Cardiopulmonary Resuscitation and Emergency Cardiac Care Rationale for One and Two Rescuer CPR — 352

Appendix 9. American Heart Association Cardiopulmonary Resuscitation and Emergency Cardiac Care Rationale For Complete Obstruction—Conscious Choking Infant — 354

CONTENTS   xi

Appendix 10.   American Heart Association Cardiopulmonary   356
               Resuscitation and Emergency Cardiac Care
               Rationale for Infant Resuscitation

Appendix 11.   American Heart Association Cardiopulmonary   358
               Resuscitation and Emergency Cardiac Care
               Rationale For Infant Obstructed Airway—
               Choking Infant Who Becomes Unconscious
               or Is Found Unconscious

Part V.   Multiple-Choice Questions and Answers   361

Index   399

Preface

Refinements in anesthetic and surgical techniques permit the successful undertaking of many more and complicated operative procedures. Disease processes considered in the recent past to be either too advanced or not amenable to surgical intervention are now encountered daily in the operating room suite. Optimal outcome depends not only on precise intraoperative monitoring and prompt, appropriate action but uninterrupted maintenance of this care well into the recovery period.

All too often, the surgeon and anesthesiologist, required by tight scheduling to return immediately to the operating room, must leave the patient semiconscious and in critical condition in the recovery room. Slight changes in vital signs may develop at any time and forewarn of the development of serious complications. Thus, in this area, perhaps more than in any other part of the hospital, a clear understanding of the underlying pathophysiology of the postoperative period and the ability to recognize and avert any physical deterioration can prevent disaster and help to ensure a good outcome.

The importance of the role of the recovery room nurse in the care of the surgical patient cannot be overemphasized. She (and increasingly by now, he) must be able to assess promptly the status of the patient just returned from the operating room; quickly and accurately take several measurements and act appropriately; deal with problems related to a new pain, anxiety, and fear; maintain a clear and accurate record; make sense of the many orders, which are occasionally conflicting, if several specialties are involved; and assist in minor procedures. All this must often be done under intense pressure as several patients are admitted or discharged simultaneously.

Recognition of the unique skills required by recovery room personnel has spurred the development of new organizations. At both the national and state levels, recovery room nurses have joined to form associations dedicated to defining standards and providing forums for education and exchange of ideas. There is no doubt that recovery room nursing is a recognized, indeed an essential entity within the nursing profession.

This basic textbook, divided into three parts, is intended mainly for nurses and other personnel in the recovery room. The contributors are clinical anesthesiologists and nurses who have been instrumental in underscoring the necessity for impeccable postoperative care. The first part deals with basic and specialized nursing requirements in the recovery room and current management of acute surgical pain. An understanding of available equipment for respiratory therapy is essential in the daily activity of the recovery room nurse as is a precise knowledge of appropriate fluid management. Generally, the nurse determines when discharge from the recovery room is appropriate, and the rigorous standards which must be met are detailed. Patients requiring special attention such as children, outpatients, neurosurgical and chest cases, those who were operated under regional techniques, and those with kidney disease are considered in the second part. A review of the management of cardiopulmonary arrest is included, again because recovery room nursing is characterized by prompt action in the event of emergency.

The third part, on administration, is concerned with the physical structure of the recovery room and nursing and educational requirements. The final chapter, written by a patient advocate, defines the legal considerations which are involved in nursing care.

As obstetrical patients and those who have undergone open heart procedures are usually nursed in other areas, these two groups of patients have not been considered.

As a means of self-evaluation, questions, grouped by chapter, are included at the end of the book.

Countrywide, there are great differences in the patient requirements, staffing, and physical structure of recovery rooms. Contributors have based their experience on working in both academic and private practice settings and in large university and small community hospitals. It is our hope, therefore, that those who read this book will find some common ground and standards that can be applied to their specific setting.

Contributors

Jeffrey Askanazi, M.D.
Department of Anesthesiology
Columbia University
College of Physicians and Surgeons
630 West 168th Street
New York, NY 10032

Walter Backus, M.D.
Department of Anesthesiology
Columbia University
College of Physicians and Surgeons
630 West 168th Street
New York, NY 10032

Nirmala Balan, M.D.
Department of Anesthesiology
Albert Einstein College of Medicine
Bronx, NY 10461

Margaret De Franco, R.N.
5066 East Henrietta Road
Henrietta, NY 14467

Elizabeth A.M. Frost, M.D.
Department of Anesthesiology
Albert Einstein College of Medicine
Bronx, NY 10461

Patricia Hartwell, M.D.
Department of Anesthesiology
Albert Einstein College of Medicine
Bronx, NY 10461

Ashok Kumar, M.D.
Department of Anesthesiology
Albert Einstein College of Medicine
Bronx, NY 10461

Rhoda D. Levine, M.D.
Department of Anesthesiology
Albert Einstein College of Medicine
Bronx, NY 10461

Richard B. Lilly, Jr., M.D.
Attending Anesthesiologist
Hartford Hospital
80 Seymour Street
Hartford, CT 06511

Cedric Prys-Roberts, M.A., D.M.,
   Ph.D., F.F.A.R.C.S.
Department of Anaesthetics
Royal Infirmary
Bristol, England

Stefanie Putkowski, R.N.
Risk Control Coordinator
1348 Midland Avenue, Apt. 4-K
Bronxville, NY

Marilyn Schneider, R.N.
Assistant Clinical Supervisor
Post Anesthesia Care Unit
Doctor's Hospital of Prince
   George's County
8118 Good Luck Road
Lanham, MD 20801

Karen D. Spadaccia, R.N.
Staff Development Instructor
P.O. Box 195
Loundsburg Drive
Baldwin Place, NY 10505

Ann Marie Terra, R.N.
1662 Crescent Drive
Thiells, NY 10989

Somasundaram Thiagarajah
Beth Israel Medical Center
Nathan D. Pearlman Place
New York, NY 10003

Dorothy M. Williams, R.N.
Recovery Room
Sloan Kettering Memorial Hospital
1275 York Avenue
New York, NY 10021

Marcelle Willock, M.D.
Department of Anesthesia
University Hospital
75 East Newton Street
Boston, MA 02118

I
GENERAL CARE

1
Admitting Assessment and Monitoring
Elizabeth A. M. Frost

All patients who have received a general or regional anesthetic should be nursed in the recovery room until the anesthetic effect is sufficiently reversed. The anesthesiologist or physician in charge of the recovery room determines which patients shall be admitted.

Obstetrical units usually have separate recovery areas and generally only use the main postanesthetic recovery room (PARR) under emergency situations or use separate areas of that room.

Occasionally patients may be transferred directly from the operating room to the ward if:

1. Local anesthesia only was used and the patient's condition is stable.
2. The patient is an infection risk and no isolation area is available.
3. There is an intensive care unit specially designed for particular care (e.g., after cardiac surgery or for premature care).
4. By agreement with the surgeon and anesthesiologist, the patient wishes to make arrangements for special care in the wards.

If the patient is to be returned directly to his room postoperatively, it is essential that the standards of ward nursing care during this period equal those pertaining to the PARR.

The main functions of the PARR nurse are:

1. to promptly recognize and treat respiratory problems
2. to maintain stability of the cardiovascular system
3. to monitor for hemorrhage
4. to adequately and safely treat postoperative pain

ADMISSION ASSESSMENT

The recovery room and operating room should be in close proximity. Five minutes transfer time is a maximum safe limit. Two individuals must accompany the patient during transfer, one of whom must be part of the anesthesia care team. Availability of adequate monitoring, oxygen, and all resuscitative measures is recommended during transportation of any patient whose consciousness is impaired.

The basic information that the anesthesiologist should give the nurse for admission assessment includes:

1. Brief personal history: diagnosis, name, age, sex, native language, physical impairments (e.g., deaf, blind)
2. Surgical procedure: operation performed, surgeon involved, surgical complications
3. Anesthetic technique: anesthesiologist of record, agents, dosages, drug reversal, complications, estimated time to return of consciousness or reversal of regional block
4. Intraoperative course: vital signs, fluid balance
5. Relevant medical history: maintenance medications, allergies, previous hospitalizations and illnesses
6. Anticipated problems

On accepting the patient to the PARR, a short form can be inserted or rubber stamped in the medical record (Figure 1-1). Recovery room orders are either included on a routine form or may be written by the surgeon or anesthesiologist (Figure 1-2).

Recovery Room Admission

Vital Signs: temperature _____ BP _____ PR _____ RR _____
Anesthesia: regional _____ general _____ other _____
Regional: level of analgesia _____
General: unresponsive _____ drowsy _____ awake _____
           airway oral _____ nasal _____ none _____
           endotracheal tube _____ tracheostomy _____

Figure 1-1. Short form which the recovery room nurse may complete to record patient data at time of admission. BP = blood pressure; PR = pulse rate; RR = respiratory rate.

Routine Recovery Room Orders

1. O₂ administration: Give O_2@ _____ 1./min. _____ mask _____ cannula
2. Vital signs q 15 minutes
3. Endotracheal tube care
   a. Suction p.r.n.
   b. Administer O_2 mist/T tube @ _____ %
   c. May be extubated when PARR written scoring criteria are met
   d. Obtain ABGs _____ minutes following admission to unit
4. Continue operating room IV _____ unless otherwise ordered by surgeon
5. Cardiac monitor _____ Yes _____ No
6. Medications
   a. Atropine 0.5-1 mg IV bolus if cardiac rate is less than _____
   b. Lidocaine 50 mg IV bolus stat for development of PVCs 6 per minute Ventricular tachycardia or bigeminy: call anesthesiologist.
   c. _____ IV for pain
7. Notify anesthesiologist if:
   Blood pressure _____ or _____
   Respiration _____ or _____
   Heart rate _____ or _____

Figure 1-2. Postoperative orders to be completed by anesthesiologist in consultation with the recovery room nurse.

Assessment of recovery from anesthesia may be made by applying the Aldrete score, which is based on the Apgar score. The range is 10 for complete recovery to 0 in comatose patients. The five categories of evaluation in the postanesthetic recovery score (PARS) are

1. Activity
   Voluntary movement of all limbs to command 2
   Voluntary movement of 2 extremities to command 1
   Unable to move 0
2. Respiration
   Breathe deeply and cough 2
   Dyspnea, hypoventilation 1
   Apneic 0
3. Circulation
   Blood pressure   20 percent of preanesthetic level 2
   Blood pressure   20-50 percent of preanesthetic level . 1
   Blood pressure   50 percent of preanesthetic level 0

4. Consciousness
   - Fully awake — 2
   - Arousable — 1
   - Unresponsive — 0
5. Color
   - Pink — 2
   - Pale, blotchy — 1
   - Cyanotic — 0

The score should be recorded on admission and at 15- to 30-minute intervals to document improvement or deterioration. Limitations of the score are clear when patients receive 10 but have oliguria or are severely nauseated or actually vomiting or have developed cardiac arrhythmias.

The patient's status should be judged by the nurse and anesthesiologist immediately upon arrival in the PARR and at a minimum of 15-minute intervals until discharge. Documentation is essential.

MONITORING

The anesthesiologist should review with the nurse the patient functions that have been monitored and should indicate which areas require further observation. Respiratory, cardiovascular, neuromuscular, thermoregulatory, and renal systems, in addition to state of consciousness and fluid and electrolyte balance, are routinely measured in the recovery room.

Respiratory System

Common measurements of respiratory function are listed in Table 1-1. Good, careful auscultation is irreplaceable in the initial assessment of adequate respiration. Rate should be recorded on admission and at 15-minute intervals. Respiratory pattern, which normally has a regular inspiratory to expiratory ratio of 1:3, should be noted. Abnormalities such as phasic variations (Cheyne-Stokes respiration), use of accessory muscles, diaphragmatic breathing, and sternal retraction indicate excess anesthetic effect, neurologic complications, or obstruction. Prompt therapy requires reestablishment of an adequate airway which may mean simply supporting the chin, insertion of an oral or nasal airway, or may require reintubation and assisted ventilation. The anesthesiologist and surgeon should be notified.

Tidal volume should be measured if the endotracheal tube is still in place or if any difficulty is suspected. Minute ventilation (normally about 5 to 6 liters) is obtained by multiplying respiratory rate by tidal volume.

Table 1-1. Common Indicators Used to Assess Respiratory Function in the Recovery Room

Indicator	Normal Range
1. Auscultation	bilaterally equal
2. Rate	10-35/min
3. Pattern	regular
4. Tidal volume	4-5 ml/kg
5. Vital capacity	20-40 ml/kg
6. Inspiratory force	-40 cm H_2O
7. Arterial blood gases at 30% O_2	PaO_2 100 mm Hg $PaCO_2$ 35-45 mm Hg

Vital capacity measurement is particularly valuable as it indicates the patient's ability to respond to commands, the adequacy of respiratory drive, and the coordination of the chest wall and lung mechanics.

Inspiratory force is obtained by connecting a manometer through a one-way valve to the endotracheal tube or to a close-fitting mask. The airway is thus temporarily blocked so the force generated is negative. Values of -40 cm H_2O are necessary to cough effectively and prevent atelectasis.

Probably the best measurement of the adequacy of ventilation is obtained from blood gas analyses. Accurate interpretation must take the inspired oxygen concentration into consideration.

Cardiovascular System

In assessing the adequacy of the circulation, blood pressure, pulse, and heart sounds are monitored. Blood pressure variations up or down of more than 25 percent of preoperative values should be reported to the physician. The quality of the pulse and heart sounds decreases with myocardial depression.

Continuous electrocardiographic recording coupled with a writer to obtain a permanent record as necessary should be a routine for all patients. Not only does this monitor afford a visual and auditory indication of rate and rhythm, but it may indicate hypoxia of cardiac muscle if the ST segment is deflected more than 1 mm from baseline. Any arrhythmia should be noted and reported to the physician. Electrolyte abnormalities (especially potassium) may cause wave changes (e.g., T wave) although serum estimations of such changes are more accurate.

GENERAL CARE

Central venous pressure gives an indication of volume status and myocardial function. An upward or downward trend is of far greater significance than single values. Increasingly, pulmonary artery and pulmonary capillary wedge pressures and cardiac output are now measured perioperatively through a flow-directed balloon catheter. Normal values for cardiac measurements are listed in Table 1-2.

Neuromuscular Transmission

Two types of neuromuscular blockade can persist into the recovery period. Pattern 1 is phase 1 block or depolarizing block and is produced by succinylcholine. Using a nerve stimulator, it is characterized by sustained tetanus, equal train-of-four responses, and no posttetanic potentiation. Phase 2 block develops after prolonged use of succinylcholine or as a residual effect of nondepolarizing relaxants (e.g., d-tubocurarine, pancuronium, metocurine). It is associated with tetanic fade, fade of train-of-four responses, and posttetanic potentiation. While there is no specific antidote for phase 1 block, which usually resolves quickly, phase 2 block may be reversed with anticholinesterase drugs such as edrophonium, neostigmine, or pyridostigmine.

Tests for residual nondepolarizing block include assessing the patient's ability to lift his head, open his eyes, grasp a hand, and extrude his tongue. Factors that may prolong neuromuscular blockade include acidosis, hypothermia, inhalation anesthetic agents (especially isoflurane), antibiotics (except penicillin G, cephradine, and cephaloridine), hypermagnesemia,

Table 1-2. Approximate Range for Cardiac Measurements Obtained in the Recovery Room

Measure	Normal Range
Pulse	55–120/min
Blood pressure	$\frac{90}{50} - \frac{160}{100}$ mm Hg
Central venous pressure	3–8 mm Hg
Right atrial pressure	1–6 mm Hg
Right ventricular pressure	$\frac{20}{0} - \frac{30}{5}$ mm Hg
Pulmonary artery pressure	$\frac{20}{8} - \frac{30}{12}$ mm Hg
Pulmonary capillary pressure	4–12 mm Hg
Cardiac output	4–8 liters/min
Cardiac index (cardiac output/body surface area)	2.5–3.5 liters/min/m^2

hypocalcemia, renal failure (especially with metocurine and pancuronium), and furosemide.

Temperature

Intraoperatively, temperature is altered by administration of cold fluids, exposure of both the interior and exterior of the body to a cool environment, and obtunding of the thermoregulatory center by anesthetic agents. Many anesthetics cause vasodilation with further heat loss, which is particularly problematic in children. Hypothermia of itself may be protective by decreasing oxygen demand. However, if rebound shivering occurs, oxygen consumption may increase by 400 percent, which may cause a hypoxic state, critical to patients with cardiac or cerebrovascular disease.

Oral recordings are influenced by the temperature of exhaled gases. The rectal temperature is an indicator of core temperature and only changes slowly in relation to other parts of the body. Esophageal temperature, although a good indicator of average body temperature, is usually not feasible in the awake or semiconscious patient. A ceramic bead placed in the tympanic membrane measures the temperature closest to the hypothalamus or thermoregulatory center. Axillary temperature should be used only as a rough indication and is of more value if trends are recorded. Skin temperature is valuable only in very small infants or in assessing continued circulation to a limb at risk of vascular occlusion.

Renal Function

Urinary volume is the most commonly recorded estimate of adequate renal function. However, as discussed in Chapter 11, this is only one of many predictors of an intact urinary system. Other measurements include specific gravity, electrolytes, and osmolality.

Level of Consciousness

Cerebral function is estimated postoperatively by the patient's state of awareness. Several scoring systems (Aldrete, Apgar, Carignan, and Glasgow coma scale) developed for different situations depend on estimations from clinical observations (respiration, eye opening, response to command and motor function).

If coma persists, an overall pattern of cerebral function may be recorded by the electroencephalograph. Regional recordings may indicate abnormal foci. In selected patients, intracranial pressure monitoring and computing of cerebral perfusion pressure (mean systemic arterial pressure minus intracranial pressure) may be indicated.

Pupillary reflexes in response to light should be monitored and the change in each eye recorded for all neurosurgical patients. The absence of clonus in the ankles after spinal operations may be a sign of trauma or surgical injury to the cord. Monitoring of brain and spinal evoked potentials during the recovery phase, although not yet a routine technique, may well become generally available in the near future.

Fluid and Electrolyte Balance

Fluid balance is frequently assessed most accurately first in the recovery room. After considerable loss and replacement, the relative stability of the postoperative period allows time to compute the patient's fluid volume status — a task which often falls to the nurse. It is extremely important to record both input and output in the recovery phase and equate these volumes with the intraoperative fluid shifts.

Electrolyte determination in the postoperative period is generally done by laboratory analysis, although the capability for on-line measurement exists. Indications for early and possibly repeated electrolyte analyses postoperatively include:

1. Major physiologic fluid loss (diarrhea, vomiting)
2. Administration of large fluid volumes (burns, transurethral resection of the prostate)
3. Bowel surgery (resection of obstructed large bowel)
4. Patients with preoperative electrolyte abnormalities (chronic diuretic administration, hypothalamic disturbances)

Glucose is easily measured at the bedside. Dextrostix determinations are simple and give a qualitative estimate of the need for emergency therapy or more accurate laboratory analysis.

CONCLUSION

The close monitoring afforded the patient in the operating room must be continued into the recovery room and individualized according to the needs of the patient.

Noninvasive techniques are preferable as the invasive approach carries the potential for infection. The computer age allows an almost limitless ability to assemble data. However, the objective of monitoring — to ensure a safe and smooth postoperative course — must be remembered. It is as important to look at the patient as it is to survey the numbers.

SUGGESTIONS FOR FURTHER READING

Aldrete JA, Kronlik D. A postanesthetic recovery score. Anesth Analg 1970; 49:924-933.

Carignan G, Keeri-Szanto M, Lavellie JP. Post anesthetic scoring system. Anesthesiology 1964; 25:396-397.

Cullen DJ. Recovery room care of the surgical patient. In: Refresher courses in anesthesiology. Vol 8. SG Hershey, ed. Philadelphia: Lippincott, 1980.

Fischer TL. Responsibility for care in recovery rooms. Can Med Assoc J 1970; 102: 78-79.

Teasdale G, Jennett B. Assessment of coma and impaired consciousness: A practical scale. Lancet 1974; 2:81-83.

2
Treatment of Postoperative Pain
Cedric Prys-Roberts

Pain is an almost inevitable consequence of surgery. Pain is a fiction; that is, as a subjective experience it can only be described qualitatively and cannot be quantified. The severity of pain following surgery varies with the perception of the individual and the nature of the injury. Relief of postoperative pain must therefore be directed at the needs of each individual. Traditional approaches to pain relief are inadequate: physicians tend to write inadequate orders, nurses tend to misinterpret these orders, and both underestimate the variety of patient requirements.

Not only does the severity and duration of pain differ from one surgical site to another, the consequences of pain also differ. Pain from the extremities, however severe, does not interfere with breathing, but the pain from upper abdominal and thoracic surgery limits the ability of the patient to breathe deeply and to cough effectively. Both these limitations contribute to the higher morbidity and mortality associated with major surgery. Adequate and continuous relief of such pain undoubtedly influences the quality and speed of postoperative recovery. By contrast, pain from lower abdominal incisions, especially from transverse rather than vertical incisions, causes less morbidity than that from upper abdominal surgery.

Muscle spasm, which may be considered a protective mechanism to restrict movement of an injured site, also contributes to the severity of postoperative pain. The relief of muscle spasm may in itself improve the comfort of a patient. Most severe postoperative pain is triggered by movement, and provided such movement can be restricted without compromise to other causes of morbidity, this too can relieve pain. Positioning of the patient is also important in order to avoid placing incisions or operated sites under tension or pressure.

ORIGIN AND TRANSMISSION OF PAIN IMPULSES

Three types of receptor are recognized in most tissues: mechanoreceptors, thermoreceptors, and nociceptors. There is also evidence of specific visceral and muscle nociceptors. Action potentials generated in these receptors are transmitted by two classes of nerve fiber to the posterior columns of the spinal cord.

Two types of pain are recognized. The sharp, transient, pricking pain associated with skin trauma is classified as fast pain, as it is transmitted by myelinated Aδ fibers (1-5 μm in diameter). The more prolonged and unpleasant burning pain, classified as slow pain, which results from tissue damage, is mediated by unmyelinated C nerve fibers (0.5-1.0 μm). Visceral pain and pain from deep somatic structures is also mediated through unmyelinated C nerve fibers and is characteristically difficult to localize and associated with autonomic disturbances, especially nausea. The Aδ fibers project centrally through the neospinothalmic tracts to the thalamic nuclei which project directly to the cortex. The unmyelinated C fibers, which are predominant in the peripheral nerves, synapse in the substantia gelatinosa of the dorsal horn. The ensuing neurons cross the midline and continue to the paleospinothalmic tract to the thalamus.

Numerous other fibers converge in the substantia gelatinosa, both descending fibers and collateral fibers (Lissauer's tract), all of which can modulate the transmission of impulses in the pain pathway. The general concept of a neuronal gate, as described by Melzak and Wall in their gate-control theory, is relevant to this area of the spinal cord. There are numerous synapses in the various pain pathways, each of which involves at least one chemical transmitter. These transmitters have not been specifically localized to individual synapses, but over the past 6 years a number of endogenous peptides having opioid characteristics have been identified.

ENDOGENOUS OPIOIDS AND THEIR RECEPTORS

Three types of endogenous peptides have been identified and classified according to the gene sequences which lead to their synthesis (Table 2-1). *Encephalins* are short-chain peptides, based on a five amino acid chain (TYR-GLY-GLY-PHE-LEU, or -MET), which are widely distributed throughout the central nervous system in association with short neurons. *Beta-endorphins* are long-chain peptides found only in the arcuate nucleus of the hypothalamus and its neuronal projections. *Dynorphins* are the most recently volume of distribution and a slow clearance from the body. Lidocaine and mepivacaine are much less lipophilic than bupivacaine and are more rapidly eliminated from the plasma.

These pharmacokinetic qualities are also important in determining the mode of action of the drug at the site of neural blockade. When lidocaine is injected close to a nerve, little of the drug is absorbed into the lipoprotein structure of the nerve sheath, and most of the drug is available for producing the membrane-stabilizing effect at the nodes of Ranvier. When lidocaine is injected into the epidural space, little of the drug is taken up by the fat depots within the space, and most of the drug is available at the active site and for uptake into the epidural veins and transport to the liver. Thus the onset of action is rapid and the duration is short, unless epinephrine is used to minimize the uptake of the drug into the bloodstream. By contrast, bupivacaine injected in the epidural space is rapidly taken up into lipid stores, either in the epidural space or in the nerve sheaths, and the onset of neural blockade is delayed and the duration of blockade extended. Epinephrine as a local vasoconstrictor has little effect on the onset or duration of blockade. To maintain blockade, bupivacaine should be given in a high concentration (0.5-0.75 percent) initially, to saturate the lipid stores of the epidural region, and thereafter as an infusion of lower concentration (0.125 percent). This approach ensures the most rapid onset of blockade and prevents a waning of the block. The least efficient but sadly, the most common, way of using bupivacaine is to wait until the effect of the initial block has finished before injecting a further dose.

PRACTICAL ASPECTS OF POSTOPERATIVE PAIN RELIEF

Postoperative pain relief should be planned at the preoperative visit and should be carefully adjusted to take account of the patient's age and constitution, the site of surgery, and the availability of recovery room and subsequent care. Use of opioids as part of premedication and intraoperative medication influences the subsequent use of these drugs postoperatively. Combinations of opioid with local anesthetic techniques must also be planned. The influence of general anesthetics and benzodiazepines, which also depress ventilation, must be borne in mind when predicting the appropriate dose of opioids postoperatively.

Postoperative Administration of Opioids

The ideal objective in the use of opioids for postoperative pain relief is to produce the highest and most constant concentration at opioid receptors consistent with adequate ventilation. It is adequacy of ventilation that finally determines the safety of any method. By employing either the intrathecal or epidural approach, *appropriate* opioids can attain the spinal opioid receptors with minimal distribution to other tissues. Parenteral administration of opioids can only achieve the appropriate concentration at spinal receptors by perfusion through the bloodstream. Thus the attainment of a stable plasma concentration is best achieved by giving a continuous infusion of the drug or by frequent injections of small doses.

Routes of Administration

Sublingual

Buprenorphine (0.2-0.4 mg) provides adequate analgesia for moderate postoperative pain. Absorption is rapid, and the effect is prolonged because buprenorphine has a strong affinity to opioid receptors.

Intramuscular

Most opioids can be administered intermittently by this route, which allows rapid onset and predictable effects. This route should be avoided in hypovolemic hypotensive patients in whom cardiac output and muscle perfusion may be impaired. For the management of severe postoperative pain, morphine (0.15 mg/kg) or meperidine (1.5 mg/kg) are the most suitable drugs for administration by this route. The disadvantage of this route is that the doses normally used are too low to provide adequate pain relief and too intermittent to sustain it.

Subcutaneous

Morphine can be administered by a continuous infusion of 1-2 mg per hour together with hyaluronidase to provide excellent relief of pain. The drug can be administered through a 20-gm teflon cannula placed in a suitable subcutaneous site such as the lateral aspect of the thigh or the deltopectoral region. Each infusion site can be used for 24 to 36 hours. The drug can be delivered either by an infusion pump or by a burette system. The total drug dose per 24 hours should be comparable with that accumulated by intermittent intramuscular injections.

Intravenous

The main advantage of the intravenous route for administration of opioid drugs is that the distribution phase is relatively short (5 to 10 minutes); thus, repeated small doses can be given at 10-minute intervals until either the desired degree of analgesia is achieved, or the slowing of breathing (to less than 10 breaths per minute) limits further dosage. Morphine should be given in 1-2-mg increments, meperidine in 10-15-mg increments.

Intravenous Infusion

By using infusion regimes designed to achieve a stable plasma concentration of narcotic analgesic in the shortest possible time, the maximal degree of analgesia consistent with acceptable ventilatory depression can be maintained for long periods of time. The most suitable agents for intravenous infusion are those which have a rapid clearance ($>$ 1000 ml per minute) and a short elimination half-life. Morphine, meperidine, and fentanyl have been used in this context, but most clinical reports give little more than dose-infusion rates and indications of the adequacy of pain relief.

Morphine diluted to 0.2 mg/ml can be infused at a rate of 12.5 ml per hour, but the infusion rate could be halved, or doubled, to meet the requirements of individual patients. This regime would allow a daily dose of 60 mg, which is equivalent to 10 mg administered regularly at 4-hour intervals. Meperidine diluted to 2 mg/ml can also be infused at the same rate (12.5 ml per hour) to provide a similar degree of analgesia. Infusion of either of these drugs should be preceded by a bolus injection equivalent to 1 hour's requirement.

Fentanyl administered as a bolus of 5 μg/kg at the commencement of anesthesia and followed by an infusion of 3 μg/kg per hour during and after anesthesia produces consistent plasma concentrations of 2.7 ± 0.3 ng/ml. Such an infusion is compatible with depression of CO_2 responsiveness to about 50 percent of the patient's preoperative awake value. This is the limit of acceptable ventilatory depression in that $PaCO_2$ levels of 44-46 mm Hg are achieved. Such limits must be regarded as the measured upper limits of safety, and in clinical practice an infusion rate of 2 μg/kg per hour may be considered as providing a greater margin of safety.

Alfentanil, a new synthetic analog of fentanyl, has a much shorter elimination half-life (90 minutes) than morphine or fentanyl. It has been administered as an infusion of 50 or 100 μg/kg per hour during surgery and at a rate of 20 μg/kg per hour during the postoperative period. This produces comparable degrees of analgesia and ventilatory depression to those found during fentanyl infusion.

Patient-demand Analgesia

Patient-controlled analgesic therapy with intravenous opioids is based on a system which dispenses a preset dose of opioid intravenously from a syringe pump activated by a press button. By administering small doses frequently, with appropriate programming to limit the number of doses in a given period, the patient is able to titrate the drug to control his pain. Although commercial systems have been available for many years, they have not achieved popularity. The sophisticated apparatus which is necessary for such therapy is too expensive to allow this type of approach to be used in all patients, but one patient-demand system per ward can be effectively used for patients with severe pain. The total doses consumed by individual patients are remarkably constant over periods between 6 and 24 hours. Requirements for meperidine have been described as 26 ± 10 mg per hour, and for morphine 2.6 mg per hour.

Epidural

Opioids injected into the epidural space are partly (20–40 percent) absorbed into the plexus of veins contained therein and distributed throughout the rest of the body. This part of the administered dose is distributed and metabolized in the same way as a similar dose administered intramuscularly. Depending on the lipid solubility and molecular size of the opioid, a variable proportion of the remainder will cross the dural membranes to reach the cerebrospinal fluid and, again depending on lipid solubility, will bind to the lipoproteins of the spinal cord and to opioid receptors in the dorsal horn.

Morphine was the first opioid to be injected by Behar in 1979 into the epidural space. However, although morphine has been widely used as an epidural analgesic, and its effects widely studied, it is perhaps the least suitable drug for this purpose on account of its low lipid solubility (oil to water solubility is 1.4). The reports of delayed ventilatory arrest have largely attributed this adverse effect to the longevity of morphine in the cerebrospinal fluid. Unfortunately diacetyl morphine (heroin), the most suitable opioid for epidural use and widely used in the United Kingdom, is unavailable to anesthesiologists in most countries.

Meperidine, fentanyl, and buprenorphine have been used by the epidural route but suffer from the disadvantage that their analgesic effects are short-lived (1 to 3 hours) when administered intermittently. Table 2–4 summarizes the range of doses of these drugs suitable for epidural or intrathecal analgesia, and the side effects produced.

In patients who come to the recovery room with an indwelling epidural catheter in either the lumbar or mid-thoracic region, the appropriate opioid should be dissolved in the same volume of saline that would be used for a segmental local anesthetic block. Nursing staff should realize the importance of recognizing changes of ventilatory frequency and to record these accurately, at 15-minute intervals for the first hour after opioid injection, and at half-hour intervals subsequently. A ventilatory frequency less than 10 breaths per minute is potentially dangerous if the

Table 2-4. Opioids Suitable for Intrathecal (I) or Epidural (E) Analgesia

Drug	Route	Dose Range	Duration (hours)	Pruritus (%)	Nausea and Vomiting (%)
Morphine	E*	2.0–7.5 mg	22	22	26
Meperidine	E	25–75 mg	3.5	0	5
Fentanyl	E*	50–200 µg	2.0	0	9
Buprenorphine	E	0.15–0.3 mg	12–24	0	15–20
Diamorphine	E	2.5–5.0 mg	8–18	0	5
Morphine	I	0.5–1.0 mg	18–24	50–70	25

*Duration of action enhanced by epinephrine 1:200,000.

patient is not carefully watched. Below 6 breaths per minute, minute ventilation becomes inadequate and $PaCO_2$ will rise to unacceptable levels.

Intrathecal

At the time that local anesthetics are injected into the cerebrospinal fluid to produce spinal anesthesia, opioids can be injected at the same time to provide prolonged postoperative analgesia. Morphine (0.5–1.0 mg) has been more widely used than other opioids. While it produces profound segmental analgesia, intrathecal morphine has also been associated with undesirable side effects such as pruritus (50–70 percent), nausea and vomiting, and urinary retention. Pruritus does not respond to antihistamine therapy but can be completely obtunded by small doses of naloxone. More serious have been reports of delayed ventilatory arrest, presumed to occur as a result of diffusion of the hydrophilic morphine from the spinal to the medullary regions of the cerebrospinal fluid. To allow early recognition of such ventilatory depression, nursing staff must record ventilatory frequency at 30 to 60-minute intervals.

TREATMENT OF OPIOID SIDE EFFECTS

Narcotic Overdose

Ventilatory arrest, or profound slowing of breathing (< 10 breaths per minute), is the main side effect of opioids. This may be precipitated by simple overdose, or the predicted effect of a given dose may be enhanced by the ventilatory depressant effects of other drugs such as benzodiazepines, barbiturates, and general anesthetics. Ventilatory arrest may also be enhanced by sleep and antagonized by pain and wakefulness. Two approaches can be used to reverse ventilatory depression.

Naloxone is a specific antagonist acting at both μ- and κ-receptors, which displaces other agonist opioids from these receptors. Intravenous naloxone (2–5 µg/kg) should be given slowly in patients whose ventilatory frequency has dropped below 6 breaths per minute. Its peak effect is reached within 2 minutes, but the duration of its antagonism is much shorter (60 to 90 minutes) than that of many opioids, especially morphine. If ventilatory frequency subsequently decreases to an unacceptable level, a further dose of naloxone must be given.

Doxapram is a nonspecific ventilatory stimulant which may be used either as a single dose (1 mg/kg) to initiate spontaneous breathing, or an infusion of 3.0 mg/kg per hour. Many patients find the effects of a larger, single dose unpleasant, and an infusion at an initial rate of 30 mg/kg per hour for 10 minutes may be more acceptable. Although doxapram stimulates ventilation, it also increases CO_2 production; thus, it may not be very effective in decreasing $PaCO_2$ to normal levels.

Nausea and Vomiting

Nausea and vomiting in the recovery room can be due to a number of factors of which previous administration of opioids is the most common. Patients who have experienced severe nausea or vomiting after previous anesthetics are more likely to suffer the same problems on subsequent occasions, irrespective of the type of anesthesia administered. The best prophylaxis is to use a powerful butyrophenone antiemetic as part of the anesthetic technique. Droperidol (5–7.5 mg) is a much more potent and dependable antiemetic than the others mentioned below, and is more effective when given at the beginning of the anesthetic rather than in the recovery room. Its antiemetic action lasts about 12 to 18 hours.

Many patients feel nauseated and retch within the first 5 to 10 minutes after waking, especially after a nitrous oxide anesthetic administered by mask. This is because of retention of nitrous oxide in the stomach cavity. Provided care is taken to turn the patient on the side to protect the airway, no specific therapy is required.

Persistent nausea and vomiting of clear or bile-stained material is best treated in the recovery room by the intravenous administration of one of the following drugs (given in order of cost).

Metoclopramide

Metoclopramide is an effective antiemetic with a spectrum of activity similar to the phenothiazines, but it also increases propulsive activity in the stomach and closes the lower esophageal sphincter. It has little anticholinergic effect. It may cause severe extrapyramidal reactions, including oculogyric crisis, especially in children. The normal dose is 5 mg intravenously in young adults (up to 21 years of age), but more may be given to older patients.

Prochlorperazine

This phenothiazine is a potent antiemetic which acts primarily on the chemoreceptor trigger zone and is therefore particularly useful to inhibit opioid-induced nausea and vomiting. It is most effective when given as an intravenous injection of 6.25 mg, but its effect is more prolonged when given as an intramuscular injection of 12.5 mg. Dystonic reactions may occur in patients who have previously been taking other phenothiazines.

Perphenazine

The cheapest, and equally effective antiemetic to those mentioned above, perphenazine is given either by intravenous injection of 2.5-5.0 mg, or by intramuscular injection of 5-10 mg. As with all phenothiazines, dystonic reactions may occur in response to overdosage.

REGIONAL AND LOCAL ANESTHETICS

Supplementation of regional anesthetic techniques used during surgery to provide postoperative pain relief can be more effective than the use of opioids, especially after intraabdominal or thoracic surgery. For many purposes the intraoperative dose provides adequate initial pain relief in the recovery room, and further injection techniques are inappropriate.

Caudal Analgesia

Children having prolonged genitourinary procedures, such as plastic surgery for hypospadias or epispadias, can be given excellent postoperative pain relief by a further injection of bupivacaine (0.25 percent) into the caudal space at the end of surgery, while the child is still anesthetized. This will provide many hours of excellent analgesia.

Intercostal Block

Intercostal nerve blockade can be established by the surgeon, under direct vision, prior to closing a thoracotomy wound. Three milliliters of 0.5 percent bupivacaine can be accurately placed alongside each of the two intercostal nerves above and below, and at the level of the interspace used for the thoracotomy.

For unilateral operations such as cholecystectomy, intercostal block can be achieved by placing a fine catheter through a Tuohy needle, or a teflon intravenous cannula (18 g) into one intercostal space (T8) posteriorly (at the rib angle). An initial injection of 12-15 ml 0.5 percent bupivacaine followed by a slow continuous infusion of 0.125 percent bupivacaine will provide blockade of the intercostal nerve at the site of injection and allow spread to adjacent intercostal nerves by diffusion through the paravertebral space.

Epidural Blockade

Lumbar epidural blockade is highly suitable for postoperative pain relief after surgery of the lower abdomen, the pelvis, and the legs. The main disadvantage of sustained analgesia by continuous infusions into the lumbar epidural space is the arterial hypotension consequent on sympathetic nervous blockade. Provided the block does not extend above the T10 level, the degree of hypotension can be minimized. This is rarely sufficient to provide adequate pain relief after major intraabdominal procedures when using local anesthetics. The principle of injecting a single dose of 0.5 percent bupivacaine followed by intermittent repeat doses of 0.25 percent bupivacaine or an infusion of 0.125 percent bupivacaine should be followed.

Thoracic segmental epidural blockade can be achieved by placing a catheter in the seventh or eighth thoracic interspace by the paraspinous approach. In the mid-thoracic region the spinous processes of the vertebrae are steeply inclined in a caudad direction, making the midline approach difficult and uncertain. A Tuohy needle can be inserted about one finger's breadth lateral to the lower margin of the spinous process of T7 and advanced perpendicular to the skin until the tip encounters the lamina of T8. The needle is then angulated toward the midline and the tip walked along the lamina until one can feel the tip of the needle slipping over the edge. The tip is then in the ligamentum flavum, and entry into the epidural space can be identified with standard loss of resistance techniques. A catheter placed at this, the T7-T8 interspace and advanced about 2 cm only, can be used to provide segmental blockade limited to the range T4-T12, thus providing excellent pain relief after intraabdominal or thoracic surgery. Bupivacaine (0.5 percent) should be injected slowly, in a volume of 1 ml per segment (5-8 ml) and supplemented by a slow infusion of bupivacaine (0.125 percent) at a rate of 6-7 ml per hour. Alternatively, appropriate opioids can be dissolved in a similar volume of saline to provide analgesia over the same segmental distribution.

For patients with severe respiratory disease who require total analgesia after intraabdominal surgery, combined opioid and local analgesia through a thoracic epidural catheter is most effective.

SUGGESTIONS FOR FURTHER READING

Bromage P. The price of intraspinal narcotic analgesia: basic constraints. Anesth Analg 1981; 60:461–463.

Bullingham RES, ed. Opiate analgesia. Clinics in anaesthesiology. Vol 1, No 1. London: WB Saunders, 1983.

Frost EAM, Andrews IC, eds. Recovery room care. International Anesthesiology Clinics. Vol 21, No 1. Boston: Little, Brown, 1983.

Kitahata LM, Collins JG, eds. Narcotic analgesics in anesthesiology. Baltimore: Williams & Wilkins, 1982.

Prys-Roberts C, Hug CC Jr, eds. Pharmacokinetics of anaesthesia. Oxford: Blackwell Scientific Publications, Inc. 1984.

3
Respiration: Mechanical Ventilation and Oxygen Therapy
Elizabeth A. M. Frost

Ventilatory difficulties are common postoperatively. The recovery room nurse must be able to promptly recognize and initiate therapy of such potentially catastrophic complications as hypoxemia, cyanosis, airway obstruction, and residual neuromuscular paralysis. Respiratory failure may be due to O_2 failure or CO_2 failure.

O_2 FAILURE

O_2 failure causing inadequate oxygenation is due to:

1. Intrapulmonary or intracardiac shunting. If blood flows past nonventilated alveoli or passes through a cardiac defect without alveolar exposure, oxygen cannot be added to the pulmonary artery blood.
2. Breathing an hypoxic gas mixture. Since O_2 enters the blood by diffusing down a concentration gradient, arterial PO_2 (PaO_2) cannot exceed alveolar PO_2 (PAO_2). If the inspired gas mixture has a low O_2 content, PAO_2 is low and therefore arterial oxygenation is even lower.
3. Hypoventilation. The relationship between O_2 and CO_2 in the alveolus is reciprocal; if ventilation is inadequate and hypercarbia occurs, $PACO_2$ rises, PAO_2 falls, and therefore PaO_2 falls.

4. Alveolar-capillary block. If the distance between the gas in the alveolus and the blood is increased, as may occur with pulmonary edema or pulmonary interstitial fibrosis, transfer of O_2 across the alveolus to the pulmonary capillary blood is less efficient. However, this effect is less important than (1) in causing arterial hypoxemia.

CO_2 FAILURE

When breathing gas mixtures free of CO_2, $PaCO_2$ is determined by CO_2 production ($\dot{V}_{CO_2}$) and alveolar ventilation ($\dot{V}A_{CO_2}$ elimination).

In most individuals, major changes in $\dot{V}_{CO_2}$ are matched by similar changes in $\dot{V}A$ and therefore produce little net change in $PaCO_2$. The patient in the recovery room, however, may be unable to appropriately increase CO_2 elimination. Conditions that suppress normal compensation include: (1) decrease in the spontaneous respiratory rate (residual narcosis); (2) decrease in V_T (as may occur when gross abdominal distension limits diaphragmatic excursion); (3) an increase in dead space (although V_T may remain unchanged, an increasingly large portion of the inspired gas is distributed to alveoli lacking perfusion); (4) an increase in CO_2 production, e.g., hypermetabolic states; or (5) any combination of the above.

Both O_2 failure and CO_2 failure are caused by hypoventilation. Hypoxia and hypercarbia result and, if untreated, may lead to respiratory failure, even in patients with normal lung function.

Hypoxia is suspected if there is undue agitation in unconscious or semiconscious patients, cyanosis, or an ashen gray color, combined with deteriorating vital signs. Diagnosis is made by arterial blood gas analysis.

Other essentials in monitoring respiration are listed in Figure 3-1. The nurse must be aware of relevant details of the past history including lung disease, smoking, or cardiovascular problems. A report must be obtained from the anesthesiologist emphasizing any intraoperative complications which occurred and especially noting routes of insertion of central cannulas (particularly if the placement was unsuccessful). Charting and trend recording of respiratory rate and character provide essential information. Breath sounds should be clear and equal bilaterally. Simple bedside measurements such as tidal volume, vital capacity (VC), and negative inspiratory force should be documented. Normally, VC is 70 ml/kg. Approximately 15 ml kg is barely sufficient for spontaneous sighing, coughing, and clearing of secretions. Accurate measurement of this volume depends on an alert cooperative patient (i.e., a patient must be capable of making a maximum expiration after a maximum inspiration). Thus, early values may not be reliable if the patient has not fully recovered from the effects of anesthetic agents. However, this test may be used to assess the appropriate time for extubation or weaning from a ventilator, as an accept-

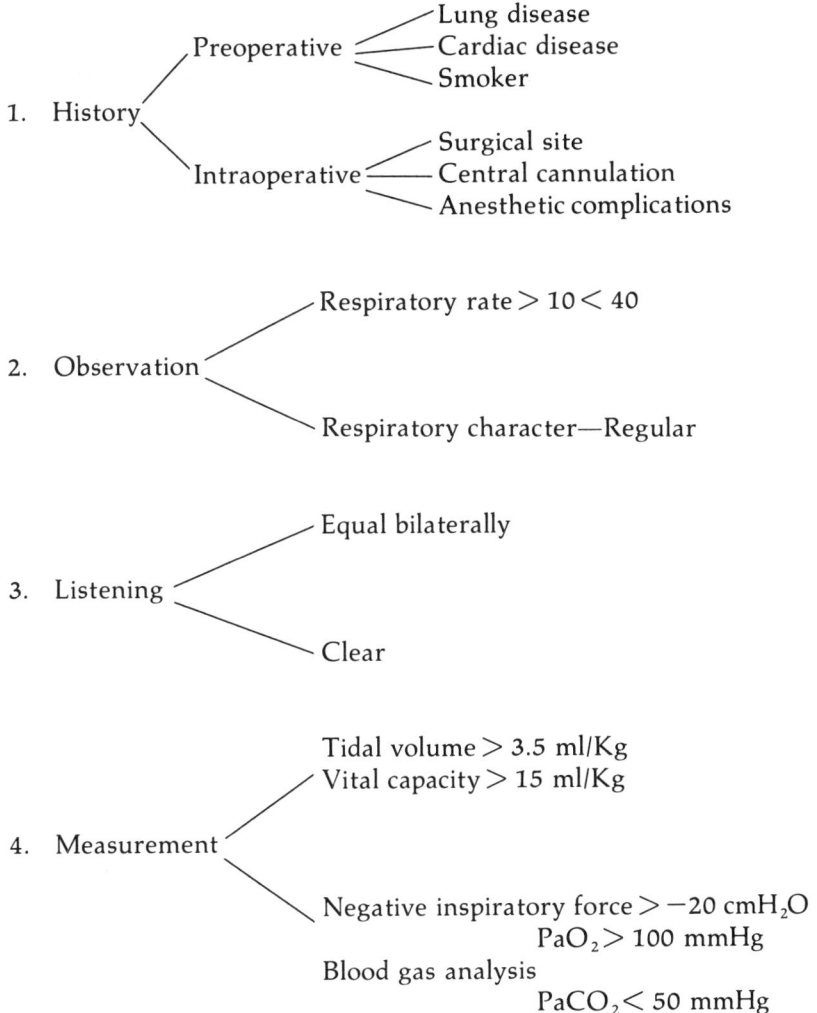

Figure 3-1. Essentials of monitoring ventilation. Deviation from the values listed means therapeutic intervention is necessary.

able value signifies adequate coordination of chest wall movement and pulmonary mechanics with minimal pulmonary dysfunction. Abnormalities of arterial blood gases should be reported promptly to the anesthesiologist. Correct interpretation requires knowledge of the inspired O_2 concentration (FiO_2) and the mode of respiration (especially if end expiratory pressure is applied). It is often necessary to measure blood gases repetitively and to establish certain ranges for PaO_2 and $PaCO_2$ that are appropriate for the individual patient. Mechanical ventilation and FiO_2 may be varied to produce acceptable values. It is desirable to standardize conditions as much as possible; to alter only one parameter at a time, and to allow sufficient time to elapse between sampling for stabilization.

As signs and symptoms of oxygen toxicity (restlessness, chest pain, increasing shunting of blood in the lungs) may develop rapidly (i.e., over a few hours), it is important to use the lowest inspired concentration of oxygen which is compatible with adequate blood exchange.

The alveolar-arterial oxygen tension gradient $P(A-a)O_2$ is a conveniently calculated number that may be used to assess the ability of the lungs to transfer oxygen. Alveolar PO_2 may be estimated from the following:

$$PAO_2 = FiO_2 \times (\text{Barometric pressure, usually } 760 \text{ mmHg} - PaCO_2 - PAH_2O)$$

where $PaCO_2$ = partial pressure of CO_2 in arterial blood (equals pressure in alveolus) and PAH_2O = partial pressure of water vapor in the alveolus (usually 47 mm Hg). Subtracting the arterial oxygen tension from this number gives the $P(A-a)O_2$.

$$P(A-a)O_2 = PAO_2 - PaO_2$$

The lower the value thus obtained, the better the pulmonary function and the higher the efficiency of exchange of oxygen from the alveolus to the arterial blood.

The ideal value should be below 50 mm Hg. Higher values indicate shunting within the lungs, which represents increasing discrepancy between the area of the lung which is ventilated and the area which is perfused by blood (i.e., $\dot{V}/\dot{Q}$ abnormality).

CAUSES OF RESPIRATORY DYSFUNCTION

Factors that contribute to early postoperative respiratory difficulties are listed in Figure 3-2.

Low Inspired Oxygen

Intraoperatively, the patient has had intensive cardiovascular and respiratory monitoring. With the conclusion of the operation, this vigilance is often relaxed, and during transfer to the recovery room, the patient frequently does not receive supplemental oxygen and may become significantly hypoxic.

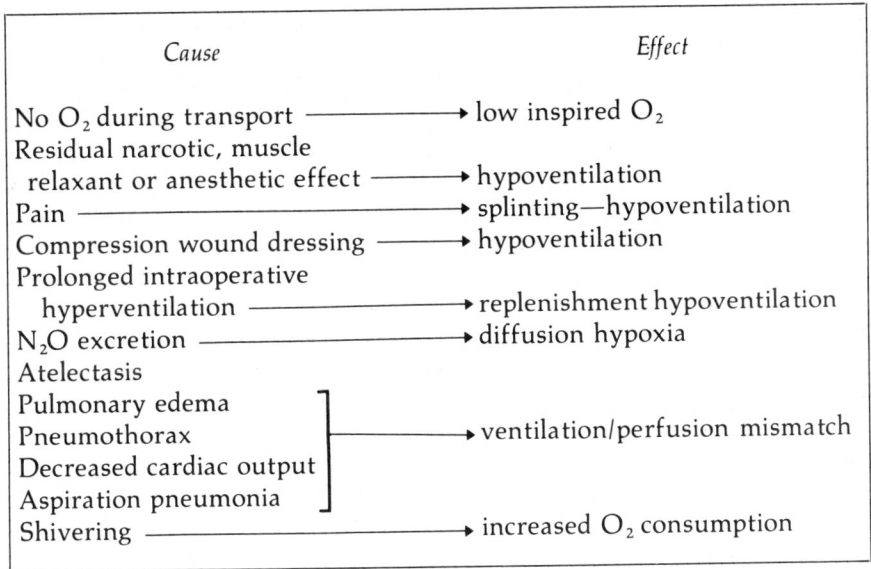

Figure 3-2. Common treatable causes of early postoperative respiratory dysfunction.

Residual Anesthetic Effect

All anesthetic agents cause respiratory depression. Inhalation agents, depending on their solubility, accumulate in tissues and may delay return to consciousness and the ability to breathe deeply and prevent atelectasis. Prolonged respiratory depression may be seen, especially in obese patients who have undergone long procedures (more than 4 hours). Sodium thiopental, although initially a short-acting drug, is not only very soluble in fat but is also reabsorbed in the kidney tubules. Thus prolonged infusion results in delayed return to consciousness and postoperative hypoventilation.

At the end of painful procedures (circumcision, spinal instrumentation) or when early postoperative immobility is necessary (cleft palate repair, skin grafting), small doses of narcotics are given intravenously in the operating room. Although the analgesic effect may be appropriate, significant ventilatory depression may result. Use of narcotic antagonists is specific in reversing the respiratory depression, but the prompt associated return of pain appreciation is less than ideal. Therefore, in these circumstances, supplemental oxygen should be given and ventilation supported.

Both nondepolarizing (pancuronium, atracurium) and depolarizing (succinylcholine) muscle relaxants are frequently used intraoperatively. The former group of drugs is fairly long acting, and effects often last well into the recovery period. Moreover, drug interaction, especially with inhalation agents such as isoflurane and antibiotics, can markedly increase the intensity of neuromuscular blockade.

This paralyzing action may be further accentuated by acidosis, and a vicious cycle of respiratory acidosis → increased drug action → decreased ventilation → more respiratory acidosis may quickly become established.

Diagnosis of residual effects of neuromuscular paralysis is made by reviewing the anesthetic record and the use of a peripheral nerve stimulator. Therapy is specific for nondepolarizing agents. After correction of acidosis, the drug action may be reversed using neostigmine and atropine. Abnormal response to succinylcholine (i.e., prolonged paralysis) is very rare and is treated by supportive measures.

Pain

Upper abdominal surgery (e.g., cholecystectomy) may cause considerable pain, provoking diaphragmatic splinting. Careful use of small doses of narcotics will relieve the distress and regain the patient's cooperation in performing adequate breathing exercises. Occasionally pain may provoke hyperventilation, which may also result in hypoxia due to increased work of breathing combined with a shift of the O_2 dissociation curve to the left because of respiratory alkalosis (i.e., less O_2 available for the tissues).

Compression Dressing

As soon as the patient is admitted to the recovery room the nurse should check all dressings. Circumferential chest or abdominal bandages may restrict respiratory movements and cause hypoxia. It should be possible to insert two or three fingers easily between a dressing and the patient's skin.

Prolonged Intraoperative Hyperventilation

After a long period of controlled hyperventilation (e.g., neurosurgical procedures), total body carbon dioxide stores are reduced. Relative hypoventilation occurs as these stores are spontaneously replenished. However, there are no "oxygen stores" which can accumulate during periods of high inspired oxygen intake, so hypoxia may develop rapidly in the recovery room as minute ventilation decreases. Therapy includes supplemental oxygen administration and, occasionally, brief periods of supported ventilation.

Diffusion Hypoxia

Diffusion hypoxia is the term applied to the reduction in alveolar oxygen tension when nitrous oxide is excreted rapidly from the tissues into the alveoli and dilutes other alveolar gases. This is a short-lived phenomenon and is avoided by ventilating the patient with 100 percent oxygen at the end of surgery. Usually this effect is not apparent in the recovery room unless it is exaggerated by the respiratory depressant effects of other anesthetic agents. Therapy involves ventilation with a high concentration of oxygen.

Ventilation/Perfusion Mismatch

Normally blood flow to an alveolus is appropriately oxygenated by the gas passing through that lung segment. Should areas develop in the lung which are ventilated and not perfused or perfused without adequate ventilation, the respiratory mechanism of exchange becomes inefficient and hypoxia develops.
    An increased shunting of blood from the right, desaturated side of the vascular system to the left side occurs. The commonest causes of right to left shunt are as follows: (1) Atelectasis is a common cause of postoperative hypoxia due to secretions, mucous plugs, splinting, endobronchial intubation, or bronchial obstruction. (2) Pulmonary edema is recognized by pink, frothy secretions from the endotracheal tube. This complication is most likely to occur in patients with a history of cardiovascular disease, or in those who have received an infusion of a hyperosmolar solution such as mannitol. It is most frequently seen in the first hour following surgery. (3) Pulmonary embolism may occur after prolonged surgery, in obese patients, or in patients with a previous history of embolism, or following trauma to the lower limbs. (4) Decreased cardiac output from shock, depressant effects of drugs, and allergy increases right to left shunt. (5) Aspiration pneumonia is most likely to occur after emergency surgery in patients with a full stomach or in patients with a history of hiatus hernia or intestinal obstruction. Silent aspiration may also occur following surgery around the brain stem when damage to the cranial nerves responsible for pharyngeal and laryngeal protective mechanisms may have occurred. (6) With shivering, O_2 consumption may be increased by 3 to 500 percent, causing venous desaturation and hypoxia. Whatever the cause of the

hypoxia, management requires administration of supplemental oxygen, encouraging the patient to breathe deeply and to cough, informing the attending physician, and treating the underlying cause.

OXYGEN THERAPY

Regardless of the cause of hypoxia in the recovery room, the administration of humidified oxygen is now routine. Many means of oxygen therapy are available.

Nasal Cannulas

Nasal cannulas are flexible disposable vinyl tubes with two short prongs inserted into the nares and held in place by an elastic strap (Figure 3-3).

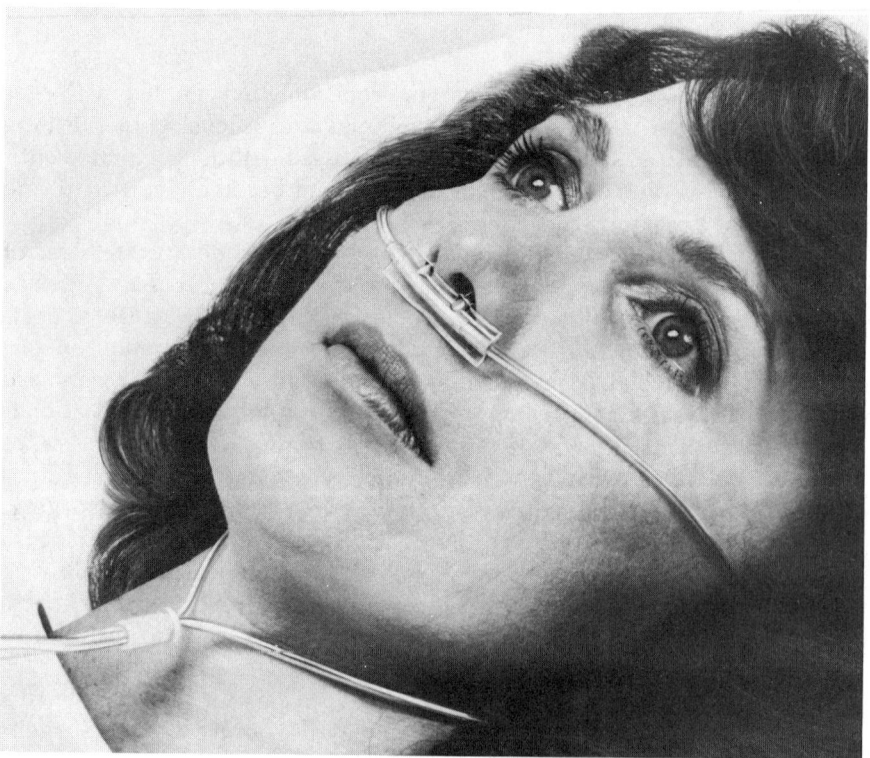

Figure 3-3. A cannula with curved flared tips is a simple, comfortable, and effective means of increasing oxygen administration to a patient who is alert enough to breathe nasally.

Flared nasal tips diffuse the flow of oxygen. Flowmeters supply oxygen at 1-6 liters per minute and deliver low oxygen concentrations (FiO_2 0.24-0.44). This technique is simple and relatively effective for patients with mild pulmonary dysfunction. However, the FiO_2 achieved is low and because the patient's minute ventilation may vary considerably, an unknown amount of oxygen dilution with room air may occur, making interpretation of blood gas results difficult.

Simple Masks

Several disposable plastic masks which are inexpensive, convenient and relatively comfortable are available for short-term use when higher concentrations of oxygen (FiO_2 0.4-0.6) are desired. Adjustable nose clips provide a more comfortable fit, and the masks may be molded to fit under the lower lip or underneath the chin (Figure 3-4). These devices have neither valves nor reservoir bags. Thus, atmospheric air may be inspired if the inspiratory flow rate of the patient exceeds the oxygen flow from the source. Again, administration of a known FiO_2 is difficult. The gas is exhaled through holes in the side of the mask.

Face tents are designed to be used with large bore tubing for high humidity aerosol therapy (Figure 3-5). Tracheostomy masks made of soft vinyl material are available in adult and child sizes (Figure 3-6). Fixed concentrations of humidified oxygen may be administered through a venturi humidifier system. The tubing adaptor can swivel for use at different angles.

Partial Rebreathing Mask

A high inspired concentration of O_2 can be achieved by combining a simple mask with a reservoir bag (Figure 3-7). Part of the patient's exhaled air enters the bag where it mixes with source oxygen and is inspired with the next inhalation. An FiO_2 of 0.6-1 can usually be achieved at oxygen flow rates of 6-10 liters per minute. Valves on the side of the mask which open during exhalation prevent total rebreathing. Difficulty arises in maintaining the mask in its proper position, especially if the patient is restless.

Nonrebreathing Mask

Figure 3-8 demonstrates an under-the-chin vinyl mask designed to deliver high oxygen concentrations without rebreathing. A low resistance check valve prevents rebreathing while low resistance flap or flutter exhalation valves on the sides allow exhaled gas to escape.

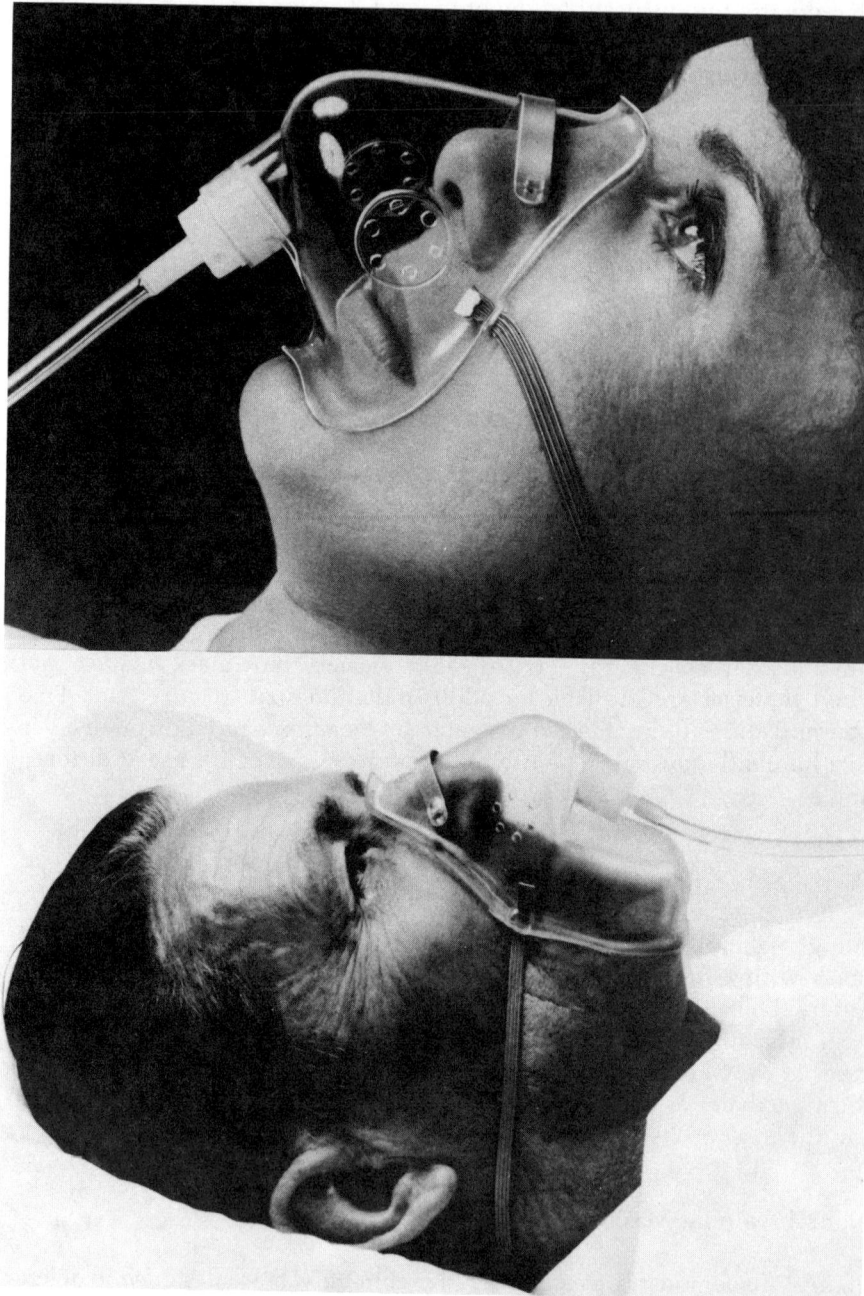

Figure 3-4. Soft vinyl masks molded to fit either under or over the chin provide higher inspired oxygen concentrations to patients breathing orally or nasally.

RESPIRATION: MECHANICAL VENTILATION AND OXYGEN THERAPY

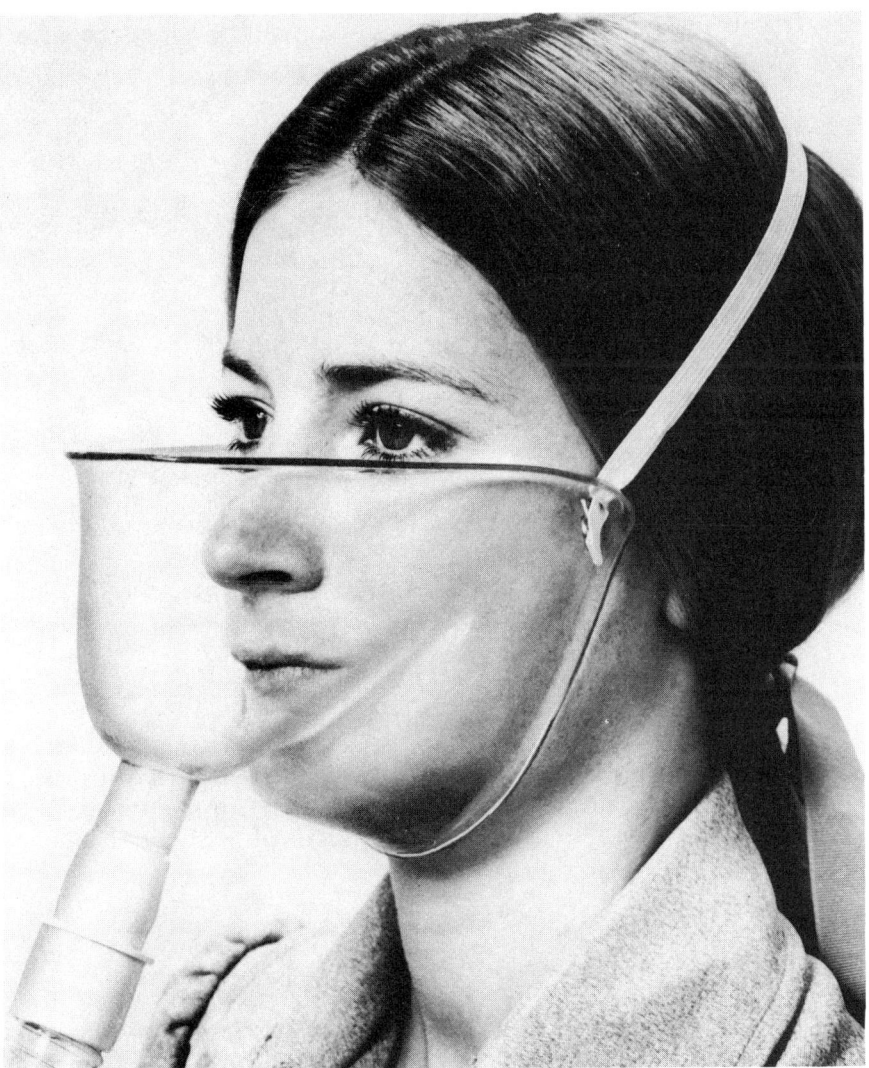

Figure 3-5. Face tents are used with large bore (0.75-inch ID) tubing to provide high humidity.

40 GENERAL CARE

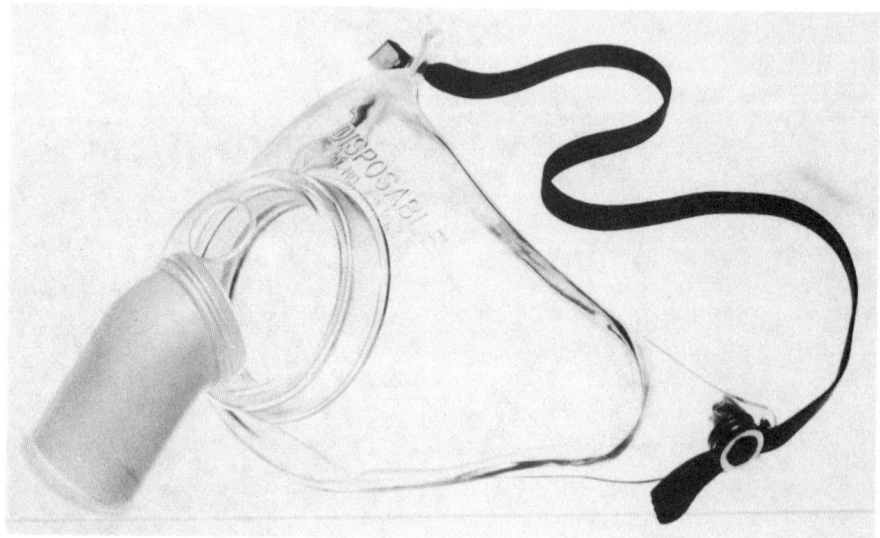

Figure 3-6. Adult disposable tracheotomy masks are molded of soft vinyl material and may be used for both tracheotomy and laryngectomy patients.

Oxygen flows into the bag during exhalation and flows into the mask during inhalation. If the fresh gas flow is inadequate, the patient may breathe atmospheric air via the inlet safety valve. With this system at an oxygen flow rate of 10 liters per minute, an FiO_2 of 1 may be maintained for prolonged periods of time.

Venturi Mask

The venturi mask allows delivery of precise concentrations of oxygen at low flow rates (4-8 liters per minute) (Figure 3-9). A known volume of air is entrained secondary to the flow of oxygen through a venturi jet. The high flow of air and oxygen overcomes the feeling of suffocation which often accompanies the use of simple masks. CO_2 rebreathing is also eliminated. The system allows improvement in arterial oxygenation without the concomitant depression of the hypoxic control of respiration associated with chronic lung disease.

Two systems are available. Lower concentrations (24, 26, 28, and 30 percent) may be achieved by setting a dial control. Higher concentrations (35, 40, and 50 percent) may be administered by changing the dial control. The desired percentage can be locked into place by a ring mechanism. Pediatric venturi masks are also available to deliver oxygen at both the low and medium concentration ranges.

Continuous Positive Pressure Masks

Silicone elastomer masks have been designed which mold closely to the face and allow oxygen delivery to the patient with exhalation through positive expiratory pressure valve assemblies. Up to 20 cm H_2O end-expiratory pressure may be used. Complications include gastric distension at high pressures, skin erosion where the mask makes tight contact with the face, and general patient discomfort. However, in some instances, this therapy may effectively avoid the need for intubation, especially in infants.

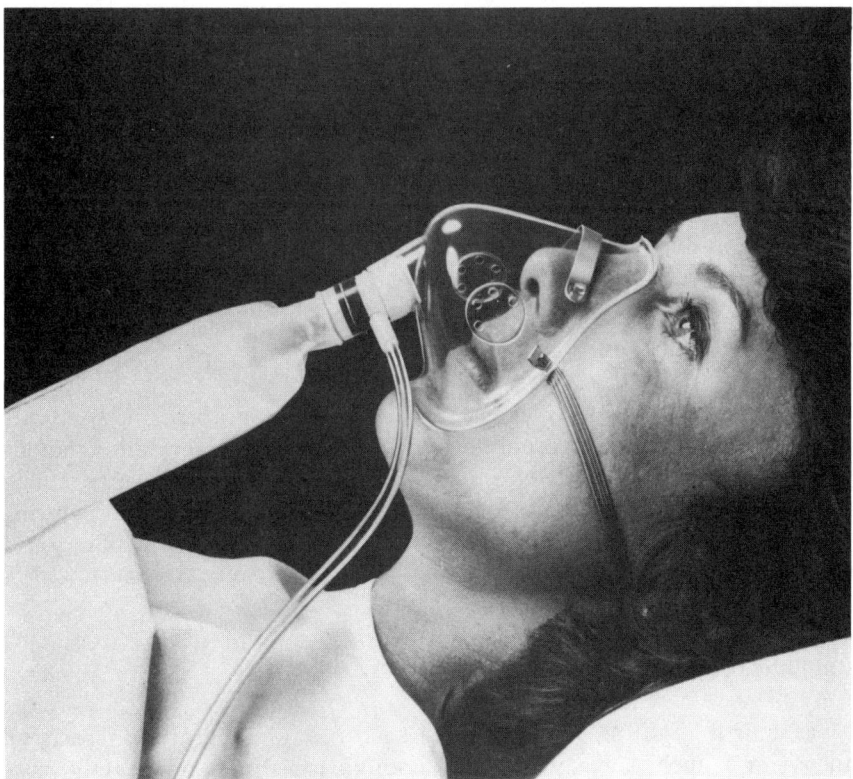

Figure 3-7. Combination of a simple mask and a reservoir bag provides higher inspired O_2 concentrations.

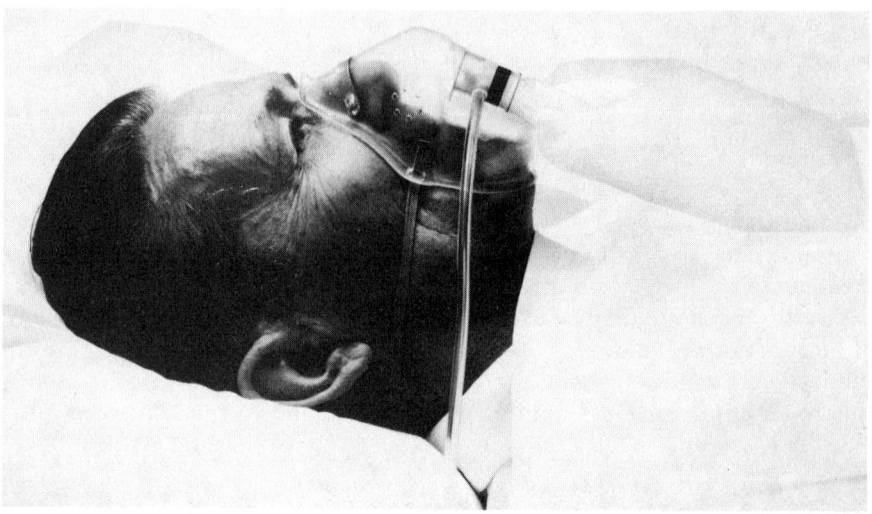

Figure 3-8. An under-the-chin mask is combined with a reservoir bag. A low resistance check valve prevents rebreathing. Flap valves on the side of the mask allow normal exhalation.

Oxygen or Croup Tents

Oxygen tents provide an oxygen-enriched and temperature and humidity controlled environment, generally by an electrically operated, canopied device (Figure 3-10). Usually only a 50 percent oxygen concentration is possible. This is probably the most suitable technique for administering oxygen to children. It is, however, costly, requires a high flow of oxygen, and affords limited patient access.

Humidification Systems

Inspired air is about 45 percent saturated at room temperature. The nasal mucosa and upper airways provide enough moisture and heat to raise humidity to 100 percent at body temperature. But, as moisture is removed, secretions become thicker and the mucous blanket does not move as efficiently to expel foreign particles. Ciliary and surfactant activity is depressed and mucous membranes become irritated. It is essential therefore

RESPIRATION: MECHANICAL VENTILATION AND OXYGEN THERAPY   43

to humidify inspired gases. The two methods which are available to provide humidity include delivery of water in a gaseous form (e.g., bubble and cascade humidifiers) or in a particulate form (e.g., venturi type and ultrasonic nebulizers).

Simple humidifiers which pass oxygen through water are made more efficient by increasing the temperature to 37°C. A filter may be added to form small bubbles which increase the surface area of contact between the gas and water. However, as the gas leaves the humidifier, heat is lost and the water vapor condenses in the tubing before it reaches the patient. Increased heating in the main chamber or heating the tubing will prevent this problem. Care must then be taken to ensure that the vapor reaching the patient is not above body temperature. Prefilled and refillable humidifiers are available.

Nebulizers produce water vapor and aerosol droplets. Gas is forced at high pressure through a restricted orifice and crosses the end of a fine capillary tube, the other end of which is immersed in the solution to be nebulized (usually water). The fluid is drawn up the capillary tube and blown off by the jet stream. It then impacts on the container walls or any

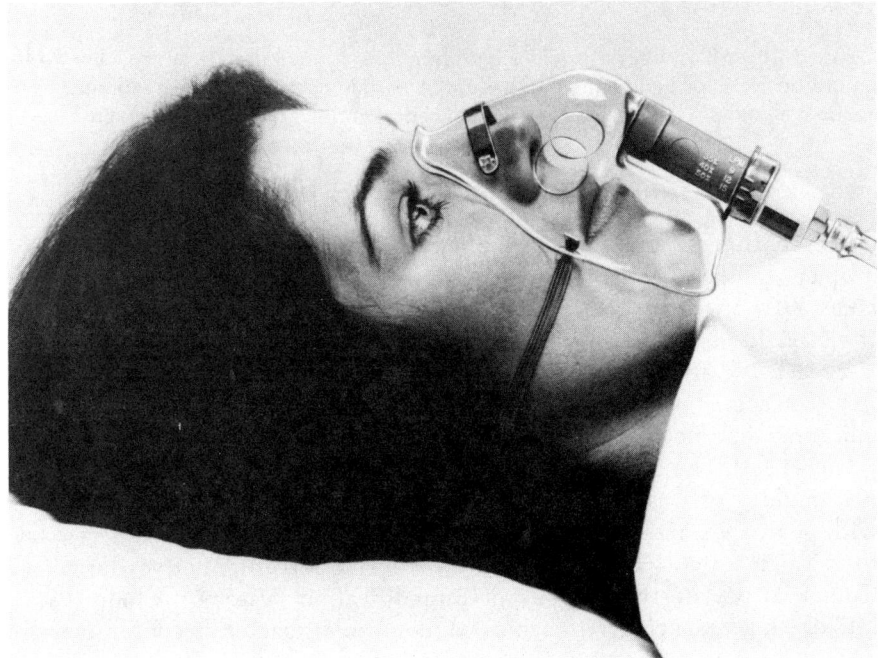

Figure 3-9. A venturi mask allows delivery of more precise concentrations of oxygen. Using the dial control, concentrations of 35, 40, or 50 percent may be given. Other controls allow concentrations of 24, 26, 28, or 30 percent.

44   GENERAL CARE

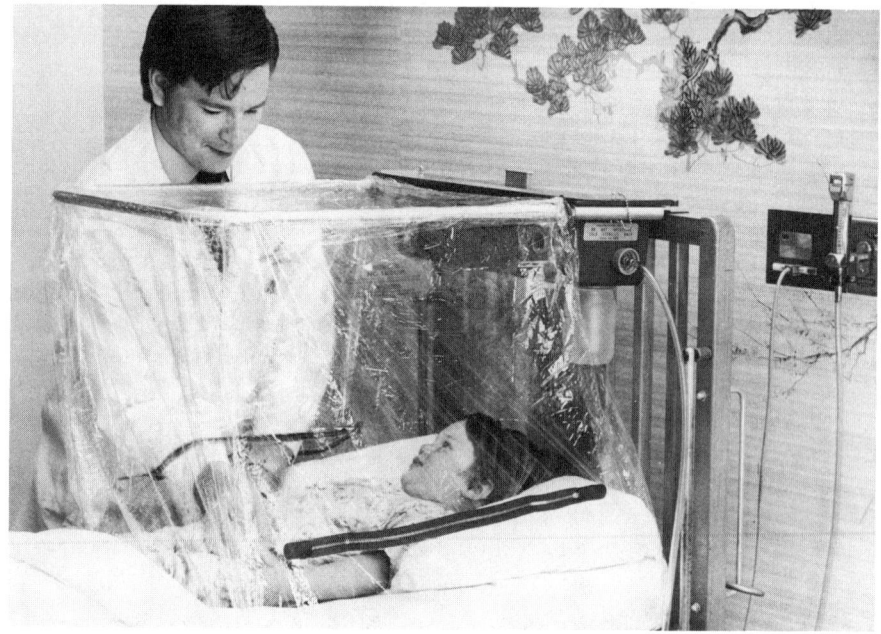

Figure 3-10.   Croup tent provides high humidity for children. It can be adjusted to mount on a crib or bed frame and has zippered side openings. An ice storage chest ensures a cool environment. Oxygen concentration is about 30-40 percent.

other "baffle" where it is broken into a high-density fog. The larger droplets fall back and the smaller ones continue in the stream. Droplets about 40 μ are deposited in the mouth and trachea; 15-μ droplets settle in the bronchi; 8-μ droplets remain in the bronchioles; and those measuring 2 μ reach the alveoli (about 35 percent of the initially inhaled vapor).

Ultrasonic nebulizers use ultra-high-frequency sound by means of a vibrating ceramic disk to produce a high-density mist of uniform particle size (1-10 μ). The droplet density obtained by this means may be as high as 550 mg/liter of carrier gas which is 10 times greater than that obtained with heated jet nebulizers and 10 times more than the amount necessary to raise dry air at body temperature to 100 percent relative humidity. Complications of these types of humidification systems include water intoxication (especially in babies) and alveolar bacterial contamination (especially *Pseudomonas*).

Apart from humidification, nebulizers provide a vehicle for administration of drugs. Table 3-1 lists some agents usually given by this route. Side effects include central nervous stimulation (anxiety, restlessness, and

Table 3-1. Inhalation Drugs Used as Bronchodilators

Generic Name	Trade Name	Inhalation by IPPB	Inhalation from Metered Nebulizer	Peak Response (minutes)	Duration of Action (minutes)
Isoproterenol preparations	Isuprel Hydrochloride Solution; Isuprel Mistometer (metered dose)	0.5 ml (0.5%) in 1.5 ml N saline	2-3 doses; 125 µg/dose	10-15	60-90
Racepinephrine	Vaponefrine	0.5 ml (2.25%) in 1.5 ml N saline		5-10	120-180
Isoetharine HCl	Bronkosol	0.5 ml (1%) in 1.5 ml N saline	1-2 doses; 340 µg/dose	10-15	90-120
Metaproterenol sulfate	Alupent	0.5 ml (5%) in 1.5 ml N saline	2-3 doses; 0.65 mg/dose	10-15	180-240
Atropine sulfate		2 mg in 1 ml N saline; 0.05-0.1 mg/kg. No more than t.i.d.		5-10	240-360
Albuterol	Ventolin; Solbutamol		2 doses; 90 µg/dose	10-15	240-360

IPPB = intermittent positive-pressure breathing; N = normal; t.i.d. = three times daily.
Reprinted with permission from International Anesthesiology Clinics, 21:1, Little, Brown.

tremor) and cardiovascular effects (tachycardia, arrhythmias, or hypertension).

RESPIRATORY ASSISTANCE

Should simple increase of FiO_2 be insufficient to correct postoperative respiratory dysfunction, intubation and ventilatory assistance may be necessary.

Endotracheal Intubation

Benefits of intubation include:

1. Patency of the airway
2. Reduction of dead space
3. "Prevention" of aspiration (decreased likelihood)
4. Easier tracheobronchial toilet
5. Facilitation of ventilation
6. Safer positioning of the patient

Intubation is most easily accomplished in the sedated, relaxed patient. Factors which may cause technical difficulties include protruding teeth, large tongue, small mouth, limited mandibular movement, short neck, and a struggling patient. Prior to attempting intubation, it is important to check all equipment (functioning largyngoscope, variety of tubes). Preoxygenation with an Ambu bag is essential. Sufficient air should be instilled into the cuff of the endotracheal tube until it just seals the airway. The cuff should be deflated every 15 minutes for a few seconds to ensure adequate perfusion of the tracheal mucosa. Endotracheal tubes must be taped or tied securely after it has been ascertained that breath sounds are equal bilaterally. Only humidified gases should be given through an endotracheal tube as the upper airway is no longer accessible to add water to the inspired air.

Complications of intubation include:

1. Transient hypertension
2. Bucking, which increases intrathoracic pressure
3. The need for continued sedation and thus the inability to assess accurately the mental status of the patient
4. Decreased ventilation (because tubes are smaller than airways)
5. Increased risk of pulmonary infection
6. Trauma

Assisted Ventilation

Just as it is not enough to simply lead the horse to water because it may then not drink, so it is following intubation. Simply securing the airway does not mean that adequate oxygenation will follow. There are several means of mechanically increasing alveolar ventilation.

Pressure Cycled Ventilators

Positive pressure ventilators produce lung inflation directly by generating and applying positive pressure to the airway. When a preset pressure is reached the inspiratory cycle stops irrespective of the volume delivered. Because this pressure is applied intermittently, this form of mechanical ventilation is often referred to as intermittent positive pressure ventilation (IPPV) or intermittent positive pressure breathing (IPPB). An example of this type of ventilator is the Bird. The principal advantage of this machine is that, as it is powered by a compressed gas source rather than an electrical supply, it can be conveniently used during transport. However, as a mainstay for ventilatory support it is unsatisfactory because of adverse effects on cardiovascular, pulmonary, and intracranial dynamics.

Volume-cycled Ventilators

The common type of ventilator used in the recovery room is a primarily volume-cycled machine. Tidal volume is preset. If the patient has no spontaneous respiratory action, rate is also set (control mode ventilation). This machine may also be used to assist ventilation. On sensing a drop in airway pressure as the patient begins a spontaneous breath, the ventilator delivers a mechanical breath. The sensitivity required to trigger the ventilator is predetermined. In this mode, if the patient becomes apneic, no ventilation occurs. The pure assist mode has been largely supplanted by assist control ventilation (A/CV), in which a minimal respiratory rate is set. As with the pure assist mode, the patient may trigger mechanical breaths by decreasing airway pressure, but even if the patient is apneic or paralyzed, a preset number of breaths are delivered. In both controlled and assisted ventilation, the $PaCO_2$ frequently falls below the apneic threshold. Deleterious effects which may result include:

1. Decreased coronary blood flow
2. Decreased cardiac output
3. Decreased myocardial contractility
4. Increased O_2 consumption
5. Decreased lung compliance
6. Increased airway resistance
7. Increased absolute shunt

8. Left shift of the oxyhemoglobin dissociation curve
9. Decreased cerebral blood flow
10. Inhibition of hypoxic pulmonary vasoconstriction

Intermittent mandatory ventilation (IMV) is a combination of mechanical and spontaneous ventilation. Tidal volume and respiratory rate are preset, but the patient is allowed to breathe spontaneously between ventilator breaths either from an independent gas supply or by means of a demand valve. Normal ventilation is more readily achieved and respiratory alkalosis, induced for the purposes of diminishing respiratory drive, is unnecessary.

The most recently developed ventilator modality is synchronous IMV (SIMV), otherwise known as intermittent assisted ventilation (IAV) or intermittent demand ventilation (IDV). With this ventilator modality, unlike conventional IMV, mechanical breaths are delivered when the ventilator senses an inspiratory effort on the part of the patient.

Expiratory Pressures

If pulmonary dysfunction is associated with alveolar collapse (especially adult respiratory distress syndrome), positive expiratory pressure may be applied to the airway during exhalation to prevent expiratory alveolar collapse. Positive expiratory pressures have been shown to increase functional residual capacity (FRC), pulmonary compliance, and arterial oxygen tensions (PaO_2). Ventilation perfusion matching is improved, and intrapulmonary shunt and the work of breathing are decreased.

Therapies, which are similar in their effectiveness, have been termed continuous positive airway pressure (CPAP), positive end-expiratory pressure (PEEP), continuous distending airway pressure (CDAP), continuous expiratory distending pressure (CEDP), and expiratory positive airway pressure (EPAP). This terminology may be dealt with simply: any positive expiratory pressure generated when the patient is being mechanically ventilated is termed PEEP and any positive expiratory pressure provided to a patient breathing spontaneously is termed CPAP.

High-frequency Ventilation

High-frequency jet ventilation has been shown to reduce barotrauma while maintaining cardiovascular stability. At rates of 60–100 breaths per minute, arterial oxygenation is well maintained. High-frequency oscillation, employing even higher rates, has been used in the treatment of respiratory insufficiency due to failure of conventional modes of gas transport and distribution.

High-frequency ventilation can maintain oxygenation and CO_2 elimination indefinitely. Other benefits include lower peak airway pressures, reflex inhibition of spontaneous respiratory drive, and minimal ventilatory effects on the cardiovascular or intracranial systems.

The technique is not without hazards including problems of humidification and temperature maintenance, overpressure with lung rupture, air trapping, hyperventilation, and CO_2 retention.

Cardiovascular Effects of Mechanical Ventilation

Respiratory acidosis stimulates the sympathetic nervous system initially, but eventually myocardial depression occurs. Changes in intrathoracic pressure caused by mechanical ventilation affect the heart and great vessels. Cardiac output is inversely related to the directional change in intrapleural pressure. During spontaneous inspiration, intrathoracic pressure is decreased by respiratory muscle activity which causes gas to flow into the lungs and creates a pressure gradient favoring return of blood to the right atrium ("the thoracic pump"). During mechanical ventilation, the opposite occurs, i.e., an increase in pressure tends to impede venous return. Thus cardiac output decreases to a degree dependent on the amount of imposed airway pressure. Hypotension may result, especially in the hypovolemic patient.

If spontaneous breathing can be maintained, mean airway pressure is lower with IMV than with other forms of positive pressure ventilation as fewer mechanical breaths are required during a given time interval, and intrathoracic pressure decreases each time a spontaneous inspiratory effort occurs. It is obvious that intrathoracic pressure is further increased by the institution of positive expiratory airway pressure, and, as would be expected, the use of PEEP in conjunction with mechanical ventilation has been observed to produce greater decreases in cardiac output than with either modality alone. The cardiac depressant effects of PEEP and CPAP may be minimized by lowering mechanical ventilatory rates or by allowing a significant decrease in airway pressure to occur during each spontaneous inspiration.

Setting the Ventilator

In choosing ventilator settings, the lowest oxygen concentration necessary to maintain adequate oxygenation should be employed. Volumes approximately twice the estimated tidal volume are appropriate with controlled rates of about 10-16 per minute or IMV rates of 4-6 per minute. Frequent recording of cardiorespiratory function (blood pressure, pulse, spontaneous respiratory rate, tidal volume, respiratory pattern, and arterial blood gas analyses) should be made.

Extubation

If the patient is conscious, ventilating adequately, and not vomiting, extubation may be considered. Other criteria include the ability of the patient to lift his head, bucking, breath holding, vital capacity over 10-15 ml/kg and a peak inspiratory force over -20 cm H_2O.

Technical considerations before extubation include good suctioning of the trachea and oropharynx, administration of oxygen, emptying the tube cuff, and generating positive pressure immediately prior to removing the tube.

Laryngospasm may occur immediately after extubation and can usually be reversed by positive pressure ventilation. If necessary, a small dose of succinylcholine (0.2-0.5 mg/kg) may be given in addition to ventilation. Following prolonged intubation, hoarseness, laryngeal edema, or croup may occur. Treatment includes reassurance, high humidity oxygen inhalation, and local anesthetic lozenges. If signs of upper airway obstruction increase (sternal retraction, nasal flaring), reintubation may become necessary.

CONCLUSION

There are many different types of equipment to treat respiratory insufficiency postoperatively. It is essential that nurses assigned to the recovery room familiarize themselves with endotracheal intubation kits, oxygen therapy apparatus, and ventilators used in their hospitals. In this area, perhaps more than in any other, "hands on" experience is essential in learning how to immediately provide optimal patient care.

SUGGESTIONS FOR FURTHER READING

Bowe EA, Klein EF. Postoperative respiratory care. In: Recovery room care. Frost E, Andrews IC, eds. International Anesthesiology Clinics, Vol 21, No 1. Boston: Little, Brown, 1983.
Comroe JH. Physiology of respiration, 2d ed. Chicago: Year Book Medical, 1966.

Dripps RD, Eckenhoff JE, Vandam LD. Introduction to anesthesia. Philadelphia: WB Saunders, 1977.

Eng UB, Eriksson I, Sjostrand U. High frequency positive pressure ventilation (HEPPV): A review based upon its use during bronchoscopy and for laryngoscopy and microlaryngeal surgery under general anesthesia. Anesth Analg 1980; 59:594-603.

Greenberg AG, Peskin GW. Monitoring in the recovery room and surgical intensive care unit. In: Monitoring in anesthesia, 2d ed. Saidman LJ, Smith NT, eds. Boston: Butterworth, 1984.

Israel JS, DeKornfeld TJ. Recovery room care. Springfield, IL: Charles C Thomas, 1982.

Lough MD, Doershuk EF, Stern RC, eds. Pediatric respiratory therapy. Chicago: Year Book Medical, 1974.

Miller NJ, Winter PM. Clinical manifestations of pulmonary oxygen toxicity. Internat Anesth Clin 1981; 19(3): 179-199.

Nunn JF. Applied respiratory physiology, 2d ed. London: Butterworths, 1977.

Shapiro BA. Clinical application of blood gases. Chicago: Year Book Medical, 1976.

Vuori A, Jalonen J, Laaksonen V. Continuous positive airway pressure during mechanical and spontaneous ventilation. ACTA Anaesth Scand 1979; 23: 453-461.

West JB. Blood flow to the lung and gas exchange. Anesthesiology 1974; 41:124-138.

4
Cardiovascular Action: Too Much, Too Little, or Irregular
Cedric Prys-Roberts

Recovery from anesthesia can be associated with marked instability of the cardiovascular system. Extremes of arterial hypotension or hypertension, bradycardia or tachycardia, and dysrhythmia are by no means uncommon and require a high degree of vigilance for detection and correction. While these abnormalities may be well tolerated by younger patients, they frequently herald the onset of serious consequences such as myocardial infarction, cerebral hemorrhage or infarction, renal failure, and acute cardiac arrest. Recognition, decision making, and action must follow in short succession.

MONITORING

The key to success in recognizing disturbances of cardiovascular function lies in continuous monitoring of as many variables as are consistent with the patient's preexisting medical state and the nature of the surgery. The more unpredictable the condition of the patient in the recovery room, the more variety of monitoring techniques and the greater emphasis on continuity of monitoring are required.

Arterial Pressure

Monitoring of arterial pressure can be considered under three headings: (1) continuation of direct intraarterial pressure recording used during surgery, (2) automatic, discontinuous, noninvasive measurements, and (3) intermittent, manual recordings.

Direct Intraarterial Pressure Measurement

This provides the most continuous and potentially the most accurate information. The observer derives a number of subsidiary indices of performance. Figure 4-1 shows how the arterial pressure pulse may be interpreted, and how abnormal conditions may be identified. These patterns can only be clearly and accurately identified if certain simple principles are

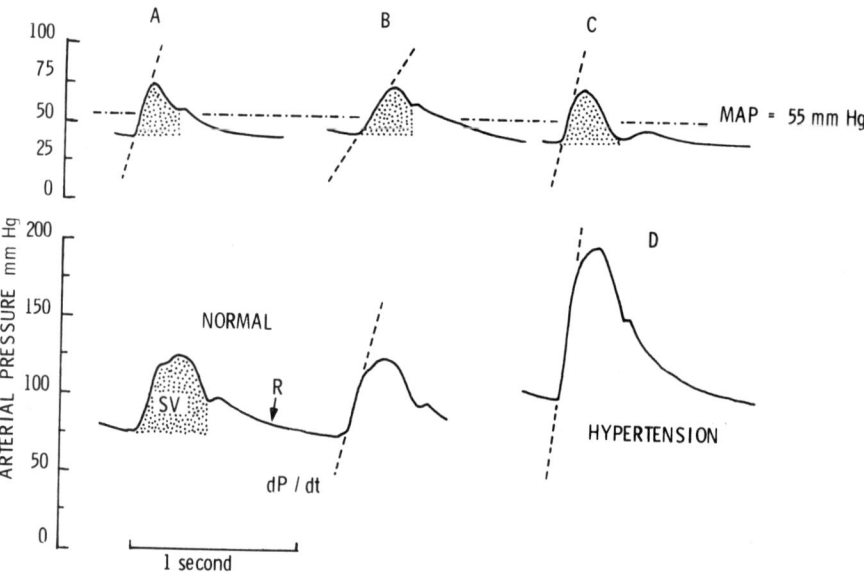

Figure 4-1. Arterial pressure waveforms as seen on a monitor screen or oscillograph tracing. The normal tracing shows that over and above the systolic and diastolic arterial pressure values, three additional pieces of information can be derived: (1) the area (shaded) under the systolic ejection curve is proportional to the stroke volume, (2) the rate of change of arterial pressure (dP/dt) is proportional to the contractile performance of the left ventricular muscle, (3) the diastolic decay of pressure is an exponential, whose time constant is the product of resistance and compliance of the systemic vasculature. Hence, the steepness of the diastolic pressure decay is proportional to the systemic vascular resistance. (A) Arterial pressure waveform during hypovolemia. (B) Arterial pressure waveform during myocardial depression by halothane anesthesia. (C) Arterial pressure waveform during an infusion of sodium nitroprusside. (D) Arterial pressure waveform in hypertension.

adhered to in the measurement process: (1) air bubbles should be avoided in the transducer domes, stop-cock systems, and catheters connecting to the patient's artery, and (2) the catheter with connecting tubing is kept as short and stiff as possible.

For a more detailed discussion of measurement techniques, the reader should consult the literature. Systolic and diastolic pressures should be recorded from whatever display or recording system is used, as these alone are the measurements common to all three categories. A wide pulse pressure (systolic-diastolic pressure) is usually indicative of a high stroke volume, and vice-versa. A high diastolic pressure and a steep diastolic pressure run-off indicate a high vascular resistance (Figure 4-1D). Low systolic and diastolic pressures could indicate either direct myocardial depression (Figure 4-1B), inadequate cardiac filling due to hypovolemia (Figure 4-1A), or persistence of drug effects from the anesthetic period causing marked arterial dilatation with consequent low vascular resistance (Figure 4-1C). Mean arterial pressure may be useful as a means of recording a trend but has little physiological significance. In each of these three circumstances (Figure 4-1A, B, and C) mean arterial pressure would have been the same and would have given *no indication of the cause* of the low arterial pressure. Steepness of the upstroke of the arterial pressure wave (dP/dt) indicates good contractility, whereas a sluggish upstroke may indicate poor contractility (Figure 4-1B). Beware of making the latter interpretation if there is any doubt about damping of the waveform due to air bubbles in the connecting tubing.

Dysrhythmias, which cause a shortening of the interbeat interval, may cause marked diminution of stroke volume and thus arterial pressure on occasional or alternate beats (Figure 4-2).

Automatic Noninvasive Measurements

During the past few years, a number of devices have become available which automatically inflate a standard sphygmomanometer cuff on the arm and, using the oscillometry principle, detect separately the systolic, mean, and diastolic pressures and determine the heart rate. A typical machine of this type is the Dynamap. Its accuracy and reproducibility in clinical practice has been described. It can measure both systolic and diastolic pressures within the range 50-250 mm Hg with a reproducibility of ± 15 mm Hg (95 percent confidence limits for a single measurement). This and other automatic systems are valuable for repeated measurements at frequent preset intervals in the recovery room. They have two disadvantages: (1) they are relatively poor at accurately measuring pressures during a sudden increase or decrease of pressure, and (2) they can produce bruising and nerve damage if set to inflate too frequently for long periods of time.

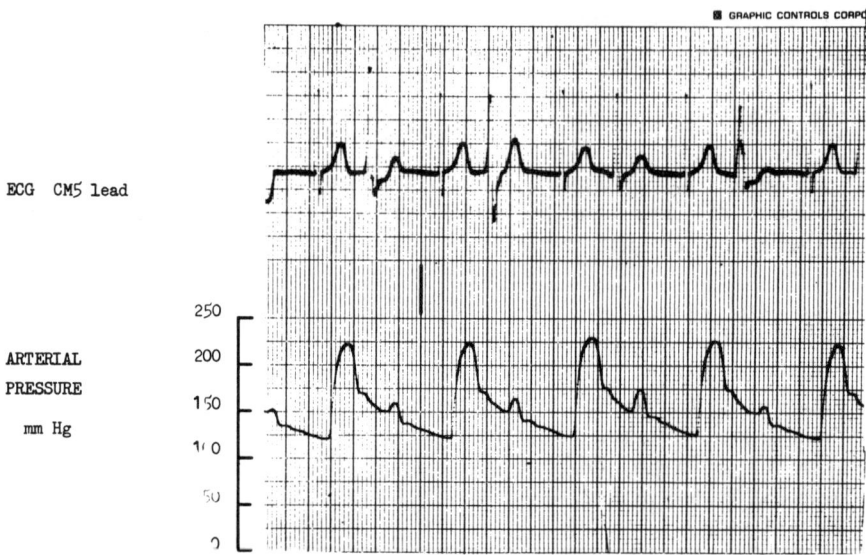

Figure 4-2. Influence of ventricular and junctional extrasystoles on the left ventricular output as manifest in the arterial pressure trace. Note that because extrasystolic beats come too early and allow inadequate time for ventricular filling and for the atrial kick the arterial pressure generated for these beats is almost nonexistent.

Intermittent Manual Recordings

The standard method of sphygmomanometry has been the mainstay of recovery room blood pressure measurement and is perfectly satisfactory for routine postoperative management. Detection of the onset of Korotkow sounds for measurement of systolic pressure gives poor absolute accuracy and reproducibility (95 percent confidence limits: ± 21 mm Hg) compared with the Dynamap, but better reproducibility for diastolic pressures (± 16 mm Hg) when determined as phase 5 limits (disappearance of Korotkow sounds).

Electrocardiogram (ECG)

The ECG is essential to monitor cardiac dysrhythmias, disturbances of cardiac conduction, and ischemia of the myocardium. Any of the standard 12 leads can be used to detect dysrhythmias or a prolonged P-R interval characteristic of first-degree heart block. To detect myocardial ischemia, which is commonly of left ventricular origin, either a standard V5 unipolar lead or preferably the CM5 bipolar lead (Figure 4-3) should be used. The CM5 lead consistently gives a positive R wave of good amplitude and has the highest probability, for any single lead, of detecting ST segment elevation characteristic of transmural ischemia. Continuous monitoring of heart rate is usually obtained from the ECG waveform.

Central Venous Pressure (CVP)

Catheters may be advanced to the superior vena cava or right atrium from the internal or external jugular veins, the subclavian vein or a peripheral vein at the elbow. Measurement of CVP by transducer or a simple saline manometer yields a mean value of pressure over the cardiac cycle. In the recovery room, the finding of a low CVP (< 1 mm Hg) in combination with a low arterial pressure is strongly suggestive of hypovolemia. By contrast, a low arterial pressure associated with elevated CVP (> 10 mm Hg) is more likely to represent impaired cardiac function.

Pulmonary Artery Balloon-tipped Catheters

Measurement of pulmonary artery (PA) pressures (systolic and diastolic) is normally only used in patients with severe pulmonary hypertension or right-ventricular failure and is of little value in monitoring the normal patient. In the early sixties PA catheters were floated without balloon control through the central veins and right ventricle, but could not be wedged. In 1969, Swan and his colleagues described a balloon-tipped catheter which could be placed in a distal branch of the pulmonary artery to yield an estimate of left atrial pressure when the balloon was inflated and phasic PA pressures with the balloon deflated. A thermistor placed at the tip of the catheter behind the balloon allows measurement of cardiac output by the thermodilution method. Such measurements are usually of value only in patients with severely compromised myocardial function or severe ventricular hypertrophy and those who have undergone cardiac surgery.

Pulse Monitors

Numerous methods have been devised to detect the existence of a volume pulse in a peripheral limb or digit. A photoelectric device is the cheapest and most reliable way of detecting such a pulse, whose existence implies an adequate circulation. As a purely qualitative estimate of volume flow and a

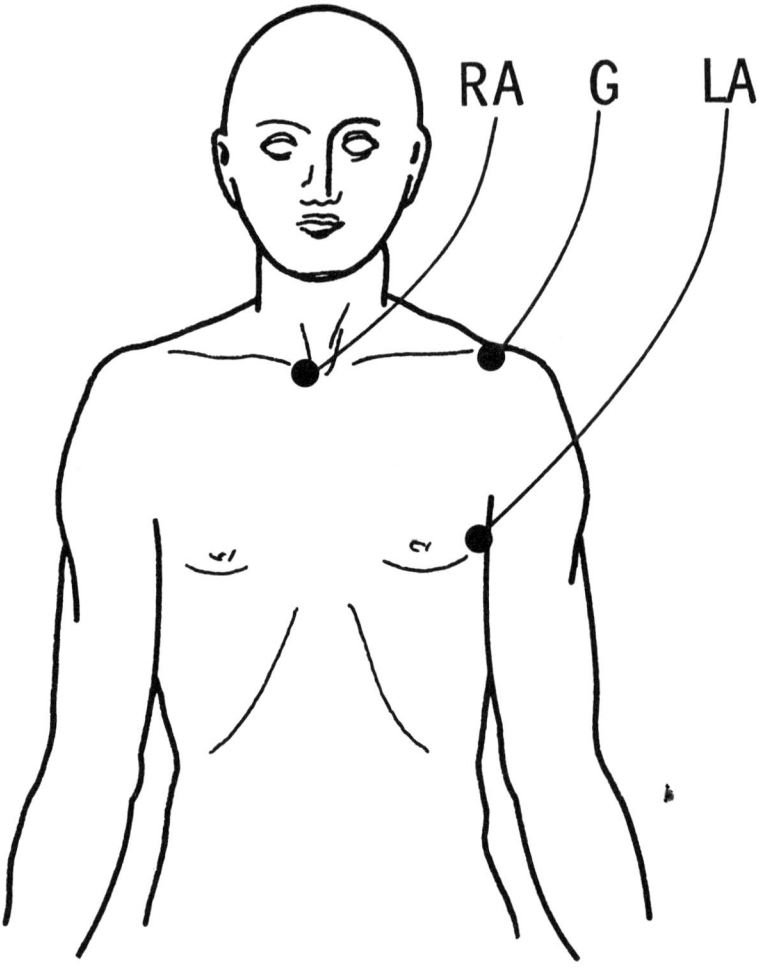

CM5 LEAD CONFIGURATION

Figure 4-3. Lead placement for CM5 configuration. When using this with a three-lead display (Lead I), the R arm lead should be placed just below the sternal notch, the L arm lead in the anterior axillary line at the fifth intercostal space (as for Lead V), and the indifferent lead on the left shoulder.

means of detecting heart rate, a pulse monitor is useful for the normal patient recovering from uncomplicated surgery.

CARDIOVASCULAR DISTURBANCES AND THEIR MANAGEMENT

This section is organized on a problem-oriented basis. Two main problems, arterial hypotension and hypertension, their recognition, causation, and management, are considered under three associated states of heart rate: normal heart rate (55–100 per minute), bradycardia (< 55 per minute), and tachycardia (> 100 per minute). Dysrhythmias and their management are considered within the context of hypotension and hypertension, as well as separately.

Problem: Arterial Pressure Too Low

Low arterial pressure can only be defined arbitrarily, depending on the preoperative arterial pressure of each patient. In the recovery room predetermined limits should be set with the anesthesiologist as to what constitutes important hypotension or hypertension. For a normotensive patient a systolic blood pressure 25 percent below the preoperative value (< 100 mm Hg in normotensive patients, < 130 mm Hg in hypertensive patients) would be considered a clinically important change requiring urgent attention. When systolic pressures fall to levels 40 percent below preoperative values, aggressive therapy is required. The nature of therapy depends on the cause of the hypotensive episode.

Causes: Decreased Cardiac Output

Normal heart rate: stroke volume decreased
• Direct myocardial depression by anesthetics. This represents a continuation of depressant effects of inhalational or intravenous anesthetics on the myocardium. Poor myocardial contractility is evident as small pulse pressure and low dP/dt of arterial pressure trace.

To treat these patients (1) encourage deep breathing to wash out any remaining inhalational anesthetics; (2) stimulate myocardial activity by infusion of isoproterenol (0.02 µg/kg per minute) or dopamine (1–2 µg/kg per minute).

• Low output failure: cardiogenic shock. The most florid clinical sign of acute left ventricular failure is pulmonary (alveolar) edema, which is the third stage of a process which starts with pulmonary congestion and proceeds through interstitial edema. Early pulmonary congestion is recognized by a history of tachypnea, orthopnea, and paroxysmal nocturnal dyspnea. Interstitial edema may be recognized by the signs of basal crepitations and rales, and by the appearance of Kerley B lines on the chest X ray. Florid pulmonary edema may occur in the recovery room when acute left ventricular failure is precipitated by sudden hypertension.

The management of low output failure is shown in Figure 4-4 in which the signs of pulmonary edema and congestion are linked to measurements of cardiac output and pulmonary artery wedge pressures.

For pulmonary congestion, the general principle is to give a diuretic and a vasodilator which exerts a venodilating effect, e.g., a nitrate: (1) furosemide 40-80 mg intravenously; (2) nitroglycerin (NTG) 0.6 mg sublingual; or (3) isosorbide dinitrate 5-15 mg sublingual; (4) intravenous infusion of NTG 0.5-5 µg/kg per minute.

For low cardiac output syndrome — cardiogenic shock — give (1) digoxin 0.25-0.5 mg intravenously; (2) combined therapy with infusions of inotropic and vasodilator drugs (dopamine 5-10 µg/kg per minute, with sodium nitroprusside 0.5-5.0 µg/kg per minute, (3) epinephrine infusion 2-10 µg/kg per minute, and (4) aortic balloon-pump counterpulsation.

• Myocardial ischemia. When arterial hypotension is caused by myocardial ischemia, it is usually secondary to some other cause of hypotension which has resulted in inadequate coronary perfusion due to a low diastolic arterial pressure. Myocardial ischemia occurs in two forms: subendocardial

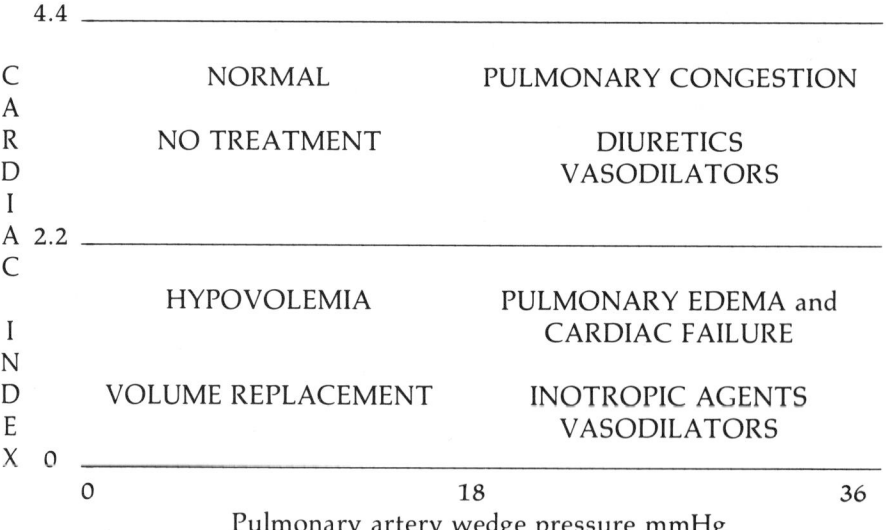

Figure 4-4. Management of low-output failure.

ischemia which is recognized by the appearance of deep ST segment depression (Figure 4-5A), or transmural ischemia characterized by ST segment elevation (Figure 4-5B). This latter type may occur after acute myocardial infarction, or more rarely as a manifestation of coronary artery spasm (Prinzmetal's variant angina).

To treat myocardial ischemia, prevent further deterioration of coronary blood flow by maintaining diastolic pressure above the critical value for that patient (usually > 80-100 mm Hg). Dopamine infusion (1-3 μg/kg per minute) can be effective, but take care to avoid a heart rate increase which will also increase the myocardial oxygen requirements. Phenylephrine infusion can also be used, but take care to avoid an excessive increase of systolic arterial pressure.

- Impaired cardiac filling. Hypovolemia without baroreflex response is due to impaired cardiac filling. Recognition of minor degrees of hypovolemia is difficult, as many other factors combined with minor blood loss can cause marked hypotension. Tachycardia in association with arterial hypotension, especially when the pulse pressure is small, is traditionally described as the cardinal sign of blood loss. One must bear in mind that when heart rate increases in response to a decreasing arterial pressure, the response is mediated through the carotid sinus baroreceptors. It has been well established that anesthesia suppresses this barostatic response, but there is little evidence available to indicate how long such depression lasts

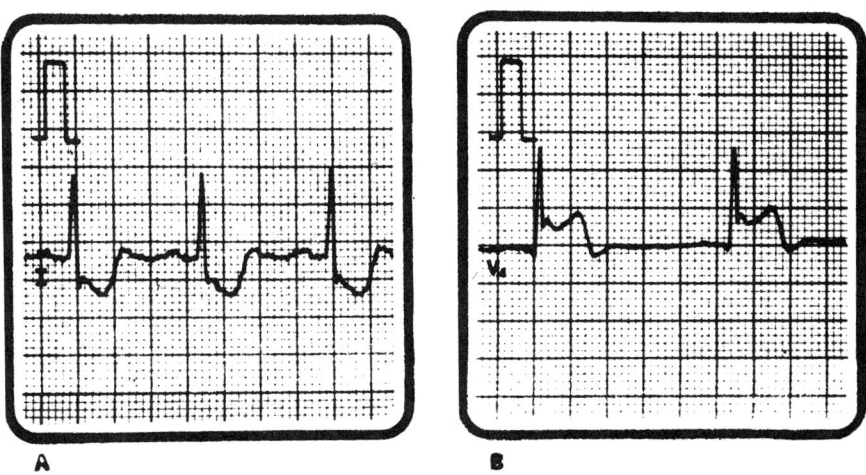

Figure 4-5. ST segment depression (A) indicative of subendocardial ischemia, and ST segment elevation (B) indicative of transmural ischemia.

after termination of anesthesia. Certainly for 30–60 minutes after the end of anesthesia, one should anticipate that modest degrees of blood loss (< 10 percent of the predicted blood volume) would not provoke a significant tachycardia. Other signs of sympathetic nervous activity in response to hemorrhage, such as sweating and pallor, may also be diminished in the first hour after anesthesia. Central venous pressure will almost always be decreased when hemorrhage exceeds 5 percent of the blood volume. In this respect, accurate setting of the reference point (mid-axillary line in the supine position) is most important. Obviously, if the reference point is set even 2 cm too high, it will give the impression that the CVP is 2 cm too low. If a CVP measurement is available, it is an easy task to test the hypothesis of hypovolemia by rapidly infusing about 200 ml of crystalloid solution, observing the response (hopefully a rapid increase) of both arterial pressure and CVP. Even in the absence of CVP measurements, an acceptable increase of arterial pressure (> 10 mm Hg) in response to such a fluid load is ample evidence.

Treatment is as follows: (1) Raise legs or tip bed head down. (2) Give 250–500 ml lactated Ringer's solution, giving the first 250 ml rapidly and watching the response of both arterial pressure and CVP. (3) If there is a marked increase of arterial pressure in response to this amount of fluid, consider expanding the patient's blood volume with 250–500 ml whole blood or an alternative colloid solution such as plasma protein factor (PPF), salt-poor albumin, or dextran.

Cardiac tamponade. This is evident as hypotension with decreased pulse pressure, paradoxical effect of breathing on arterial pressure (decrease of arterial pulse during inspiration), and distention of neck veins. Causes are pericardial effusion or hemopericardium, for instance, knife wounds to the chest or upper abdomen. Pericardial drainage is performed by insertion of an 18-g needle in the midline behind the xiphisternum, toward the base of the heart.

Bradycardia

• Sinus bradycardia. This is usually a residual effect of neostigmine given at the end of anesthesia to reverse muscle relaxation and may be very marked in patients receiving beta-receptor blockers. This is also a common finding after spinal anesthesia or thoracic epidural blockade and is common in patients with body temperatures below 32°C. To treat, give atropine 0.6 mg, repeated at 5 minutes if heart rate is still below 50 per minute.
• Junctional bradycardia. No P waves are visible on ECG (Figure 4-6). This is usually caused by interaction of volatile anesthetics and their effect on cardiac conduction, with the effect of neostigmine. To treat, give (1) atropine 0.6 mg intravenously; (2) calcium chloride 5 ml of a 10 percent solution, to aid and improve cardiac conduction; (3) isoproterenol infusion

(0.02 μg/kg per minute) if the use of atropine and calcium chloride has been ineffective.

• Heart Block (Figure 4-7). In first-degree heart block, the ECG P-R interval is greater than 0.12 seconds. In Möbitz Type I (Wenkebach) second-degree heart block, the ECG P-R interval lengthens with successive beats until one QRS complex is then dropped. In Möbitz Type II second-degree heart block, the P-R interval is constantly long, but occasional beats are dropped. There is also 2:1 or 3:1 block with an atrial rate 2 or 3 times that of the ventricular rate. In third-degree heart block, there is complete dissociation of P and QRS waves, usually with a slow heart rate.

To treat give isoproterenol infusion (0.02 μg/kg per minute). Take care not to increase the infusion rate above 10 μg per minute in the absence of a reversal of heart block, as this may increase ventricular irritability and precipitate ventricular fibrillation. Insert a transvenous pacemaker catheter. In all cases of severe refractory bradycardia or heart block, call a physician immediately.

Tachycardia

• Sinus tachycardia. The commonest cause of sinus tachycardia is increased sympathetic nervous activity stimulated by pain, bladder distention, or by apprehension. If heart rate is greater than 150 per minute,

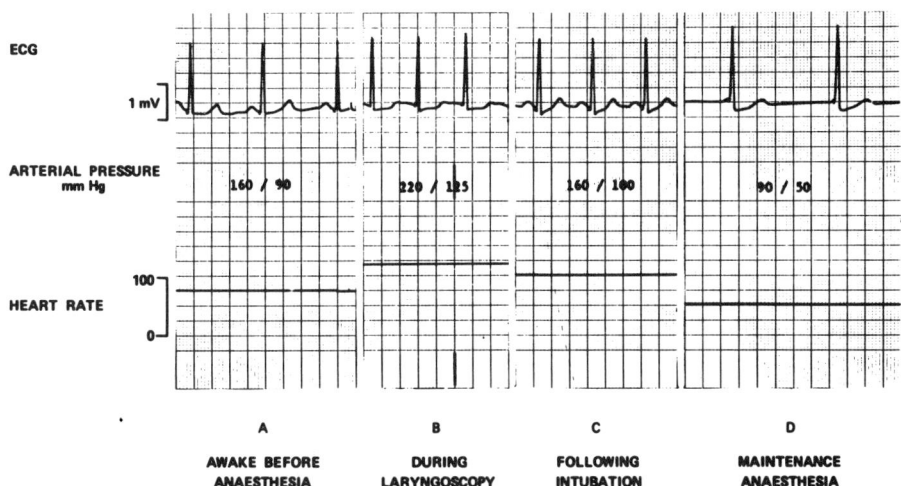

Figure 4-6. Episodes of junctional tachycardia (B) and bradycardia (D) occurring during anesthesia. Compare with the normal ECG awake (A), and note that ST segment has occurred on both occasions.

1st degree heart block

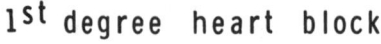

2d degree heart block

a. Möbitz I (Wenckebach)

b. Möbitz II

c. 2/1 block

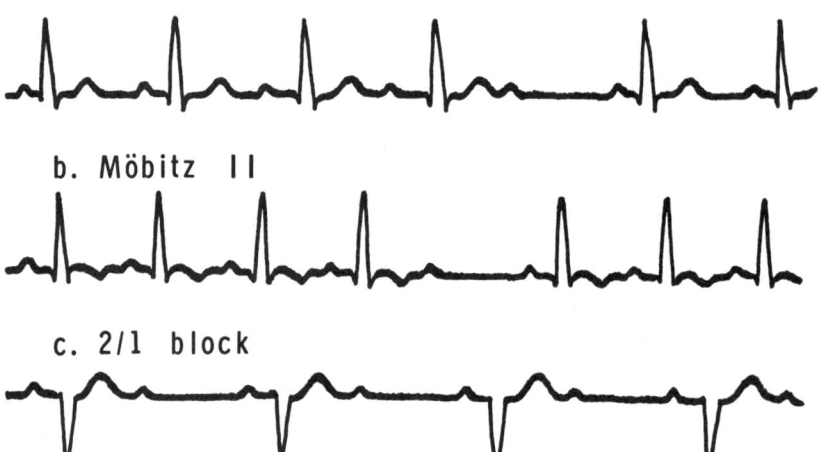

3d degree heart block

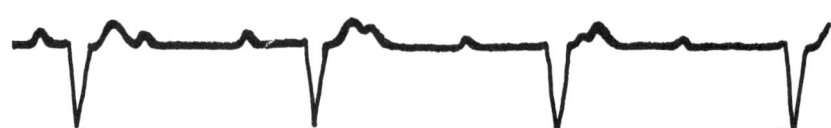

Figure 4-7. Heart block: different ECG patterns.

cardiac filling may be inadequate and may cause myocardial ischemia in susceptible patients. To treat, give propranolol 1-2 mg, or metoprolol 2-5 mg intravenously if heart rate is greater than 120 per minute.
• Junctional tachycardia. This is commonly caused by increased sympathetic nervous activity in patients with depressed cardiac conduction, either due to the effects of anesthetics or digitalis toxicity. If the patient has

not been receiving digitalis, give propranolol 1–2 mg intravenously, or verapamil 5 mg intravenously can be used to control the heart rate. When junctional tachycardia is a complication of digitalis overactivity, many authorities advise the use of DC countershock.

• Atrial fibrillation. When this is associated with a ventricular rate more than 120 per minute, cardiac output falls markedly due to poor filling. This may occur due to inadequate treatment with cardiac glycosides.

If the heart rate is greater than 150 per minute, propranolol may be given in small increments (0.2 mg intravenously every minute) until the rate can be decreased to about 100 to 110 per minute. DC countershock may also be used in these circumstances if propranolol or metoprolol are in any way contraindicated. Digoxin may be given to patients with rapid atrial fibrillation, but the peak effect is slow in onset and a satisfactory decrease of heart rate may take a few hours to achieve. Digoxin 0.25–0.5 mg may be given intravenously.

• Wolff-Parkinson-White Syndrome. Recurrent atrial tachycardia associated with this condition may cause impaired ventricular filling. Heart rate should be controlled with small doses of propranolol or verapamil.

Causes: Decreased Systemic Vascular Resistance (SVR)

Normal heart rate: no baroreflex response to low blood pressure

• After spinal or epidural anesthesia. When there is evidence that somatic blockade is still effective, low arterial pressure is usually the result of arteriolar dilatation coupled with expansion of the venous capacitance vessels. Treatment is as follows: (1) Raise patient's legs or tip bed head-down. (2) Give 250–500 ml lactated Ringer's solution intravenously. (3) Give methoxamine 1–2 mg intravenously, repeated at 5-minute intervals if necessary. Do not give methoxamine to patients with heart rates less than 55 per minute. (4) Give ephedrine 5–10 mg intravenously followed by another 5 mg intramuscularly.

• Persistent effects of vasodilator drugs given during the course of anesthesia. Drugs such as trimetaphan, hydralazine, or sodium nitroprusside may produce delayed and protracted arteriolar dilatation after the end of anesthesia. To treat, give methoxamine 1–2 mg intravenously, repeated at 5 minutes if necessary.

Tachycardia. Low arterial pressure associated with tachycardia may imply a normal baroreflex activity, in which case, treatment of the hypotension should follow the pattern described above for hypovolemia.

• Septicemia (endotoxic shock). In patients who have undergone elective or emergency intraabdominal surgery, the possibility of endotoxemia should be considered when hypotension and tachycardia are found in the recovery room. Characteristic features are: arterial pressure wave with little or no diastolic run-off, a warm, dry skin (in the early stages), a high cardiac output, and low CVP.

Treatment is as follows: (1) Infuse colloid solutions (salt-poor albumin or fresh frozen plasma) to counteract the loss of protein from the extracellular blood. (2) Give methylprednisolone 1 mg/kg, dexamethasone 8 mg, or hydrocortisone hemisuccinate 500–800 mg. (3) Give antibiotic therapy effective against *Escherichia coli* and other gram-negative organisms: gentamycin 1 mg/kg and metronidazole 500 mg intravenously.

• Hemodilution. Inadequate red-cell replacement despite an adequate volume replacement with crystalloid or colloid solutions can lead to excessive hemodilution, especially in patients who start with mild to moderate anemia. To treat, transfuse whole blood or red-cell concentrates.

Problem: Arterial Pressure Too High

The definition of hypertension is quite arbitrary. For the purposes of patient care in the recovery room we can define hypertension as systolic pressure greater than 180 mm Hg with diastolic pressure greater than 90 mm Hg in previously normotensive patients, and systolic pressure greater than 220 mm Hg with diastolic pressure greater than 110 mm Hg in previously hypertensive patients.

Causes: Cardiac Output Increased

The common finding is of a patient with a high pulse pressure, resulting in systolic hypertension with normal or low diastolic pressure. These conditions are commonly found in patients with arteriosclerosis (rigid arterial disease) in whom a small change of the stroke volume ejected into the rigid arterial system results in large changes of pulse pressure. Pain or bladder distention are the most frequent causes of such systolic hypertension.

Normal heart rate: no baroreflex response to hypertension
• Arteriosclerotic patients. Treatment is as follows: (1) Give morphine sulfate 5–10 mg intravenously slowly to relieve pain. (2) Catheterize patient if the urinary bladder is distended and the patient cannot void urine. (3) Give propranolol 1–2 mg intravenously if systolic pressure is greater than 250 mm Hg.
• Hypertensive patients. Awakening after anesthesia and surgery may be associated with sudden and severe hypertension in patients with preexisting hypertension, both treated and untreated. Because of the adaptive hypertrophy in the arterioles of hypertensive patients, their arterial pressures show exaggerated responses to stimuli which generate

vasoconstriction. These patients may develop systolic arterial pressures between 200 and 300 mm Hg and diastolic pressures between 130 and 160 mm Hg during the first 30 to 60 minutes after the end of anesthesia. Such pressures pose a serious threat to the well-being of the patient and can cause (1) cerebral hemorrhage, (2) acute left ventricular failure with pulmonary edema, (3) acute myocardial ischemia, and (4) disruption of recently grafted arteries.

Treatment is as follows: (1) Infuse sodium nitroprusside 0.5–5.0 µg/kg per minute to reduce arterial pressure to 160/100 mm Hg. (2) To maintain this pressure, give propranolol 2 mg intravenously repeated at 10 minutes if heart rate is greater than 100 per minute or the rate-pressure product stays above 18,000. Also give hydrallazine 5–10 mg intravenously, repeated at 20-minute intervals if diastolic pressure is over 100 mm Hg.

• Carotid endarterectomy patients. Carotid surgery is often performed in arteriosclerotic patients. Excessive hypertension in the postoperative period may be associated with transient or permanent neurologic deficit, myocardial ischemia, or acute pulmonary edema. This requires aggressive therapy to bring systolic arterial pressure into a range (150–170 mm Hg) compatible with adequate cerebral perfusion, but with diminished risk of a local hematoma, intracranial hemorrhage, cerebral edema, and other problems created by hypertension.

For treatment of hypertension, see above, but select propranolol or hydralazine as the first line of treatment rather than sodium nitroprusside. If sodium nitroprusside is used, beware of suddenly reducing the arterial pressure too much. Sodium nitroprusside increases intracranial pressure and thus cerebral perfusion may become inadequate.

Tachycardia. Hypertension combined with tachycardia is a manifestation of increased sympathetic nervous activity, usually in response to noxious stimuli, of which pain is the most important to recognize. Distension of the urinary bladder is also a common cause in patients who have undergone genitourinary surgery. Misplacement of urinary catheters, so that the balloon is inflated in the prostatic bed or the urethra of the male, is also an uncommon but important cause of postoperative hypertension. Sympathetic storms are uncommon, but some unusual causes should be borne in mind: thyrotoxicosis, tetanus, and the Landry-Guillain-Barré syndrome.

The combination of hypertension and tachycardia increases the work of the heart dramatically. Rate-pressure product (RPP) was introduced to highlight this combination effect. RPP is the product of systolic arterial pressure (SAP) and heart rate (HR). Normal values are in the range 7200 (SAP 120 × HR 60) to 12,000 (SAP 120 × HR 100, or SAP 150 × HR 80). Values in excess of 24,000 (SAP 240 × HR 100, or SAP 200 × HR 120) clearly represent a very high myocardial oxygen requirement in order to fulfill the required work. Such a demand can easily be met for the normal heart by increased coronary blood flow; for instance, exercise may increase the RPP to at least the same extent. For the patient with coronary artery disease, such a requirement may precipitate acute subendocardial ischemia, manifest as depressed ST segments in the ECG (see Figure 4-5A) or, more rarely, elevated ST segments indicating transmural ischemia (Figure 4-5B). Aggressive therapy to reduce both systolic arterial pressure and heart rate must be begun as soon as possible to avoid the consequences of prolonged ischemia — acute myocardial infarction.

Treatment is as follows: (1) Ensure adequate analgesia (see Chapter 2). (2) Give propranolol 1-2 mg, or metoprolol 2-5 mg intravenously, at 10-minute intervals until heart rate is less than 100 per minute. (3) Give hydralazine 10-20 mg intravenously in patients with a known history of treated or untreated hypertension. Hydralazine may cause tachycardia and require propranolol therapy. (4) If the patient has a history of recent clonidine therapy, adopt a more aggressive regimen for controlling arterial pressure using sodium nitroprusside.

Bradycardia. The combination of hypertension (blood pressure greater than 220/110 mm Hg) and bradycardia (HR less than 50 per minute) is unusual and requires less aggressive therapy provided the patient is in sinus rhythm. It implies active baroreflexes. The commonest cause is a hangover effect of neostigmine in a previously untreated or poorly treated hypertensive patient. Such a large pulse pressure indicates an adequate stroke volume, which, despite the bradycardia, should be enough for the patient's requirements.
• Raised intracranial pressure (ICP). Hypertension at slow heart rates may represent the attempt of the vascular control system to maintain cerebral perfusion in face of raised ICP. Management is considered in Chapter 9.
• Hypertensive patients. The commonest cause of systolic or diastolic hypertension with bradycardia is unrelieved pain.

Problem: Dysrhythmia without Hypotension or Hypertension

Many dysrhythmias occur during the patient's recovery from anesthesia which are not associated with hypotension or hypertension (as defined at the beginning of this chapter). Provided these occur at heart rates between 50 and 90 per minute, they are unlikely to require treatment. Examples are unifocal ventricular extrasystoles occurring less than five times per minute (especially in patients known to have such a dysrhythmia preoperatively) or atrial fibrillation which is clearly well controlled either with or without digitalis therapy.

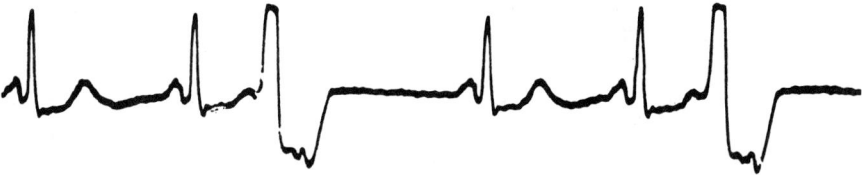

Lead I

Figure 4-8. Ventricular extrasystoles: R on T phenomenon.

However, there are some dysrhythmias which precede one of four life-threatening conditions: complete heart block with syncope, asystole (cardiac standstill), ventricular tachycardia, and ventricular fibrillation.

Ventricular extrasystoles. If these occur with every other beat, the cardiac rhythm is said to be coupled (synonymous with *bigeminy*). Coupled ventricular extrasystoles are not dangerous in themselves and occur commonly in association with hypercapnia (Figure 4-2 is a good example of a coupled rhythm). Check arterial blood gases and if these indicate a $PaCO_2$ higher than 55 mm Hg, take steps to improve the patient's ventilation or to establish artificial ventilation. If there is no apparent cause, adopt the decision process outlined below.

Multifocal ventricular extrasystoles. When there is more than one aberrant pacemaker, there is a danger of precipitating either ventricular tachycardia or fibrillation. Another serious precursor of these conditions is the existence of an R on T phenomenon (Figure 4-8) when the R wave occurs during the T wave (a time when part but not all of the ventricular muscle is no longer refractory).

To treat, give lidocaine 1 mg/kg intravenously followed by an infusion at 2-4 mg per minute, or a repeat dose in 15 to 20 minutes. Ventricular tachycardia should be managed in exactly the same way as multifocal ventricular extrasystoles. Ventricular asystole or fibrillation constitutes cardiac arrest and the general process of cardiopulmonary resuscitation (CPR) should be set in motion (see Chapter 14).

SUGGESTIONS FOR FURTHER READING

Frost EAM, Andrews IC, eds. Recovery room care. International Anesthesiology Clinics. Vol 21, No 1. Boston: Little, Brown, 1983.
Kaplan JA, ed. Cardiac anesthesia. Vol 2. Cardiovascular pharmacology. New York: Grune & Stratton, 1983.

Mason DT, ed. Cardiac emergencies. Baltimore: Williams & Wilkins, 1978.

Prys-Roberts C, ed. The circulation in anaesthesia. Oxford: Blackwell Scientific Publications, Inc, 1980.

Prys-Roberts C, ed. Hypertension, ischemic heart disease and anesthesia. International Anesthesiology Clinics. Vol 18, No 4. Boston: Little, Brown, 1980.

Prys-Roberts C, ed. Vascular disease and anaesthesia (Postgraduate Educational Symposium). Br J Anaesth 1981; 53(7):673-776.

Saidman LJ, Smith NT, eds. Monitoring in anesthesia. 2d ed. Woburn: Butterworths, 1983.

5
Postanesthetic Fluid Management
Walter Backus and Jeffrey Askanazi

The evolution of fluid therapy for surgical patients to a large degree reflects changing attitudes toward the handling of sodium in injury. Attention has shifted from plasma and the renal handling of salt and water to the extracellular space and the overall behavior of sodium. This change in attitude has resulted in marked changes in fluid therapy of acute surgical patients. Isotonic saline, which once was felt to be contraindicated in the immediate postoperative period, is now regarded as essential. However, it is clear that excesses can result in complications.

Essential to proper fluid therapy is an understanding of body composition and of the changes that occur in injury. The abnormal body composition of the injured patient after resuscitation is the result of the therapy superimposed upon the body's response to the injury. The daily fluid and electrolyte therapy for such a patient is the sum of normal requirements and additional needs, which are associated with the stage of convalescence after injury.

NORMAL BODY COMPOSITION

The adult body is composed of three functional components: fat, cell mass, and extracellular structures. The amount of each varies as a function of age, sex, and body size.

Total body water (TBW) is the largest single component of body weight, being greatest in the young muscular adult male (over 60 percent) and least in the elderly obese female (under 45 percent). In general, total body water is considered to be distributed into two major fluid spaces: intracellular fluid (ICF), consisting of 25–30 percent of average body weight, and extracellular fluid (ECF), consisting of 20–25 percent of normal body weight.

The body content of electrolytes is discussed in terms of their exchangeable components, when measured with an isotope dilution technique. Body stores of potassium can be measured by whole body counting of the naturally occurring isotope. Neutron activation has recently been used to measure many tissue components. Minerals that are incorporated into bone, collagen, and connective tissue exchange very slowly with plasma and generally are not considered in determining the composition of parenteral fluid therapy needed to achieve daily balance.

The total exchangeable potassium can be considered as equivalent to the body stores of potassium for clinical purposes. A healthy man (70 kg) has a pool of exchangeable potassium of 2700–3400 mmol; a woman, 2100–2300 mmol. The major fraction of this pool is intracellular, the small extracellular portion approximating 1–2 percent of the total.

In contrast to potassium, exchangeable sodium is only 65 percent of total body sodium. Men contain approximately 2800 mmol (70 kg); women, approximately 2600 mmol. The fraction of sodium in the skeleton is only slowly exchangeable. A normal 70-kg man contains approximately 2100 mmol of chloride.

NORMAL DAILY BALANCE

Water

The daily amount of water and dilute liquids required by the normal individual varies widely with habit and climate, but in temperate climates the average adult exchanges 2500–4500 ml of water daily with a body pool of 25–45 liters. Fluid intake averages 1000–2500 ml per day. Water in foods averages 1000–1500 ml. Water of oxidation adds 200–400 ml per day.

Losses take place by three routes: evaporation from the respiratory tract and skin, urinary output, and the water content of stool. The first two are termed "insensible losses." In the normal individual, water intake and losses balance each other very closely. Daily body weight usually fluctuates by less than 2 percent, and often by less than 1 percent if measured at the same time of day. Insensible losses depend on body size, physical exertion, environmental temperature, and humidity. Surface evaporation and sweat together average 600–800 ml per day. Total insensible water loss is between 300 and 500 ml per meter of body surface area per day, with minimal activity in a temperate environment. Sweat volume is small in a temperate climate except with vigorous activity, but may reach several liters a day, with serious losses of both water and sodium chloride in warm humid environments with exposure to the sun. Markedly obese patients have an increased water loss largely due to sweat. Such patients show marked changes in daily weight consistent with unusually large fluctuations in ECF.

Electrolytes

The daily sodium intake of the normal individual varies between 50 and 100 mmol. Normal body composition is maintained primarily as the result of the renal capacity to excrete any excess intake. When there is a low intake, or extrarenal losses, the kidney has the capability of reducing sodium excretion to as low as 1 mmol per day. As renal function is lost in disease, the capability of this extreme reduction in sodium excretion may be lost, and certain renal disorders have a wasting of sodium considerably in excess of the daily intake.

The daily intake of potassium varies from 40 to 80 mmol per day. However, potassium metabolism is strongly influenced by acid-base balance and the normal kidney does not respond to a reduction in intake by prompt conservation of potassium in the way that it does for sodium.

SERUM ELECTROLYTE CONCENTRATIONS

Several studies have reviewed the electrolyte composition of body fluids. A definite relationship exists between the serum concentration of sodium and potassium and the total exchangeable sodium and potassium. There is poor correlation between the serum sodium and total body sodium.

$$\text{Serum sodium} = \frac{(\text{total exchangeable sodium}) + (\text{total exchangeable potassium})}{(\text{total body water})} - 26$$

Thus serum sodium can be increased by additional potassium or sodium or restriction of free water. Retention of water in excess of sodium can lead to hyponatremia even with an excess of total body sodium. Administration of potassium can raise the serum sodium concentration in hyponatremic patients.

Most potassium is contained in the intracellular fluid, leaving only a small fraction of body potassium in plasma. Thus the absolute reduction of serum potassium which occurs with depletion can be expected to reflect a very large total body potassium deficit. However, a change in acid-base status may alter the serum potassium levels quite markedly as H^+ is exchanged for K^+. Thus, alkalosis may lower serum K^+ markedly, particularly if there is a preexisting total body deficit.

To maintain electroneutrality:

serum $(Na^+) + (Ca^{2+}) + (Mg^{2+}) + (K^+) = (Cl^-) + (HCO_3^-) +$ (protein) + (sulphate) + (phosphate) + (organic acids)

Thus:

$(Na^+) + (K^+) = (HCO_3^-) + (Cl^-) + 14$

The factor of 14 is commonly termed the anion gap. If (sodium + potassium) − (bicarbonate + chloride) exceeds 18, the substantial addition of an anion must be suspected.

These are (1) HPO_4^{2-} and SO_4^{2-}, as in renal failure; (2) lactic acid, as in hypoxia, shock states, and salicylate intoxication; (3) keto acids, as in diabetic ketoacidosis. If the anion gap is less than 5, hypoproteinemia is the most likely cause.

GASTROINTESTINAL TRACT LOSSES

The normal daily volume of secretion into the gastrointestinal tract is not precisely known but has been estimated to be 8000–10,000 ml per day, of which saliva constitutes 1–2 liters, gastric juice, including body acid and mucoid secretions, about 2500 ml, bile 500–750 ml, and pancreatic juice in the range of 100 ml. In addition, secretion of the upper small-bowel mucosa contributes between 2000 and 3000 ml. All but 100–200 ml of the secretions are normally reabsorbed by the small bowel and the colon.

Abnormal losses from the gastrointestinal tract include water and electrolytes and varying amounts of protein. The electrolyte content of fluid from the gastrointestinal tract varies significantly with the level from which most of the fluid is derived. Table 5-1 shows the average value and the range of variation of sodium, potassium, chloride, and bicarbonate in fluids from different levels of the intestine. It is important to note that, of all the secretions, only bile and pancreatic juice are approximately isotonic in their electrolyte content. The average calculated osmolality of saliva is about 160 mOsml; of upper small-bowel content, 220 mOsml; and of fluid from the distal ileum about 240 mOsml. Other substances including mucoproteins, other polysaccharides, urea, calcium, and phosphate add to these approximations of the total osmolality.

The values shown in Table 5-1 may be used for semiquantitative replacement of gastrointestinal tract losses. When volumes of these losses exceed 2000 ml in 24 hours or when substantial losses (1 l or more per day) continue for more than a few days, it is wise to send an aliquot of the

Table 5-1. Electrolyte Content of Gastrointestinal Secretions (mmol/liter)

Source of Fluid	Na^+	K^+	Cl^-	HCO_3^-
Saliva	60	20	16	50
Gastric	30–90	4·0–12	50–155	0
Upper small bowel	70–120	3·0–7·0	70–120	10
Ileum	90–140	3·0–8·0	80–125	15–20
Bile	145	4·0–7·0	80–110	50
Pancreas	120–140	5–8	60–80	

From Randall HT. Fluid, electrolyte and acid base balance. Surg Clin N Am 56:1019.

24-hour drainage to the laboratory for measurement of electrolytes and protein and to determine the pH of a freshly obtained specimen. More precise replacement can be made with this information. It is important to note that replacement of abnormal losses should be provided in addition to baseline requirements.

The data listed in Table 5-2 are intended only as approximate guidelines in fluid replacement. Fluid therapy should be individualized for a given patient. In general, urinary output serves as a useful guide to fluid therapy and should be maintained at levels of 600 ml per day or more. If output decreases below 600 ml per day in association with a decreasing central venous pressure or a decrease in body weight, an increase in fluid requirements is indicated. A decrease in urinary output, associated with a rising central venous pressure and weight gain, may indicate the onset of interstitial pulmonary edema, and diuretic therapy should be instituted.

The common use of the term "dehydration" can lead to confusion since two different clinical syndromes may each be referred to as dehydration. One syndrome is due to the loss of sodium and chloride with contraction of the extracellular volume, causing decreased skin turgor, a rapid pulse and a lowered blood pressure. Laboratory findings are related to increased hemoglobin and hematocrit with lower sodium and chloride values in the plasma while the urine volume and concentration is not remarkable. Another syndrome is associated with the primary loss of water without loss of electrolytes. Skin turgor, together with circulatory signs and symptoms, are usually normal even though thirst becomes intense. Oliguria with maximal urine concentration is associated with elevated plasma sodium and chloride. When referring to dehydration, sufficient description should be provided to clarify which of these two syndromes is under discussion.

Table 5-2. Baseline Fluid Requirements

	Age (years)	Fluid (ml/kg per day)
Average adults	25–55	35
Young active adults	16–30	40
Older patients	55–65(±)	30
Elderly	65	25

Adult values are based on ideal weight for height and age. Modified from Randall HT. Fluid, electrolyte and acid base balance. Surg Clin N Am 56:1019.

FLUID AND ELECTROLYTE CHANGES IN INJURY

Normal individuals usually tolerate large amounts of intravenously administered sodium chloride. In the immediate postoperative period these same individuals will tend to retain some of the administered fluid and may even develop respiratory symptoms from relatively modest excesses of sodium chloride. This observation of postoperative salt tolerance was recognized as early as 1911. As complications secondary to salt loss were increasingly observed, an era of postoperative saline administration ensued. The studies which emphasized the dangers of salt deprivation led to a period where many surgeons administered saline whether or not losses had occurred and the manifestations of fluid overload sometimes became evident. Reports soon followed cautioning against excessive salt administration. In 1944, Coller retracted his previously published formula for fluid administration and stated that no salt solution should be given for the first two postoperative days.

In 1950, Ariel and Kremen performed salt tolerance tests prior to and following elective operation. They noted that, postoperatively, a great fraction of the administered salt load shifted into the interstitial space. Lyon et al determined that postoperative preservation or restoration of blood or plasma volume appeared to be dependent on a state of positive fluid balance. Patients in negative fluid balance following an operation had delayed recovery of the available fluid until a state of positive fluid balance was established. In 1953, Aronstam demonstrated an expansion of the extracellular space which followed major thoracic operations.

Wiggers noted that animals which did not survive hemorrhagic shock demonstrated hemoconcentration even though the shed blood was returned. Gilman demonstrated that animals which were deficient in extracellular fluid were sensitive to relatively small degrees of hemorrhage.

Reynolds demonstrated that dogs in hemorrhagic shock treated with saline alone could survive with a return of cardiac output.

A series of studies by Shires et al emphasized the disparate reduction of functional extracellular fluid volume (as measured by the ^{35}S space) induced by hemorrhagic shock. This deficit is not alleviated by return of the shed blood alone or by moderate overexpansion of the intravascular volume with plasma. Rather, the reduction in ECF could be alleviated by use of a balanced salt solution as an adjunct to shed blood replacement. It must be emphasized that these measurements of a reduced function ECF were made either during, or soon after, the period of injury or shock.

The changes in the ECF following injury or shock vary with time. Table 5-3 demonstrates that during shock there is a reduction in the ECF, while following resuscitation the ECF is expanded.

Pluth et al and Moore et al demonstrated an expansion of the extracellular space following injury and resuscitation which did not appear to be due to excessive fluid administration. Roth et al also reported an increase in ECF following injury and suggested moderation in the use of Ringer's lactate for resuscitation. Elwyn and Shoemaker reported an expansion of the extracellular space in postoperative patients which was similar to that seen in nutritional depletion. The changes seen in nutritional depletion resolved with adequate nutrition (Tables 5-1 and 5-2).

The weight gain due to fluid administration as immediate treatment for operation or injury is variable and a function of the severity of the injury, as well as the preexisting clinical state of the patient. Elective operations such as total hip replacement or colon resection are commonly associated with a 3-5 percent weight gain, while major trauma may be associated with a 10-15 percent gain in body weight after resuscitation. In our view, such acute weight gains are difficult to avoid. Fluid administration should be guided by parameters such as blood pressure, central venous pressure, and urinary output. It is important to note that from the 3rd to

Table 5-3. Changes in Membrane Potential and Extracellular Water Following Shock

	ECF (% body weight)	Membrane potential (MV)
Control	13.9	−91
Shock	7.7	−65
Resuscitation	18.4	−90

Modified from Shires GT. Fluid and electrolyte therapy. In: Inney JM, Egdahl RH, and Zuidema GD eds. Manual of preoperative and postoperative care, 2nd ed. Philadelphia: WB Saunders, 1971.

the 6th day following injury a diuresis will ordinarily develop. Failure to return to the initial weight by the 10th day after operation or injury should be regarded as a warning of an impending complication (congestive heart failure, sepsis, renal failure, etc).

It has been suggested by Flear et al that the postinjury changes in ECF and ICF probably reflect a change in permeability of cell membranes and disturbance in ionic exchange. Thus injury is thought to lead to an increased escape of nondiffusible solutes into the ECF. This causes a decrease in the osmolality of cell fluids, while increasing the osmolality and resultant volume of the ECF.

Skeletal muscle represents the major component of lean body tissue and can be safely sampled by needle biopsy. Studies performed by Bergstrom et al and Askanazi et al using the needle biopsy technique have evaluated the role of nutrition and activity level in muscle fluid sequestration. Patients undergoing total hip replacement were assigned to receive a daily intravenous infusion of either 5 percent dextrose solution or 5.5 percent amino acid solution (with appropriate electrolytes and vitamins) for the first four postoperative days. Muscle biopsies were performed in the nonoperated thigh preoperatively and on the fourth day postoperatively. These studies demonstrated that an increase in muscle sodium and chloride occurs in noninjured portions of the body. These changes are not affected by the form of nutritional support administered. There was an increase in muscle ECF in these patients, which was unaffected by the nutritional support system administered. In normal subjects on bedrest, receiving either a regular diet or a 5 percent dextrose solution, there were no comparable changes in muscle composition.

With increasing severity of injury and injury complicated by sepsis, there is a progressive increase in muscle ECF, sodium, and chloride, while the intracellular space is decreased. Muscle potassium and magnesium tends to decrease with increasing degrees of injury.

These studies suggest that there is an obligatory expansion of the ECF following injury. This is associated with characteristic changes in muscle membrane potential (Table 5-3). This expansion requires fluid and sodium administration above maintenance levels and results in an increase in body weight. The physiological effect of this weight gain is variable and depends upon the underlying clinical state of the patient. In a young healthy individual a 10–12 percent weight gain (7 liters positive fluid balance) may be well tolerated, whereas a much smaller weight gain may be poorly tolerated by the elderly patient with decreased cardiopulmonary system reserve.

Hyptertensive patients receiving chronic diuretic therapy are somewhat vasoconstricted and often salt-depleted. These patients often are dehydrated and require additional fluid. Fluid restriction can result in severe dehydration and possible irreversible renal failure and is contraindicated. These patients may be hypokalemic and should be given potassium.

Urologic Concerns

The trans-urethral resection of the prostate (TURP) syndrome is often observed following urologic procedures. This is a vascular overload caused by the rapid absorption of irrigating fluid into open venous channels within the prostate. The diagnosis and treatment of this disorder often begins in the recovery room. The major concern is hyponatremia secondary to the absorption of irrigating fluid and associated with the length of operative time. Hypotension, bradycardia, an elevated central venous pressure, and seizures may accompany the hyponatremia. The first set of postoperative electrolytes received in the recovery room may provide a clue to the diagnosis. Treatment varies with the severity of the hyponatremia and water intoxication. If hyponatremia with an associated volume deficit is present, isotonic sodium chloride or Ringer's lactate may be used. When the hyponatremia is severe (Na^+ 90 mEq in the hypoosmotic patient), hypertonic saline (3 percent) can be used to correct the serum sodium.

Type of Anesthetic

There is an association between the type of anesthetic given and the amount of fluid and blood given. With regional anesthetics the area anesthetized and agent used generally will guide fluid requirement. For example, an axillary block covers the area of the upper extremity and the extent of vasodilation is smaller than with a subarachnoid block which would cover a larger area and have a larger fluid requirement. With resolution of the anesthetic the affected area may vasoconstrict and lead to fluid overload.

Burns

Care of the burn patient is quite complex. Some general guidelines are noted below. Relatively easy to remember is the rule of nines to calculate the percentage of the burn. Basically the surface area of each upper extremity is 9 percent of body surface area. The rest of the body is broken down as head, lower extremity front, 9 percent; lower extremity back, 9 percent, front and back torso, 18 percent each. There are several formulas for fluid replacement in burn patients, and they are generally calculated from the percentage of the burn. The Parkland formula is as follows: (per 24 hours)

$$\text{Colloid amount} = \frac{\% \text{ burn} \times \text{weight in kg} \times 0.5 \text{ ml}}{24 \text{ hours}}$$

$$\text{Lactated Ringer's} = \frac{\% \text{ burn} \times \text{weight in kg} \times 1.5 \text{ ml}}{24 \text{ hours}}$$

$$\text{D5W} = \frac{2000 \text{ ml}}{24 \text{ hours}}$$
(Dextrose 5% in water)

USE OF COLLOID IN FLUID RESUSCITATION

The use of albumin in resuscitation of injured patients is a controversial issue. The proponents of the use of colloid as part of fluid therapy argue that resuscitation with crystalloid alone dilutes plasma proteins, thereby reducing plasma oncotic pressure. Reduced oncotic pressure favors fluid movement from the intravascular to the interstitial compartment and thereby predisposes the patient to the development of interstitial pulmonary edema. In contrast to these findings, Lowe et al, Moss et al, and Virgilio et al found no advantage to the administration of colloid solutions. Lucas et al demonstrated that patients receiving large quantities of albumin had a greater dependency on ventilator support with a detrimental effect on renal function.

Our own policy is to use a balanced salt solution together with whole blood for resuscitation of postoperative and injured patients. Albumin infusions are generally confined to patients whose serum albumin is below 2·5g·% and who are also receiving nutritional repletion. In the absence of infection, the capillary bed is considered to be intact; therefore, a rise in serum albumin level may be expected with albumin infusion.

FLUID AND ELECTROLYTE REQUIREMENTS IN CONVALESCENCE

The purpose of administering parenteral fluids and electrolytes is to prevent deficiencies that otherwise result from inability of the patient's gastrointestinal tract and kidneys to fulfill their normal function. Also, in acute trauma or when there has been a substantial loss of water, electrolytes, or both from the body without adequate replacement, parenteral fluid therapy is required to restore a normal distribution of body fluids.

The requirements for parenteral therapy can be considered in three categories:

1. *Normal requirements.* What does the patient require in water, electrolytes, basic calories, and micronutrients to minimize the effects of dehydration and of starvation due to cessation or reduction of oral

intake? The calculation of baseline requirements disregards any preexisting losses, but baseline volumes may require modification in patients with extracellular fluid expansion associated with dilutional hyponatremia.
2. *Preexisting deficits or excesses.* What deficits (or excesses) does the patient have in water, electrolytes, blood volume, plasma proteins, and micronutrients? What should be done to correct these abnormalities?
3. *Abnormal losses.* What does the patient require in order to replace ongoing abnormal fluid and electrolyte losses resulting from the disease or its treatment? This includes ECF sequestration.

A part of this requirement will be obtained through metabolism of body tissue in a semistarving state. Endogenous water is derived from the shrinkage or breakdown of protoplasm which is roughly 75 percent water, as well as the water of oxidation which results from fuel oxidation. Other endogenous water derived from muscle breakdown approximates 800–850 ml/kg of body cell mass lost. This water is almost completely sodium-free but is rich in potassium, magnesium, phosphate, and sulphate.

Oxidation of fat provides approximately 1 ml of water per gram of fat oxidized. Moore estimated that about 100 ml of water is available for each 100 kcal which is derived from the burning of body tissues, part of which is fat and part body cells. The daily caloric requirement of the surgical patient depends in part upon sex and age but much more upon the extent and type of trauma, the presence of infection, the degree of immobilization, and the amount of energy required to maintain body temperature in the presence of abnormal evaporative water losses, either from hyperventilation or from evaporative cooling which occurs as the result of extensive thermal injury.

The daily caloric requirement of the afebrile patient of average size, at bed rest, will vary from 1300 to 1900 kcal, 400–500 kcal of which are often provided by the administration of isotonic glucose into a peripheral vein. The baseline production of endogenous water of oxidation in this situation will be from 150 to 200 ml, or about 10 percent of the total daily requirement. However, fever, trauma, and infection will increase endogenous water production along with the increased oxidation of tissue fuel.

CLINICAL EVALUATION OF THE PATIENT

External abnormal loss may be in the form of excessive loss of water and electrolytes by normal routes of excretion or secretion, or losses which may occur from intraluminal tubes, drains, fistulas, or wounds. The most common source of abnormal external loss in surgical patients is the gastrointestinal tract; next in frequency are the losses from surgical wounds, increased evaporation from the skin and respiratory tract, and from direct injury to the skin. Sequestration of extracellular fluids into areas of traumatized or infected tissue produces a decrease in the usual distribution of extracellular fluid without external loss or change in body weight.

Body Weight

Daily changes in body weight present the most practical index of the changing state of hydration. The daily weight of a patient on conventional fluid therapy by peripheral vein should reveal a loss of approximately 0.2–0.4 percent body weight per day until adequate oral nutrition is instituted. Exceptions occur with blood transfusions or deliberate changes in hydration, as well as during the first 48 hours following trauma or operation when local sequestration of fluid occurs and parenteral fluid is given to compensate for it. The patient who gains weight in other circumstances while on routine fluid therapy is usually being overhydrated or may have developed some complication, most often sepsis. The patient who loses weight at a faster rate, except during a temporary posttraumatic diuresis, is in need of more aggressive fluid therapy. Frequent measurements of body weight are probably the single most important method of recognizing changes in water balance.

Factors That Modify Fluid Requirements

Factors that increase baseline requirements for fluid intake are essentially those which increase the insensible water loss. Fever increases the water requirements to a variable degree. Hyperventilation results in increased water loss by evaporation in addition to cutaneous losses. A patient with a fever of 103°F (39.4°C) will require an average of 500 ml of additional water per day. The endogenous water production associated with the hypermetabolism of fever is also increased, but not enough to offset the increased losses.

Sweating will increase the average adult water requirements by 500 ml per day for each degree Fahrenheit of ambient temperature above 85°F (29.5°C), depending on the humidity. Sweat is about one-half normal sodium chloride, so that additional salt must be provided in the therapy. The potassium content of sweat is negligible. When the environmental temperature rises above 90°F (32°C), the seriously ill febrile patient should be cooled, preferably by air conditioning, because the insensible loss of water from evaporative cooling becomes very large.

Increased Metabolism

Hyperthyroidism increases the turnover of water substantially, in parallel with increases in caloric requirements. Hyperthyroid patients in the semi-starving state tend to consume massive amounts of lean tissue and fat, producing unusual amounts of endogenous water, and simultaneously losing water both by respiratory evaporation and skin sublimation together with sweating.

Use of Blood and Blood Products

Indications for the use of the various available blood products are listed in Appendix 1.

SUGGESTIONS FOR FURTHER READING

Ariel IM, Kremen AJ. Compartmental distribution of sodium chloride in surgical patients pre- and post-operatively. Ann Surg 1950; 132:1009.
Aronstam EM, Schmidt CH, Jenkins E. Body fluid shifts, sodium and potassium metabolism in patients undergoing thoracic surgical procedures. Ann Surg 1953; 137:316.
Askanazi J, Gump FE, Furst P, et al. Effects of nutrition and activity on muscle water and electrolyte changes following injury. JPEN 3, 24 (abstract).
Bartlett RM, Bingham DCL, Pedersen S. Salt balance in surgical patients. Surgery 1938; 4:441.
Bergstrom J, Furst P, Holstram B, et al. Influence of injury on muscle water and electrolytes: effects of elective operation. Ann Surg 1981; 193:134.
Carrico CJ, Cohn D, Lightfoot SA, et al. Extracellular fluid replacement in hemorrhagic shock. Surg Forum 1963; 14:10.
Coller FA, Dick VS, Maddock WG. The maintenance of normal water exchange with intravenous fluids. JAMA 1936; 107:1522.
Coller FA, Bartlett RM, Bingham DCL, et al. Replacement of sodium chloride in surgical patients. Ann Surg 1938; 108:796.
Coller FA, Campbell KNV, Vaughan HH. Postoperative salt intolerance. Ann Surg 1944; 119:533.
Edelman IS, Leibman J, O'Meara MP, et al. Interrelations between serum sodium concentration, serum osmolality and total exchangeable sodium, total exchangeable potassium and total body water. J Clin Invest 1958; 37:1236.
Edelman IS, Leibman J. Anatomy of body water and electrolytes. Am J Med 1959; 17:256.
Elwyn DH, Bryan-Brown CW, Shoemaker WC. Nutritional aspects of body water dislocations in postoperative and depleted patients. Ann Surg 1975; 187:76.

Evans GH. The abuse of normal saline solution. J Am Med Assoc 1911; 57:2126.
Flear CTG, Bhattacharya SS, Singh CM. Solute and water exchanges between cells and extracellular fluids in health and disturbances after trauma. Journal of Parenteral and Enteral Nutrition 1980; 4:98.
Gamble JL. Chemical anatomy, physiology, and pathology of extracellular fluid: a lecture syllabus. 5th ed. Cambridge: Harvard University Press, 1947.
Gilman A. Experimental sodium loss analogous to adrenal insufficiency: the resulting water shift and sensitivity to hemorrhage. Am J Physiol 1934; 108:662.
Gump FE, Kinney JM, Lond CL, et al. Measurement of water balance — a guide to surgical care. Surgery 1968; 64:154.
Gump FE. Fluid and electrolyte management. In: Kinney JM, Bendixen HH, Powers SR, eds. Manual of surgical intensive care. Philadelphia: WB Saunders, 1977.
Limbert EM, Power MH, Pemberton DEF, et al. Effects of parenteral administration of fluid on the metabolism of electrolytes during postoperative convalescence. Surg Gynecol Obstet 1945; 80:438.
Lowe RJ, Moss GS, Jilek J, et al. Crystalloid vs colloid in the etiology of pulmonary failure after trauma: a randomized trial in man. Surgery 1977; 81:676.
Lucas CE, Weaver DW, Higgins RF, et al. Effects of albumin vs non-albumin resuscitation on plasma volume and renal excretory function. J Trauma 1978; 18:564.
Lyon RP, Stanton JR, Freis ED, et al. Blood and 'available fluid' (thiocyanate) volume studies in surgical patients. Part 1: Normal patterns of response of the blood volume, available fluid, protein chloride and hematocrit in the postoperative surgical patient. Surg Gynecol Obstet 1949; 89:9.
Moore FD. Common patterns of water and electrolyte change in injury, surgery and disease. N Eng J Med 1958; 258:277, 377, 427.
Moore FD, Olsen KH, McMurray JD, et al. Body cell mass and its supporting environment: body composition in health and disease. Philadelphia: WB Saunders, 1963.
Moss GS, Siegel DC, Cochin A, et al. Effects of saline and colloid solutions in pulmonary function in hemorrhagic shock. Surg Gynecol Obstet 1971; 133:53.
Pluth JR, Clelland J, Meadow CK, et al. Effect of surgery on the volume of distribution of extracellular fluid determined by the sulfate and bromide methods. In: Berguer PE, Lushbough EE, eds., Medical physiology. Springfield, Ill: USAEC, 1967, pp 217-239.
Randall HT. Fluid, electrolyte and acid base balance. Surg Clin N Am 1976; 56:1019.
Reynolds M. Cardiovascular effects of large volumes of isotonic saline infused intravenously in dogs following severe hemorrhage. Am J Physiol 1949; 158:418.
Roth E, Lax LC, Maloney JV Jr. Changes in extracellular fluid volume during shock and surgical trauma in animals and man. Surg Forum 1967; 18:43.
Shires T, Williams J, Brown F. Simultaneous measurement of plasma volume, extracellular fluid volume, and red blood cell mass in man using ^{131}I, $^{35}SO_4$ and ^{51}Cr. J Lab Clin Med 1960; 55:776.
Shires T, Cohn D, Carrico J, et al. Fluid therapy in hemorrhagic shock. Arch Surg 1964; 88:688.

Shires T, Carrico CJ, Cohn D. Role of the extracellular fluid in shock. Int Anesthesiol Clin 1964; 2:435.
Shires T. The role of sodium-containing solutions in the treatment of oligenic shock. Surg Clin North Am 1969; 45:365.
Shires GT. Fluid and electrolyte therapy. In: Inney JM, Egdahl RH, Zuidema GD, eds. Manual of preoperative and postoperative care. 2d ed. Philadelphia: WB Saunders, 1971.
Shires T, Carrico CJ, Canizaro PC. Shock. London: WB Saunders, 1973, p 32.
Shoemaker WC, Bryan-Brown CW, Quigley L, et al. Body fluid shifts in depletion and post stress states and their correction with adequate nutrition. Surg Gynecol Obstet 1973; 136:371.
Shoemaker WC, Hauser CJ. Critique of crystalloid versus colloid therapy in shock and shock lung. (abstract) Crit Care Med 1979; 7:117.
Skillman JJ, Retall DS, Salzman EW. Randomized trial of albumin vs electrolyte solutions during aortic operations. Surgery 1975; 78:291.
Skillman JJ. The role of albumin and oncotically active fluids in shock. Crit Care Med 1976; 4:55.
Streeten DHP, Rapaport A, Conn JW. Existence of a slowly exchangeable pool of body sodium in normal subjects and its diminution in patients with primary aldosteronism. J Clin Endocrinol Metab 1963; 23:928.
Virgilio RW, Smith DE, Zarins CK. Balanced electrolyte solutions: experimental and clinical studies. Crit Care Med 1979; 7:98.
Weaver DW, Ledgerwood AM, Lucas CE. Pulmonary effects of albumin resuscitation for severe hypovolemic shock. Arch Surg 1978; 113:387.
White JC, Sweet WH, Hurwitt HS. Water balance in neurosurgical patients. Ann Surg 1938; 107:438.
Wiggars MD, Ingraham RC. Hemorrhagic shock: definition of criteria for its diagnosis. J Clin Invest 1946; 25:30.

6
Why Is the Patient Not Awake Yet?
Elizabeth A. M. Frost

Following general anesthesia, most patients are admitted to the recovery room at least drowsy if not unconscious. By far the majority will regain consciousness within a few minutes to an hour. However, a small percentage remain somnolent for longer periods. An understanding of the possible underlying causes of such unresponsiveness is essential to the correct management and successful outcome of the postoperative period. The commonest reasons why the patient is not awake shortly after the end of surgery are as follows:

1. Prolonged anesthetic action and overdose
2. Drug interaction
3. Respiratory insufficiency
4. Cardiovascular instability
5. Thermoregulatory dysfunction
6. Fluid and electrolyte imbalance
7. Allergic or atypical drug reaction
8. Intraoperative catastrophe
9. Preoperative state

PROLONGED ANESTHETIC EFFECT

If patients are admitted to the recovery room comatose, the most usual reason is anesthetic effect. Table 6-1 outlines the stages of anesthetic management where drug administration may give rise to difficulties postoperatively.

Table 6-1. Unresponsiveness Due to Prolonged Effects or Overdose of Anesthetic Drugs

Anesthetic Drugs	Diagnosis	Treatment
Premedication	order sheet in chart	supportive
Inhalation agents		assist ventilation
Barbiturates	anesthetic record	maintain cardiovascular stability
		maintain normothermia
Narcotics	anesthetic record	naloxone (Narcan)
Muscle relaxants	block-aid monitor	correct acid-base imbalance; give neostigmine and atropine

It is important to review premedication orders as many tranquilizer drugs such as diazepam have half-lives of 12 hours or more, which means that their effect often extends well into the postoperative period.

The commonly used inhalation agents—enflurane, isoflurane, and halothane—are usually associated with rapid awakening when they are discontinued (i.e., within 15 minutes). Studies have indicated that recovery should not be delayed even in markedly obese patients if anesthetic time was less than 3 hours. However, the anesthetic effect may persist because administration lasted more than 3 hours or because of interactions with other drugs. Delayed awakening is most marked after the very fat-soluble agents methoxyflurane and ether, both little used today.

Intravenous techniques involve the administration of several drugs (barbiturates, narcotics, tranquilizers, muscle relaxants). Several factors can combine to prolong the action of these agents. Sodium thiopental has a very short duration of action when it is used only as a single bolus for induction. However, it is extremely fat-soluble and, if it is used as a continuous infusion over several hours, return to consciousness may be considerably delayed as the drug is slowly released from the tissues. Moreover, it is reabsorbed by the renal tubules and recirculated in the body.

Following administration, barbiturates bind to protein. Only free barbiturate is effective. Thus, in patients with decreased protein levels (e.g., liver disease), more drug is available to exert a hypnotic effect. Other factors that increase the hypnotic effect of barbiturates are as follows:

1. Cardiac output
2. Blood volume
3. Fat solubility
4. Renal excretion
5. Microsomal enzyme induction

Also, if other drugs are present to competitively bind the protein sites, a greater effect is seen with average barbiturate doses (e.g., X-ray contrast material). Biotransformation of barbiturates by microsomal enzyme systems reduces the effect of these drugs. This is seen in patients who are addicted to barbiturates and in chronic alcoholics. The result is that these patients require a higher dose for the same effect. The opposite effect, i.e., a decrease in microsomal enzyme activity and delayed awakening, is seen after acute alcoholic intoxication.

Small doses of narcotics such as fentanyl (3–15 μg/kg) usually do not contribute to postoperative somnolence. However, if doubt exists, naloxone hydrochloride 0.4 mg may be given intravenously. This drug acts very quickly to reverse any analgesia, and the patient may wake suddenly in severe pain. Some techniques, such as those used in cardiac surgery or to reduce stress responses, may employ much larger doses (e.g., 50–150 μg/kg fentanyl). These patients may be markedly depressed postoperatively, requiring several hours or even days of respiratory support despite administration of narcotic antagonists.

Neuromuscular paralysis persisting into the postoperative period may be caused by several factors:

1. Atypical cholinesterase
2. Puerperium
3. Acid-base imbalance
4. Hypothermia → normothermia
5. Drug interactions
6. Overdose

If the action of muscle relaxant drugs has not been reversed at the end of surgery, the patient may appear unresponsive although he is really paralyzed and not anesthetized. The patient's condition (e.g., severe intracranial disease with raised intracranial pressure or respiratory impairment) may require continued ventilatory support postoperatively which is often best achieved by sedation and the use of neuromuscular blocking agents. Under these circumstances, the anesthesiologist may have elected not to give specific relaxant antagonists. Inadequate reversal may be due also to metabolic acidosis. Any acid-base imbalance should be corrected before withdrawing ventilatory support. A low body temperature decreases the effectiveness of d-tubocurarine but not of pancuronium. As the patient becomes warmer during recovery, neuromuscular paralysis may become more intense.

Rarely (1:2,500 individuals possess a homozygous genotype) prolonged paralysis follows average doses of succinylcholine (0.5–1 mg/kg) due to the presence of atypical pseudocholinesterase which metabolizes the drug very slowly or not at all. Increased effect of muscle relaxants is usually due to drug interaction (see below) or decreased calcium or potassium levels. The effect of succinylcholine is also increased in the puerperium because serum cholinesterase activity is decreased. A diagnosis may be made by reviewing the anesthetic record and using a nerve stimulator to measure the twitch response in the ulnar nerve. In patients with prolonged paralysis, improvement of muscle power may be followed more comfortably in the awake patient by using the train-of-four response, which is a series of four supramaximal single shocks delivered to the ulnar nerve at 2 Hz for 2 seconds. A decreased response from the first to the fourth response (ratio of 4 to 1 twitch of up to 50 percent) indicates marked nondepolarizing block. Edrophonium chloride 20 mg and atropine 0.5 mg may be used as a clinical test and as an indicator of the effectiveness of neostigmine (a longer acting drug). A train-of-four value of 75–80 percent indicates adequate neuromuscular function.

DRUG INTERACTION

During hospitalization, the average patient receives 8 drugs. An additional 5 to 10 agents are used during anesthesia. Many are multicomponent preparations. The relationship between the number of drugs administered and the incidence of reactions is not linear as one might suppose. If less than 6 drugs are used, the reaction rate approximates 4 percent. However, if more than 11 drugs are given, the complication rate increases out of proportion to the number of drugs consumed (e.g., 20 drugs have a 45 percent reaction rate). Some of the commonly used drugs which interact with anesthetic agents to cause increased sedation are listed in Table 6-2.

Table 6-2. Drugs that Interact with Anesthetics

Maintenance medications
    Cardiovascular: antihypertensive drugs, antiarrhythmic agents, digitalis glycosides
    Antibiotics
    Psychotrophic drugs: lithium, monoamine oxide inhibitors, phenothiazine derivatives, street drugs
    Cimetidine
Intravenous agents: narcotics, barbiturates, benzodiazepines, ketamine, trimethaphan
Inhalation agents: nitrous oxide, isoflurane, halothane, enflurane
Muscle relaxants

Maintenance Medications

Cardiovascular Drugs

Methyldopa (Aldomet) and reserpine reduce the effective dose of halothane. Propranolol, which is compatible with isoflurane and halothane, may cause cardiovascular collapse in the presence of cyclopropane or ether. In combination with morphine, effectiveness of histamine is increased and severe bronchospasm may occur in the asthmatic patients. Propranolol acutely potentiates neuromuscular blockade due to nondepolarizing agents. In patients maintained on moderate doses of propranolol, neostigmine may cause severe bradycardia associated with somnolence which may persist for several hours. Neuromuscular blockade is also prolonged by chronic administration of diuretics (reduced potassium levels), quinidine, procaine hydrochloride, and lidocaine. There is a narrow safety range with digitalis preparations. Hyperventilation causes alkalosis which decreases serum potassium levels and increases the effect of digitalis. During halothane administration, on the other hand, more digitalis is required which may result in an overdose as the patient wakes up, causing cardiac dysrhythmias and heart failure.

Antibiotics

Neuromuscular blockade is increased by streptomycin sulfate, neomycin, kanamycin sulfate, gentamycin sulfate, tobramycin sulfate, tetracyclines, polymyxin, colistin sulfate, lincomycin, clindamycin, and erythromycin. This interaction is usually seen when antibiotics are given intravenously or intraperitoneally during surgery, but the margin of safety of neuromuscular transmission may be reduced for many hours postoperatively. Administration of antibiotics in the early postoperative period may be particularly dangerous when respiratory assistance has been withdrawn and the effect of other depressant drugs is still evidenced. Antibiotics which do not interfere with neuromuscular transmission include penicillin G, cephradine, and cephaloridine.

Psychotropic Drugs

Lithium increases the effect of all muscle relaxants except d-tubocurarine and gallamine and increases the reversal time of pancuronium by neostigmine. It also increases the hypnotic effect of pentobarbital.

The monoamine oxidase inhibitors (pargyline hydrochloride, tranylcypromine, phenelzine sulfate, isocarboxazid) increase the effect of narcotics, barbiturates, and succinylcholine. Tricyclic antidepressants (imipramine, amitriptyline, desipramine, doxepin) increase respiratory depression and analgesia with narcotics and hypnosis with barbiturates. A similar effect occurs with the phenothiazine derivatives (promethazine, chlorpromazine, perphenazine) and butyrophenones (droperidol).

Intravenous Agents

Narcotics cause respiratory depression which decreases the rate at which inhalation agents can be excreted through the lungs. Morphine can potentiate acute alcohol intoxication (e.g., injured drunk driver). All the narcotics have a synergistic central nervous system depressant effect with inhalation agents. Morphine-induced respiratory depression is potentiated by the H_2 antagonist cimetidine. Ventilatory response to CO_2 is depressed for up to 24 hours.

Barbiturates and benzodiazepines reduce the intraoperative inhalation requirements, prolonging the hypnotic effect which may be particularly evidenced after short procedures. Barbiturates can acutely inhibit the metabolism of ketamine and increase its action. Barbiturates can be readily displaced from protein-binding sites by other drugs, thus increasing their hypnotic effect.

Drugs such as diazepam, barbiturates, hydroxyzine, and droperidol, which have been used to control the adverse central nervous system effects of ketamine, all cause delayed return to consciousness. Ketamine reduces the effective dose of inhalation agents for hours and enhances d-tubocurarine blockade.

The action of trimethaphan, a ganglionic blocking agent that also releases histamine, is potentiated by general and spinal anesthesia, diuretics, and antihypertensive medications. Profound hypotension, prolonged coma, and respiratory depression may occur. Therapy includes respiratory support, fluid administration, and phenylephrine hydrochloride infusion.

Inhalation Agents

Effective inhalation anesthetic concentration is significantly reduced by the addition of nitrous oxide. Appropriate intraoperative decrease in administration must be made to avoid postoperative depression. There is marked synergism between all the inhalation agents (especially isoflurane) and nondepolarizing muscle relaxants.

RESPIRATORY INSUFFICIENCY

Respiratory depression commonly occurs in the immediate postoperative period. All degrees of ventilatory inadequacy from mild depression to overt failure may occur and lead to prolonged unconsciousness. The diagnosis is made if one or more of the criteria listed in Table 6-3 are met. Table 6-4 lists common causes of postoperative respiratory insufficiency.

Table 6-3. Criteria Used in Diagnosis of Respiratory Insufficiency

Respiratory pattern	irregular
Respiratory rate	$<10/min > 40/min$
Tidal volume	<3.5 ml/kg
Vital capacity	<15 ml/kg
$PaCO_2$	>50 mm Hg
PaO_2	<70 mm Hg

Table 6-4. Causes of Inadequate Respiration in the Postoperative Period

Cause	Diagnosis	Therapy
Intraoperative hyperventilation	observation anesthetic record	O_2 mask
Anesthetic agents	history anesthetic record	supportive (ventilation, cardiovascular stability)
Fluid overload	chest X ray central venous pressure input-output discrepancy in anesthetic record	diuretics positive pressure ventilation
Operative site	observation patient complains of pain	narcotics regional anesthesia
Intraoperative complication	anesthetist's and surgeon's reports chest X ray	fluid replacement assisted ventilation chest tube inserted if necessary
Aspiration	observation chest X ray blood gases anesthetist's report	assisted or controlled ventilation suction antibiotics; steroids bronchoscopy bronchodilators
Preexisting disease	history	ventilatory support bronchodilators antibiotics

Adapted from: Frost E. Postoperative coma in recovery room care. International Anesthesiology Clinics. Boston: Little, Brown, 1983; 21:1;22.

Intraoperative Hyperventilation

Intraoperative hyperventilation causes alkalosis and decreases $PaCO_2$. Postoperatively the patient hypoventilates as CO_2 is stored. However, there are no oxygen stores and unless supplemental oxygen is given, hypoxia develops.

Anesthetic Agents

All anesthetic agents, especially narcotics, cause respiratory depression. Therapy is supportive until the drug effect has been reversed or worn off. Small doses of narcotics (e.g., demerol 25 mg) may cause marked respiratory depression in the recovery room if the patient is still under the influence of other anesthetic agents.

Fluid Overload

Excess intraoperative fluid administration or use of hyperosmolar solutions such as mannitol may cause congestive cardiac failure in the elderly, small babies, or in patients with a history of cardiac disease. Central venous pressure is elevated, sputum is pink and frothy, there is obvious respiratory distress and a fluffy picture is seen on the chest X ray. Therapy requires reintubation and positive pressure ventilation, furosemide (40 mg intravenously), and morphine sulfate (2-5 mg intravenously).

Operative Site

Upper abdominal and thoracic surgery are associated with considerable pain and splinting of the diaphragm. Appropriate therapy includes regional epidural blockade, intercostal nerve block, and small doses of narcotic.

Special attention must be paid to patients who have undergone anterior cervical spinal surgery. Ventilation may have been marginal preoperatively because of cord injury and spasm. Edema caused by surgical trauma and decreased function of auxiliary muscles of respiration may cause ventilatory failure postoperatively. If in doubt, ventilatory support should be continued for several days if necessary.

Intraoperative Complications

Intraoperative complications which can cause postoperative respiratory problems (pneumothorax, endobronchial intubation, hemothorax, asthmatic attack, pulmonary collapse) are uncommon but should have been included in the anesthesiologist's report.

Aspiration

Aspiration of stomach contents is rare following extubation but may occur during transfer of the comatose patient. It is more likely to occur if a nasogastric tube is present. Diagnosis is usually made by observation. Arterial blood gases are a much more sensitive indicator of lung damage than a chest X ray, which may not show changes for 24 hours. If the amount aspirated is more than a few milliliters or if the pH of the secretions obtained immediately is less than 5, the patient should be reintubated and given ventilation support. Bronchoscopy may be indicated to reexpand collapsed lung segments.

Shivering

Reduced body temperature and infusion of cold fluids may cause postoperative shivering which can increase oxygen use by 400 percent and reduce PaO_2 especially if there is ventilatory difficulty already or a fixed low cardiac output. Therapy involves oxygen administration, careful warming, sedation, and small doses of methylphenidate (Ritalin).

Preexisting Disease

Appropriate evaluation of postoperative respiratory difficulties must include a review of preoperative lung function. Additive effects of anesthetic depression and chronic obstructive pulmonary disease may precipitate respiratory failure.

CARDIOVASCULAR INSTABILITY

As with the respiratory system, instability of the cardiovascular system is not uncommon in the recovery room. Both hypotension and arrhythmias may cause coma. Hypotension may be due to inadequate volume replacement, drug overdose, intraoperative catastrophe, or acute cardiopulmonary disease. Cardiac arrhythmias may be precipitated by myocardial ischemia, hypoxia, or drugs. Diagnosis requires a careful review of the chart and examination of the patient. Therapy is determined by the underlying cause.

THERMOREGULATORY DYSFUNCTION

Regulation of body temperature is impaired during anesthesia (poikilothermic state). Core temperatures may decrease by 6°C or more, especially in children if the ambient temperature is low. At this level, the depressant effects of all anesthetic agents are exaggerated. Diagnosis is made immediately when the temperature is checked on admission to the recovery room. Rewarming should be done gradually to prevent burns in areas of low perfusion. Continuous electrocardiographic monitoring for ventricular arrhythmias is essential. Sudden body movements (especially of the extremities) should be avoided as this may push large volumes of relatively cold peripheral blood into the heart. Close attention must be paid to respiratory status if *d*-tubocurarine was used because neuromuscular paralysis may become more intense during rewarming.

Postoperative hyperthermia may be due to preexisting disease, an infective process, drug reaction, or malignant hyperthermia. This last syndrome may be triggered by pain or stress and is associated with persistent coma, high fever, supraventricular tachycardia, hyperventilation, unstable blood pressure, acute pulmonary and cerebral edema, and acute renal failure. Therapy requires cardioventilatory support, sodium bicarbonate, external and internal cooling, dantrolene sodium, procaine hydrochloride, steroids, diuretics, and insulin in glucose.

FLUID AND ELECTROLYTE IMBALANCE

Complications of fluid and electrolyte balance are most likely to occur in elderly or debilitated patients (especially after major intestinal surgery) or in severe hypertensives maintained on diuretics and in diabetics and neurosurgical patients who have received large doses of mannitol or who have disturbances involving the thalamohypophyseal pathways.

Serum electrolyte estimation should be performed shortly after admission to the recovery room and the results correlated with vital signs. Two situations deserve special attention.

Diabetes Mellitus

Patients with severe diabetes are usually stabilized for 1 to 2 days preoperatively on a regimen of a sliding regular insulin dosage determined according to urinalysis (i.e., 1+ sugar in urine—no insulin; 2+, 5 units; 3+, 10 units, 4+, 15 units). However, preoperative fasting, stress, infection, and intraoperative glucose administration may cause either a hypoglycemic or hyperglycemic state postoperatively. Urinalysis should be performed immediately on admission to the recovery room. At least a small amount of sugar should be detected. Bedside glucose determination with Dextrostix provide only a rough guide to sugar levels (± 100 mg/dl) and are no substitute for laboratory determinations in these patients. Insulin, which has a half-life of about 10 minutes, is rapidly cleared by metabolism and renal excretion. Intravenous bolus injections are short-acting and small amounts given continuously are probably more effective (e.g., 100 units in 100 ml saline over 1 to 2 hours). Potassium 20 mEq should be added to the infusion. Insulin decreases blood sugar levels at approximately 100–200 mg/dl per hour as opposed to rehydration which by dilutional effect can cause a fall of up to 700 mg/dl per hour. Ketosis is best treated postoperatively by small doses of insulin (5 units).

Patients in hypoglycemic coma will usually respond to a rapid injection of 50 ml 50 percent dextrose in water within 5 minutes. The clinical features of hypoglycemia and hyperglycemia are contrasted in Table 6-5. Hypoglycemia is most likely to occur in patients maintained on oral agents (chlorpropamide lasts for 2 days), if there is coexistent renal failure which delays insulin excretion, or in patients fasted (e.g., nonfunctioning intravenous lines) or vomiting. Hyperglycemia occurs in association with sepsis, stress, or if the patient has not received insulin or has been hydrated with dextrose solutions.

Hyperosmolar nonketotic coma is a rare cause of hyperglycemia which occurs in elderly, debilitated patients or associated with major trauma and is caused by disturbance of thirst mechanisms. Blood glucose levels are over 1000 mg/dl. Patients are severely dehydrated and coma and seizures are frequent. However, these patients respond promptly to small doses of insulin (10-20 units) and to rehydration.

Abnormalities of Antidiuretic Hormone Secretion

Oversecretion or undersecretion of antidiuretic hormone (ADH) from the pituitary can cause fluid and electrolyte complications postoperatively. Table 6-6 compares the causes and diagnostic features of overproduction

Table 6-5. Clinical Features of Hypoglycemia and Hyperglycemia

Hypoglycemia	Hyperglycemia
Coma	Dehydration
Seizures	Hypokalemia
Tachycardia	Metabolic acidosis
Low blood pressure	Hyperventilation (air hunger)
	Coma
< Blood sugar 70 mg/dl	> Blood sugar 300 mg/dl

Table 6-6. Antidiuretic Hormone (ADH) Abnormalities

Inappropriate ADH (SIADH)	Diabetes Insipidus
Causes	
CNS pathology	head trauma
Pneumonia	intracranial surgery
Pulmonary TB	(hypophysectomy)
Bronchogenic CA	
Diagnosis	
Oliguria	polyuria (300 ml/hr)
Hyponatremia	hypernatremia
UO, PO	UO, PO
Normal renal and adrenal function	urine specific gravity
Normotension	hypotension
No dehydration	dehydration
Confusion, delirium, coma	seizures, coma

UO = urine osmolality; PO = plasma osmolality.

(syndrome of inappropriate antidiuretic secretion, SIADH) and underproduction of ADH (diabetes insipidus).

Treatment of SIADH involves administration of sodium as a 3–5 percent saline solution preceded by furosemide 20 mg to promote diuresis. Fluid restriction is necessary. Diabetes insipidus should be treated over a 24-hour period with hypotonic solutions (e.g., 5 percent dextrose in 0.25 percent NaCl) with potassium chloride supplementation as necessary. Too rapid correction of hypernatremia can cause water intoxication and cerebral edema. Vasopressin tannate 5 units subcutaneously is specific therapy. 1-Desamino-8-D-arginine vasopressin (DDAVP) is rapidly effective by nasal insufflation, but obviously, its use is restricted to cooperative patients.

ALLERGIC OR ATYPICAL DRUG REACTION

Individual response to drug action is the rule. Occasionally an allergic or atypical reaction may occur which interferes with early return to consciousness. Some of the drugs which may prove problematic are listed in Table 6-7.

INTRAOPERATIVE CATASTROPHE

Rarely complications in the operating room may be the cause of prolonged postoperative coma. Some of the causes and the differential diagnosis are listed in Table 6-8. Early and close communication between all the medical personnel involved in the patient's care is essential.

Shock

Sudden loss of volume (fluid or blood) may cause shock. Multiunit transfusions are often associated with pulmonary and renal problems after a few hours. Careful monitoring is essential. Septic shock may develop rapidly after manipulation of a large abscess, infarcted bowel, or gangrenous area. The clinical picture is one of severe hypotension, tachycardia, and hypothermia without obvious bleeding. Treatment requires cardiopulmonary support, steroids, and antibiotics.

Myocardial Infarction

All degrees of cardiac ischemia may be caused by hypotensive or hypertensive episodes or by stress. Typical electrocardiographic changes develop. Diagnostic serum enzyme levels may be masked by surgical trauma. Technetium 99 pyrophosphate infarct scintigrams that become positive in 12 to 24 hours may help in making a positive diagnosis.

Table 6-7. Allergic or Atypical Drug Response

Cause	Diagnosis	Treatment
Penicillin	skin reactions bronchospasm tachycardia hypotension	antihistamines epinephrine
Droperidol	anesthetic record decreased ventilation positive Babinski sign	ventilatory support
Diazepam (Valium)	hypoventilation hypotension anesthetic record	ventilatory support fluid replacement
Muscle relaxants	hypoventilation block-aid monitor	assisted ventilation neostigmine and atropine
Narcotics	hypoventilation hypotension	naloxone
Ketamine	hallucinations	diazepam
Barbiturates	hypoventilation	assisted ventilation ritalin (?)

Adapted from Frost E. Postoperative coma in recovery room care. 6-31. International Anesthesiology Clinics. Boston: Little, Brown, 1983; 21:1; 29.

Table 6-8. Some Intraoperative Factors That Can Result in Prolonged Coma

Cause	Diagnosis	Treatment
Shock	vital signs	
Hemorrhagic	BP	fluid replacement
Septic	pulse	steriods
	temperature	antibiotics
	CVP	ventilatory assistance
	physician's report	
Myocardial infarction	ECG	cardiovascular support
	enzyme studies	(vasopressors, anti-arrhythmic agents)
		O_2 mask
Intracranial lesion	vital signs	
Blood shift	BP	support ventilation
Herniation	pulse	diuretics
		steroids
	neurologic exam; unequal pupils	barbiturates
	radiologic studies	
Hypoxia	physician's report	support ventilation
	arterial blood gases	

Adapted from Frost E. Postoperative coma recovery room care. International Anesthesiology Clinics. Boston: Little, Brown, 1983; 21:1; 24.

Intracranial Lesion

Rupture of an intracranial aneurysm prior to clipping carries a poor prognosis. If major vessels have been occluded to control bleeding or if there has been deep or extensive tumor dissection requiring prolonged brain tissue retraction, cerebral edema may cause increased intracranial pressure and coma.

Another problem which may become obvious in the recovery room is that of intracranial air. Intraoperatively, the brain size is decreased by diuretic administration and hyperventilation. Air becomes trapped within the skull. As the brain reexpands, this air may be put under pressure, resulting in a tension pneumocephalus and coma.

In any patient with altered intracranial dynamics, small increases in $PaCO_2$ may cause marked deterioration in the level of consciousness. Should hypertension, bradycardia or respiratory or cardiac abnormalities associated with decrease in sensorium occur in any neurosurgical patient, prompt therapy must include neurosurgical consultation and immediate attempts to control intracranial pressure at less than 20 mm Hg (hyperventilation, diuretics, head up position). A CT scan should be performed as soon as possible.

Patients who have undergone bilateral carotid endarterectomy either as one procedure or during two operations spaced several months apart are very sensitive to the respiratory depressant effects of small doses of narcotics. As hypoxemia develops without normal carotid body function, there is no increase in ventilation.

Preoperative State

Finally, accurate assessment of the cause of postoperative somnolence must include a review of the patient's preoperative mental status. A patient comatose before surgery will most likely remain so for some time postoperatively. As in all the several situations which contribute to delayed awakening, close communication, including a verbal report, is essential between the recovery room nurse, anesthesiologist, and surgeon.

SUGGESTIONS FOR FURTHER READING

Cullen BF, Miller MG. Drug interactions and anesthesia: A review. Anesth Analg 1979; 58:413.

Cullen SC, Larson CP. Essentials of anesthetic practice. Chicago: Year Book Medical Publishers, 1974.

Frost E. Differential diagnosis of postoperative coma. In: Recovery room care. Frost EAM, Andrews IC, eds. Internat Anesth Clin, Boston: Little, Brown, 1983.

Lichtiger M, Moya F. Introduction to the practice of anesthesia. 2d ed. New York: Harper & Row, 1978.

May FE, Stewart RB, Cluff LE. Drug use in the hospital: Evaluation of determinants. Clin Pharmacol Ther 1974; 16:834.

Rosenbaum SM. Anesthetic management of the diabetic patient. In: ASA refresher courses in anesthesiology. Vol 9. Hershey SG, ed. Philadelphia: Lippincott, 1981.

Smith JW, Seidl LG, Cluff LE. Studies on the epidemiology of adverse drug reactions. V. Clinical factors influencing susceptibility. Ann Intern Med 1966; 65:629.

Waud BE. Interaction of muscle relaxants and other drugs. In: ASA refresher courses in anesthesiology. Vol 9. Hershey SG, ed. Philadelphia: Lippincott, 1981.

7
Criteria for Discharge
Marilyn Schneider

Assessing the patient's readiness for discharge from the PACU (postanesthesia care unit) is a significant responsibility of the PAN (postanesthesia nurse). Determining the criteria to be applied in this assessment is a joint responsibility of the Department of Anesthesiology, the PACU nurse-manager, the Department of Surgery, and any designated others. Together, these individuals identify the criteria to be used by the nursing and anesthesiology staffs for evaluating the patient's response to anesthesia and surgery. These criteria should be written as departmental policy to serve as the standards against which the nurse and anesthesiologist evaluate the patient for discharge from the PACU.

Several national agencies have addressed the issue of determining the patient's readiness for discharge from PACU. These include the Joint Commission on Accreditation of Hospitals (JCAH), the American Society of Anesthesiologists (ASA), and the American Society of Postanesthesia Nurses (ASPAN).

JCAH

The JCAH *Accreditation Manual* (1983) states in its guidelines:

> The basis for the decision to discharge a patient from any postanesthesia care unit shall be made only by a physician or, in the case of a patient without medical problems admitted by a qualified oral surgeon, by that oral surgeon, and not by nursing service personnel. However, the actual release of a postanesthesia patient by a physician or, when appropriate, by a qualified oral surgeon and documentation thereof does not necessarily require the presence or signature of a specific physician or qualified oral surgeon at the

time of release. When discharge criteria are used, they shall be comprehensive, approved by the medical staff to assure the same standard of care for all patients, and rigidly enforced. When the responsible physician or qualified oral surgeon has not issued a written order or authenticated a verbal release, the name of the physician or qualified oral surgeon responsible for the patient's release shall be recorded in the medical record.

JCAH guidelines require a mechanism for releasing a patient from the PACU. The use of established discharge criteria is recognized as an acceptable mechanism. When established discharge criteria are used, the discharge order need not be signed by the physician or oral surgeon at the time of the patient's release. When no established discharge criteria are used, the physician or oral surgeon must make the decision as to when to discharge the patient from PACU. JCAH does not require that an anesthesiologist write the criteria for discharge or the discharge order.

JCAH speaks to who may make the decision to discharge a patient, not to when, how, or where. While an anesthesiologist's signature is not required to discharge a patient, under JCAH guidelines, in the absence of a physician's or oral surgeon's signed order to discharge a patient, documentation that the patient has met established discharge criteria is required.

ASA

The ASA suggests (1977) that an anesthesiologist evaluate the "status of the patient on admission and discharge from the postoperative recovery suite," and that the "anesthesiologist shall determine and document when the period of postoperative surveillance has terminated." In its *Practice Advisory* (1978) ASA said, "Patients may be discharged (from PACU) only after vital signs are stable and after an evaluation of the patient's condition by a responsible physician or designee."

ASPAN

ASPAN, in its *Guidelines for Standards of Care* (1983), states that evaluation of the following parameters are necessary prior to the discharge of a patient:

1. Airway patency and respiratory function
2. Stability of vital signs, including temperature
3. Level of consciousness and muscular strength
4. Mobility
5. Patency of tubes, catheters, drains, intravenous lines
6. Skin color and condition

7. Fluid intake and output
8. Comfort

Another aspect of discharge criteria and planning recommended by ASPAN includes communicating with the patient's family or significant others, and with the patient's care unit.

Guidelines for the nurse, according to ASPAN, are

> The post-anestheisa Nurse shall discharge the patient in accordance with written policies set forth by the Department of Anesthesiology and also in accordance with the criteria and data collected through the nursing process. A final nursing assessment and evaluation of the patient's condition will be performed and documented. If a numerical scoring system is used, the discharge order will be recorded to reflect the patient's status. The PAN arranges for the safe transport of the patient from the PACU to his or her room.

NUMERICAL SCORING SYSTEMS

The use of a numerical scoring system for assessment of the patient's recovery from anesthesia has been investigated, and widely used for the past 10 years. The first anesthesia and surgery scoring system to be suggested was developed by Gaston Carignan et al in 1964. This evaluated long-term recovery from anesthesia, measuring five physiological system parameters at the 2nd, 5th, and 15th postoperative days (Figure 7-1). The Apgar scoring system was introduced for evaluation of newborns in 1958 and formed the basis for subsequent scoring systems. Carignan's scoring system was developed because of the need for "observing, tabulating, and presenting in condensed form, the postanesthetic course of a large number of patients."

A postanesthetic recovery score (PAS) analogous to the Apgar score, and applicable to the postanesthetic period was introduced by Aldrete and Kroulik in 1970. Physical signs, which could be easily observed and commonly seen, were selected for evaluation. To simplify assessment, a numerical score of 0, 1, or 2 is assigned in each of five selected areas: activity, respirations, circulation, consciousness, and color. A maximum score of 10 indicates a patient in optimum postanesthetic condition to return to the nursing unit. It was recommended that scoring assessment be performed on admission to PACU, and hourly thereafter, until discharge from PACU. This has been modified with usage over the years, and many PACUs have added a 15-minute postadmission assessment. Figure 7-2 shows the PAS introduced by Aldrete and Kroulik. It should be noted that PACUs have adapted, modified, and condensed the graph. Figure 7-3 is an

	0	1	2	3	4	5
Circ.	BP stable. Pulse always under 100	BP-change less than 30%. Pulse 100–120	Vasopressors OR Digitalis	BP under 100 in spite of treatment	Decompensated	Severe shock
Resp.	Rate under 15, Breath-holding more than 25 sec.	Rate 15–20. Productive cough	Rate over 20, rales OR temp. up to 100°	Temp. over 100°, partial atelectasis	Major atelectasis	Pneumonia
C.N.S.	Amnesic, satisfied	Confused OR recalls induction	Dissatisfied with anesthesia for any reason	Extrapyramidal signs	Major neurological complications	Coma
G.I.	Nothing	No more than 3 episodes of nausea	Nausea, vomited once only	Vomiting	Ileus	Evisceration OR perforation
Renal	Voids over 800 cc.	Over 800 cc. per catheter	Voids 500–800 cc.	500–800 cc. per catheter	Under 500 cc.	Anuria

Figure 7-1. Carignan scoring system (Hospital of Notre Dame, Montreal, Canada).

RECOVERY-ROOM SCORE SYSTEM

ACTIVITY	SCORE	AT ARRIVAL	HOUR 1	2	3
Able to move 4 extremities	2				
Able to move 2 extremities	1				
Able to move 0 extremities	0				
RESPIRATION					
Able to deep-breathe & cough freely	2				
Dyspnea or limited breathing	1				
Apneic	0				
CIRCULATION					
BP ± 20% of preanesthetic level	2				
BP ± 20–50% of preanesthetic level	1				
BP ± 50% or more of preanesthetic level	0				
CONSCIOUSNESS					
Fully awake	2				
Arousable on calling	1				
Not responding	0				
COLOR					
Pink	2				
Pale, dusky, blotchy, jaundiced, other	1				
Cyanotic	0				
TOTALS					

SCORE MUST BE AT LEAST 7–8
FOR PATIENT'S RELEASE

PATIENT

PLEASE NOTE: This Recovery-Room Scorecard is one example of the kind of postsurgical charts in current use. Roche Products Inc. and Hoffmann-La Roche Inc. are not responsible for any decisions based on information provided by its use.

Figure 7-2. Recovery room score system.

POST ANESTHESIA SCORE

SCORE	CRITERIA	ADM	15 MIN	DIS
Activity 2 1 0	Able To Move 4 Extremities Able To Move 2 Extremities Able To Move 0 Extremities			
Resp. 2 1 0	Able To Breathe Deeply & Cough Dyspnea or Limited Breathing Apnea			
Circ. 2 1 0	Pre-anesthetic Level BP is 20% of pre-anesthetic level BP is 20%-50% of pre-anesthetic level BP is 50% of pre-anesthetic level			
Awareness 2 1 0	Fully Awake Arousable on Calling Not Responding			
Color 2 1 0	Pink Pale, Dusky, Blotchy, Jaundiced Cyanotic			
TOTAL SCORE				

Figure 7-3. Postanesthesia score (Doctors Hospital of Prince Georges County).

example of a PAS currently in use. The scoring system is employed with the following considerations:

Activity. Muscular activity may be spontaneous or on command. This assists in evaluating recovery from the effects of regional and local anesthetic techniques, as well as general anesthesia.

Respirations. The ability to breathe deeply and cough is the maximum achievable; apnea is the other extreme. Limited respiratory efforts (e.g., splinting, airway adjuncts, dyspnea) rate the median value.

Circulation. Blood pressure is rated in relation to its preanesthetic level, and circulatory function is evaluated. A percentage of the preanesthetic systolic arterial blood pressure is determined and rated. (Some PACUs have modified this and consider the pressure difference in mm HG, which is simpler and faster to calculate, instead of percentage).

Consciousness. Full alertness, orientation to person, place, and time, and the ability to answer questions and summon assistance receives the maximum value. Response to calling the patient by name is assigned the median value. If no response is elicited by oral communication, the 0 value is assigned. Painful stimulation is not employed to elicit a response.

Color. A normal skin and mucous membrane color receives the highest score; obvious cyanosis rates the lowest score. Assessments between these two — pallor, duskiness, blotchy discoloration, flushed appearance, and jaundice — receive the median value. Even if alterations in color existed preoperatively, the postoperative assessment is rated objectively.

Many PACUs use the PAS as a criterion for discharge. Departmental policy may state, "Patient may be discharged from PACU when PAS reaches 10." But a PAS may constitute only minimal criteria for discharge and other functions must be considered.

Another scoring system employed in PACU settings is the Glasgow coma scale (GCS) (Figure 7-4). This scale was developed as a prognostic indicator of outcome in head injury but has been used as a simple assessment of level of consciousness as well. When used in PACUs, it is a part of a larger assessment procedure. The GCS consists of three areas of assessment: response by opening eyes, verbal response, and motor response. Scoring at five levels is provided for verbal and motor response, and at four levels for the opening of eyes. Measurements are recorded at predetermined intervals, usually every 15 minutes in PACU, and more (or less) frequently as indicated by the patient's condition. In and of itself, the scale is not sufficient for use as the criterion for discharge, but may be a useful adjunct, particularly in assessing neurosurgical patients.

DISCHARGE BY ANESTHESIOLOGIST

Many PACUs operate under a policy which requires an anesthesiologist's assessment, discharge note, and signature prior to the release of any patient. This works well in a setting where an anesthesiologist is always readily available to the PACU; it is not a workable solution in many institutions. A short form may be conveniently used by the anesthesiologist as a discharge note (Figure 7-5). The destination of the patient is also indicated. The form may be stamped on each patient's record.

TIME		M	1	2	3	4	5	6	7	8	9	10	11	N	1	2	3	4	5	6	7	8	9	10	11
EYE	SPONTANEOUS 4																								
	TO SPEECH 3																								
	TO PAIN 2																								
OPENING	NONE 1																								
BEST	ORIENTED 5																								
	CONFUSED 4																								
VERBAL	INAPPROPRIATE 3																								
	INCOMPREHENSIBLE 2																								
RESPONSE	NONE 1																								
BEST	OBEYING 5																								
	LOCALIZING 4																								
MOTOR	FLEXING 3																								
	EXTENDING 2																								
RESPONSE	NONE 1																								

Figure 7-4. Glasgow coma scale.

```
┌─────────────────────────────────────────────────────┐
│ Recovery Room Discharge                             │
│                                         Yes    No   │
│ Vital signs stable                  ___   ___   ___ │
│ Patient awake (obeys commands)      ___   ___   ___ │
│ Laryngeal reflexes present          ___   ___   ___ │
│ Regional block: Sensation           ___   ___   ___ │
│                 Motion              ___   ___   ___ │
│ To room ___  To ICU ___  To home ___                │
└─────────────────────────────────────────────────────┘
```

Figure 7-5. Anesthesiologist's discharge assessment checklist (Hospital of the Albert Einstein College of Medicine).

DISCHARGE CRITERIA

Some hospitals have opted for an across-the-board minimum stay in PACU, generally based on length of surgical procedure: for example, 1 hour in PACU for every hour in the operating room (OR), or 2-hour minimum stay for adult patients and 1-hour minimum stay for children under 12 years of age. These arbitrary time constraints may vary between institutions and may refer exclusively to patients receiving general anesthetics. Other time restrictions may be assigned following general anesthesia or for alternate techniques of anesthesia administration.

Other factors which may be considered for imposing a waiting period prior to discharge include:

1. A minimum 30-minute observation period following administration of intravenous narcotics, antibiotics, or naloxone (Narcan)
2. A 1-hour observation period following administration of intramuscular antibiotics, antiemetics, or narcotics
3. Other medication-related observation periods as determined by the Department of Anesthesiology
4. A 30-minute observation period following discontinuance of oxygen therapy
5. A 1-hour observation period following extubation

Writing Discharge Criteria

In assessing a patient's eligibility for discharge from PACU, the nurse must consider the complete physiological response of the patient to the effects of anesthesia and surgery.

GENERAL CARE

At University Hospitals in Cleveland, Ohio, all of the following constitute criteria or considerations for discharge:

1. A minimum stay of 1 hour
2. Stability of vital signs (blood pressure, pulse rate, respiratory rate)
3. Body temperature
4. Level of consciousness
5. Complications related to:
   a. Pain
   b. Wound drainage
   c. Nausea and vomiting
   d. Urinary output
   e. Specific surgical procedure
6. Patency of tubes and catheters
7. Postoperative orders
8. Ongoing nursing care needs

Standards for each of these criteria have been developed. For example, stability of vital signs is measured by three consecutive 15-minute interval readings immediately prior to discharge, which are in the same range, as well as in the patient's normal range (as determined by preoperative and intraoperative values). Standards include written postoperative orders that have been reviewed, stat orders carried out, and parenteral medications started unless contraindicated in the immediate postanesthetic period.

In New York State, representatives of the Society of Anesthesiologists, Recovery Room Nurses Association, and Association of Nurse Anesthetists have published *Guidelines for Recovery Room Care*. In their introduction, they state, "no two hospitals are alike . . . No guidelines can possibly fit all situations." Application of the guidelines is recommended to be adapted by individual institutions.

Regarding responsibilities of the PAN at the time of discharge, the guidelines say:

> Appropriate criteria for discharge . . . should be detailed in the Recovery Room Procedure Manual. When the patient meets these criteria, an anesthesiologist or surgeon should be notified to verify and approve his or her discharge. A discharge note including time and level of consciousness should be written and signed. The individual discharging the patient should determine the type and number of personnel required for transport to the floor or special unit. The Recovery Room nurse should report to the floor nurse the patient's general condition, operation, Recovery Room progress, fluid and blood replacement, urine output, drainage, and any other pertinent information.

Each PACU is responsible for establishing written criteria for discharge and standards for these criteria.

In assessing the patient's readiness for discharge to a hospital room following general anesthesia, certain parameters seem evident and universally accepted.

1. The patient is able to maintain his own airway, clear secretions, and deep breathe and cough on command. The patient can turn to his side in the event of vomiting, and summon assistance when needed.
2. The hemodynamic status of the patient has stabilized. Blood pressure and pulse are stable and correlate with the preoperative measurements.
3. The fluid balance status of the patient is equilibrating. The patient is neither hypovolemic nor hypervolemic, urinary output is adequate according to the standards of that institution (usually 25–50 ml per hour), and electrolyte levels are within normal limits (or are being treated).
4. The postsurgical status of the patient is pointing toward recovery. There is no evidence of active bleeding. All tubes, drains, catheters, intravenous lines, etc., are patent, working properly, and connected according to physician instructions. Where indicated, the ordered fluids are infusing or irrigating.
5. The continuing care needs of the patient have been identified and implemented as indicated. Ice has been applied where ordered, stat and other medications have been administered, and the patient's responses to treatment have been observed and documented. Physician orders to be initiated in the PACU have been implemented.
6. Pain has been assessed and treated, and the patient's response to treatment documented.
7. Potential problems have been forestalled, and no active problems (i.e., any not undergoing treatment) are apparent.

Special Discharge Criteria

In the PACU, patients who have special discharge criteria needs are also seen.

Ambulatory Patients

The ambulatory surgery patient, in addition to meeting the criteria established for patients who will remain at least overnight in the hospital, must meet more stringent criteria. Persistent nausea and vomiting is unacceptable for discharge home. The patient must be able to retain oral fluids and to walk without assistance. (In some cases, minimal assistance may be necessary and acceptable). Most PACUs require a responsible adult to accompany the patient home.

Some PACUs keep ambulatory surgery patients for 4 to 6 hours postoperatively and serve a meal. Others may elect to discharge the patient home in 1 to 2 hours, provided other criteria have been met. PACUs have also reported that a first voiding is a requirement prior to discharge.

Discharge planning for the ambulatory surgery patient is integral to the care. Detailed postanesthesia and postsurgical instructions should be provided to the patient in writing. Examples of these types of instructions, as used at Doctors Hospital of Prince Georges County, Lanham, Maryland, are shown in Figures 7-6 and 7-7.

Critical Care Patients

The patient who will be transferred from the PACU to another critical care area may not achieve the levels of stability anticipated in a patient returning to a hospital room. The continued, intense nursing care provided to these patients enables the transfer of patients still intubated, of hemodynamically and surgically unstable patients, and of patients with multisystem problems. Criteria for discharge to critical care areas need to be developed by each PACU. For example, if a unit uses a PAS system as a discharge criterion, the departmental policy may state, "Patients with a PAS of 5 or below must be transferred to a critical care area." Discharge policy will also indicate who must accompany the patient during transfer, and any other precautions deemed necessary.

Pediatric Patients

Pediatric patients constitute another group with special discharge criteria needs. Further subdivision may be made into ambulatory surgery, in-house, and critical care patients. Adjustments in the discharge criteria may need to reflect the indications for measurement of blood pressure and its effect on the PAS (if this system is used). Depending on the needs of a particular PACU, all discharge criteria employed for adult patients are established with reference to pediatric patients.

The pediatric ambulatory surgery patient should have no nausea or vomiting, and, depending upon age, cry lustily, talk and be oriented, and walk. The patient should have no nystagmus. Clear fluids should be retained.

Regional Anesthetic Techniques

The patient who has received any of a variety of regional blocking techniques requires specific assessment of recovery from the effects of those agents.

**OUTPATIENT POSTANESTHESIA AND POSTSURGERY
INSTRUCTIONS AND INFORMATION**

1. Although you will be awake and alert in the recovery room, small amounts of anesthetic will remain in your body for at least 24 hours and you may feel tired and sleepy for the remainder of the day. Once you are home, take it easy and rest as much as possible. It is advisable to have someone with you at home for the remainder of the day.
2. Eat lightly for the first 12 to 24 hours, then resume a well-balanced, normal diet. Drink plenty of fluids. Alcoholic beverages are to be avoided for 24 hours after your anesthesia or intravenous sedation.
3. Nausea or vomiting may occur in the first 24 hours. Lie down on your side and breathe deeply. Prolonged nausea, vomiting, or pain should be reported to your surgeon.
4. Medications, unless prescribed by your physician, should be avoided for 24 hours. Check with your surgeon and/or anesthesiologist for specific instructions if you have been taking a daily medication.
5. Your surgeon will discuss your postsurgery instructions with you and prescribe medication for you as indicated. You will also receive additional instructions specific to your surgical procedure prior to leaving the hospital.
6. Your family will be waiting for you in the hospital's waiting room area adjacent to the outpatient surgery department. Your surgeon will speak to them in this area prior to your discharge.
7. **Do not operate a motor vehicle or any mechanical or electrical equipment for *24 hours* after your anesthesia.**
8. Do not make any important decisions or sign legal documents for 24 hours following your anesthesia.

Figure 7-6. Outpatient postanesthesia teaching information (Doctors Hospital of Prince Georges County).

DISCHARGE (TRANSFER) OF PATIENTS FROM PACU

The postanesthesia care record must contain a discharge summary and transfer note. The PAN documents how the patient has met established criteria. Areas to be documented include:

Discharge instructions:
___ Keep limb elevated, apply ice packs if ordered. Instructions given.   ___ Other instructions given by private physician.
___ If dressing on extremity is "too tight" and swelling occurs, or discoloration, loosen and contact private physician.   ___ Keep dressing dry and clean. Instructions given.
___ Reinforce dressing if necessary. Instructions given.
___ If "redness, numbness, unusual swelling" occur either in suture line or on operative extremity, contact private physician.   ___ Contact private physician if bleeding occurs. Instructions given.
___ Make appointment with private physician for postoperative visit in _____ _____ (Days or Weeks)
___ Prescription given by private physician.
Additional Comments: _____
Signature of Discharge R.N./L.P.N. _____ Date _____
I have reviewed and understand the instructions listed above:
Signature of Patient and/or Guardian _____ Date _____

Figure 7-7. Outpatient postsurgical instruction information (Doctors Hospital of Prince Georges County).

1. The patient's level of consciousness and degree of orientation
2. The patient's response to regional anesthetics, if applicable
3. Vital signs at discharge, and indication of pattern of stability
4. Cardiac rhythm(s) observed in the postanesthetic period
5. Status of all peripheral lines, i.e., amount remaining, patency, etc.
6. Status of surgical dressing(s) or operative area, i.e., drainage, swelling, etc.
7. Patient's level of pain perception, or response to pain medication, if administered
8. Voiding status of the patient
9. Continuing care to be provided during the transfer process, e.g., oxygen, cardiac monitor, traction
10. Mode of transfer, e.g., stretcher, wheelchair, ICU bed
11. Patient teaching accomplished and reinforced
12. Time of discharge
13. Signature and title of PACU nurse writing the discharge summary
14. Name and title of the nurse on the patient's care unit who has received a verbal report on the patient's status

The PACU nurse should provide a verbal report to a nurse on the patient's assigned care unit. In addition to the information on the written transfer note, the verbal report includes:

1. Medications administered in the PACU, and the patient's response to medications
2. Medications administered in the OR which have continuing implications for the patient's care
3. Equipment that will need to be obtained by the nursing unit for the continuing care of the patient
4. Interactions of the OR and PACU staff with the patient's family and significant others
5. Physician's orders, particularly those which have been clarified by the PAN
6. Any other pertinent information

Each PACU should develop written standards for documentation on the postanesthesia care record. This provides completeness and consistency and a uniform standard of care. These charting criteria also serve as the basis for an audit tool, providing quality assurance. Written standards are also a valuable teaching tool during the orientation phase of new PACU staff members, and for nursing student experiences in the PACU.

SUMMARY

Discharge criteria should be developed by each PACU to meet its own needs and standards. Several published models are available for reference. The benefits of written standards and criteria include:

1. Consistent application of quality care for all patients
2. Improved relations between the Department of Anesthesiology staff and the PACU staff
3. Professional application of abilities and accountability for the PAN
4. Fulfillment of JCAH guidelines for discharge criteria
5. Available standards and retrievable data for audit purposes

SUGGESTIONS FOR FURTHER READING

Aldrete JA. Assessment of recovery from anesthesia. Curr Rev Rec Room Nurs 1980; 1(21):161-168.
Aldrete JA. Recovery room scorecard. AORN J 1973; 17:79-83.

Aldrete JA, Kroulik D. A postanesthetic recovery score. Anesthes Analges 1970; 49:924-933.

Andrews IC. Criteria for discharge from the recovery room. Curr Rev Rec Room Nurs 1980; 2(7,8):49-64.

Bakutis AR. Assessing the anesthesia patient. J Am Assoc Nurs Anesthet 1975; June:255-268.

Bushong MW. Principles of postanesthetic recovery room management: criteria for patient discharge. Curr Rev Rec Room Nurs 1980; 1(10):75-79.

Carignan G, Keeri-Szanto M, Lavelee J-P. Postanesthetic scoring system. Anesthesiology 1964; 25(3):396-397.

Danner CA, et al. Recovery scoring revisited. S Med J 1973; 66:865-868.

Drain CB, Shipley SB. The recovery room. Philadelphia: WB Saunders, 1979.

Dripps RD, Eckenhoff JE, Van Dam LO. The immediate postoperative period: recovery and intensive care. In: Introduction to anesthesia: the principles of safe practice. 6th ed. Philadelphia: WB Saunders, 1982.

Figueroa M. The postanesthesia recovery score: a second look. S Med J 1972; 65(7):791-795.

Guidelines for recovery room care. Task Force of the Anesthesia Care Team Committee of the New York State Society of Anesthesiologists, 1983.

Guidelines for standards of care. American Society of Postanesthesia Nurses, 1983.

Hartwell PW. Discharge criteria. In: International anesthesiology clinics: recovery room care. Frost E, Andrews IC, eds. Boston: Little, Brown, 1983.

Holzgrafe RE. A postanesthesia recovery score. Wisc Med J 1972; 239-241.

Joint Commission for Accreditation of Hospitals Accreditation Manual. 1983.

Jones C. Glasgow coma scale. Am J Nursing 1979; 1551-1553.

Practice advisory for recovery room. American Society of Anesthesiologists, No 2, May 1978.

Schneider M. Meeting the criteria for discharge. Curr Rev Rec Room Nurs 1982; 4(6):41-48.

Selvin BL. Recovery room policy manual: a model. Md St Med J 1981; 56-59.

Suggestions for a record of anesthesia care to facilitate medical audit. American Society of Anesthesiologists, October 1977.

II
PATIENTS WHO REQUIRE SPECIAL CONSIDERATION

8
Children in the Recovery Room
Nirmala Balan

DIFFERENCES BETWEEN CHILDREN AND ADULTS

Anatomic, physiologic, and psychologic differences in children dictate special attention in the recovery room. Just as surgical indications differ in the pediatric setting so must nursing care be modified.

Anatomic Differences

Size

The most striking difference between adults and children is size. Though the body weight of a child is significantly less as compared to that of an adult, the body surface area is relatively greater and the potential for heat loss is increased. Besides the actual difference in size, there is also a difference in the relative proportion of body structures. For instance, the newborn has a relatively large head, with a small thorax and a protuberant abdomen.

Airway

The larynx and trachea of children under 5 years of age differ from that of older patients. The normal child has:

1. A relatively large head and a short neck.
2. A relatively big tongue.
3. A longer and stiffer epiglottis than the adult. It is U-shaped and

aimed at an angle of 45 degrees from the anterior pharyngeal wall making exposure and elevation of the epiglottis difficult.
4. A larynx located more cephalad than the adult. The rima glottidis is opposite the level of the interspace of the 3rd and 4th cervical vertebrae in infants, and 4th and 5th cervical vertebrae in adults.
5. A smaller airway. The narrowest portion of the larynx is at the cricoid ring rather than at the glottis, as in adults.

Physiologic Differences

Cardiovascular System

The cardiac output of the neonate is 2 times higher than that of adults and is dependent on heart rate. Therefore a slow rate is more worrisome than a tachyarrhythmia. The neonate has an average heart rate of 120 to 140 beats per minute, which progressively decreases to 80 beats per minute by 12 years of age. Blood pressure measurement is especially important in children because it has been shown to correlate well with the circulating blood volume. Because the heart rate response to hypovolemia is unpredictable, it is necessary to rely on blood pressure as a guide to the adequacy of intravascular volume. The right ventricle is bigger than the left ventricle in size and wall thickness, and by 6 months of age, the adult ratio of ventricular size is reached. The blood volume in children is relatively larger:

Newborn, 85 ml/kg
Infant (12 months), 80 ml/kg
Child (1–12 years), 75 ml/kg
Adult, 65 ml/kg

Respiratory System

Differences in physiologic parameters between neonates and adults are noted in Table 8-1.

Lung growth. The number of alveoli in a full-term newborn is approximately 8 percent that of an adult. There is, therefore, more than a 10-fold increase in the number of alveoli during postnatal lung growth. The adult value of 300×10^6 alveoli is reached by 8 years of age.

Anatomy. The thoracic cage of a newborn is small, with horizontally placed ribs, which limit expansion. The motion of the highly placed diaphragm is easily restricted by any increase in the volume of the abdominal contents.

Table 8-1. Differences in the commonly measured respiratory parameters

	Adult	Neonate
Respiratory rate (per minute)	20	40
Tidal volume (ml/kg)	6-7	6-7
Alveolar ventilation (ml/kg/minute)	60	100-150
Dead space (ml/kg)	2.2	2.2
FRC (ml/kg)	34	30
PaO_2 mm Hg	80-100	60-80
$PaCO_2$ mm Hg	38-40	32-35
pH	7.38	7.38

Airway resistance. Large airways contribute to 80 percent of the total airway resistance in adults, whereas small airways contribute more resistance in patients less than 5 years of age. Thus the signs and symptoms of small airway disease (bronchiolitis) are more marked in children.

Lung volumes. The tidal volume is the same in both children and adults (6-7 ml/kg), but the respiratory rate is higher in children. The alveolar ventilation of the newborn is twice that of the adult (V_A expressed as ml/kg per minute is 60 in adults and 100-150 in a newborn). The closing volume, defined as the volume at which lung units begin to close on reduction of lung volume, is relatively larger, with the closing capacity exceeding the functional residual capacity (the amount of air left in the lung at the end of tidal expiration) in patients less than 6 years of age. Children, therefore, are more prone to develop hypoxemia secondary to a higher metabolic rate (higher oxygen consumption) and a bigger closing volume.

Kidneys

The differences in renal function include: (1) Glomerular filtration rate is reduced at birth due to an increased resistance of afferent renal arteries. The permeability of the glomerular capillaries is also decreased. (2) Glomerulotubular imbalance exists secondary to a more rapid development of the glomeruli as compared to the proximal tubules. (3) The concentrating power of urine is reduced in neonates. Urine specific gravity of 1.025 compares to 1.040 in adults. This impairs the neonatal compensatory mechanisms in the face of dehydration. (4) Neonates are obligatory sodium losers, which means that they are unable to conserve sodium. These functional limitations are most marked during the first 4 weeks of life, by which time renal function is 80-90 percent of that in the adult.

Central Nervous System

Inadequate neurologic function causes instability of respiration and muscular activity. The minimum alveolar concentration (MAC) of inhalational anesthetics is higher in children, however, which means that more drug is required to reach the same depth of anesthesia. Emergence is rapid. The increased permeability of the blood-brain barrier and the lack of myelination lead to accumulation of drugs such as barbiturates in higher concentration than in adults.

Autonomic Nervous System

Parasympathetic and alpha-sympathetic innervation occurs earlier in gestation than beta-sympathetic innervation, which is incomplete at birth and continues to develop in early life. The infant responds to hypoxemia and shock by bradycardia due to vagal preponderance rather than by the initial tachycardia seen in adults. The adrenals, although oversized at birth, have little functional activity. It has been shown that norepinephrine plays a more important role than epinephrine in neonatal life, and that the norepinephrine is produced solely by the organs of Zuckerkandl along the sympathetic chain.

Fluid and Electrolyte Metabolism

The relative size of fluid compartments differ. The newborn total body water and extracellular fluid volume are larger (see Table 8-2). There is a gradual decrease in the proportion of the extracellular fluid volume so that by the time the child is 9 months to 2 years of age, adult values are reached.

Table 8-2. The Percentage of Body Weight of Fluid Compartments in the Newborn and Adult

Compartment		Newborn	Adult
ECF	Plasma Volume	5	5
	ISF	+ 35	+ 15
ICF		40 + 40	20 + 40
TBW		80% (2L)	60% (40L)

TBW = ECF (Plasma volume + ISF) + ICF. TBW = total body water; ECF = extracellular fluid; ISF = interstitial fluid; ICF = intracellular fluid.

The rate of fluid metabolism is 2 to 3 times faster in infants than in adults. Thus, following 24 hours of starvation, an adult loses 4 percent of his body weight while a newborn loses 10 percent. The metabolic rate is higher in children; the basal oxygen requirement in infancy is 6 ml/kg per minute, while it is 4 ml/kg per minute in adults. There is more danger of metabolic acidosis and hypoglycemia in children.

Temperature Regulation

Infants, particularly ex-prematures, are susceptible to developing hypothermia for the following reasons: (1) They have a large body surface area relative to body weight. The body weight of a full-term newborn is 5 percent of that of an adult's, but the body surface area is 15 percent. (2) The subcutaneous fat is thin, leading to a fourfold increase in core conductance in an infant. (3) They have a higher metabolic rate. (4) The hypothalamic temperature control center is immature. (5) Infants are dependent upon nonshivering thermogenesis as a source of heat production in response to cold. Metabolism of this fat is stimulated by norepinephrine and occurs only with adequate levels of oxygen; that is, hypoxia will prevent this response to cold. Nonshivering thermogenesis is less efficient in producing heat than a shivering response.

Psychological Differences

The child characteristically has lack of self-control, and it is usually difficult to persuade children in the preschool age to act against their will. Induction of anesthesia and the waking-up process in the recovery room are critical times. During these periods every effort must be made to minimize psychological trauma, which may have a more serious and longer lasting effect on the child than the adult.

TRANSFER FROM THE OPERATING ROOM TO THE RECOVERY ROOM

The recovery process actually begins in the operating room when the surgery and anesthetic are terminated and the patient's trachea is extubated. Transport from the operating room to the recovery room is a critical period and mandates continuous monitoring of the heart sounds and breath sounds with a percordial stethoscope. The patient should be transported on his side to prevent airway obstruction and aspiration of gastric contents and to allow secretions to escape. Upon arrival in the recovery room, the airway and ventilation should be rechecked. The nurse should receive a full report of events during surgery, the patient's medical problems, and any special measures to be taken. The anesthesiologist should remain with the patient until the vital signs have been taken and the patient is in stable condition and well attended.

MONITORING

The waking up process begins in the operating room and continues in the recovery room, where the patient regains full consciousness and cardiopulmonary stability. In the majority of cases, the patients are retained in the recovery room for a minimum of 1 hour following any general anesthetic. During this period, close observation includes monitoring of:

1. Pulse: rate, rhythm, and pulse volume.
2. Respiration: rate and depth; freedom from obstruction; good bilateral breath sounds on auscultation.
3. Blood pressure: proper width of the cuff should equal two-thirds the length of the upper arm. A narrow cuff will give an erroneously high reading and too wide a cuff will give a lower reading. In older children who have undergone relatively simple procedures, systolic blood pressure alone may be measured by the palpatory method or by watching the bounce of the needle on the pressure gauge as the cuff is deflated. In infants, blood pressure can be measured accurately with the Doppler or an Infrasonde.
4. Color of the skin.
5. Temperature.
6. Level of consciousness: awake and alert, drowsy, disoriented, or unconscious.
7. Intake (fluid and blood replacement) and output (gastric, urinary, hemovac, or active bleeding).

RESPIRATORY COMPLICATIONS

In all children the major respiratory complications encountered in the recovery room include:

1. Airway obstruction
2. Postextubation croup
3. Respiratory depression
4. Pulmonary aspiration
5. Acute respiratory failure

Airway Obstruction

In the early postoperative period, the most frequent and serious complication is airway obstruction. Etiology is as follows:

1. Soft tissue obstruction of the upper airway. Although infants are often obligatory nasal breathers, the relatively large tongue tends to fall back and produce pharyngeal obstruction.
2. Enlarged tonsils and adenoids.
3. Laryngeal spasm.
4. Laryngeal edema.

Diagnosis is made on the basis of suprasternal, subcostal, and intercostal retractions; nasal flaring; vigorous diaphragmatic and abdominal contractions; inspiratory crowing; and decreased air entry.

Airway obstruction should be relieved promptly. Arterial carbon dioxide tension ($PaCO_2$) rises 6 mm Hg during the first minute of total obstruction and then rises at a rate of 3 to 4 mm Hg per minute, along with a progressive fall in arterial oxygen tension (PaO_2) due to a decrease in alveolar oxygen tension. Airway obstruction due to pharyngeal obstruction by the tongue can be effectively overcome by hyperextension of the head with anterior displacement of the mandible. If obstruction is still not relieved, a nasal or oral airway can be inserted. The nasal airway is preferred because it is better tolerated by patients recovering from general anesthesia. The oral airway may stimulate gagging, vomiting, and laryngospasm. One hundred percent oxygen should be administered by face mask.

Laryngeal spasm is defined as laryngeal obstruction due to partial or complete spasm of the intrinsic or extrinsic muscles of the larynx. Two mechanisms are in effect: (1) Reflex closure of the glottis is due to a shutterlike adduction of the vocal cords, i.e., it involves the intrinsic laryngeal muscles. The resulting airway obstruction is incomplete and intermittent and occurs during inspiration or expiration. It usually occurs in response to somatic sensory stimulation, such as suctioning or the presence of an airway during light planes of anesthesia and during recovery. Treatment includes discontinuation of the stimulus and application of positive pressure with bag and mask, and administration of 100 percent oxygen. (2) Reflex closure of the larynx is due to a ball valve mechanism involving the extrinsic muscles and occurs in response to visceral sensory stimulation. It results in complete laryngeal obstruction.

To treat laryngeal spasm, stop the stimulus and remove any irritant from the larynx such as secretions, blood, or a long airway. Administer 100 percent oxygen. This spasm cannot be broken by positive pressure. Forcing the chin forward by strong pressure applied behind the angles of the jaw is often an effective maneuver. A small dose of succinylcholine (10–20 mg) may be necessary. Respiration must then be supported by positive pressure ventilation (e.g., Ambu bag).

Postextubation Croup

Infants are more prone to postintubation complications for the following reasons (in order of decreasing importance):

1. Small size of the larynx: In the adult, 1 mm of edema produces only slight hoarseness. In the infant the same amount of edema reduces the lumen by 75 percent and produces serious airway obstruction.
2. Loose areolar tissue in the submucosa of the subglottic area, where edema fluid easily accumulates.
3. Complete ring formed by the cricoid cartilage.

The incidence is 1 to 3.7 percent of intubated patients. It is most common in children 1 to 3 years of age. Contributory factors include:

1. Tight-fitting endotracheal tube
2. Trauma during intubation
3. Long duration of intubation (more than 48 hours)
4. Movement of the head and, therefore, of the endotracheal tube during positive pressure ventilation
5. Concomitant airway infection
6. Hypotension
7. Anticoagulant therapy

Postextubation croup usually occurs 1–2 hours postoperatively, peaks at 6–8 hours and usually subsides in the next 24 hours. The diagnosis is made on the basis of stridor, thoracic retraction, hoarseness, crouplike cough, and varying degrees of respiratory obstruction.

To treat:

1. Position patient upright.
2. Cool humidified oxygen.
3. Give racemic epinephrine (0.25 to 0.5 ml of a 2.25 percent solution is diluted with enough distilled water to reach a volume of 3.5 ml) and administer by nebulization over 15 minutes.
4. Give dexamethasone 0.2 to 0.5 mg/kg.
5. Insert artificial airway only if the child is retaining carbon dioxide, appears obtunded, or the clinical condition does not improve with the above measures.

Respiratory Depression

The etiology of respiratory depression is as follows:

1. Residual anesthetic: All inhalational agents are respiratory depressants. Barbiturates produce depression of both tidal volume and respiratory rate. Narcotic overdosage shows marked pupillary constriction and a slow rate of respiration with full tidal exchange.
2. Residual neuromuscular blockade due to inadequate reversal of muscle relaxants administered intraoperatively. This is easily diagnosed with the aid of a nerve stimulator.
3. Preexisting pulmonary disease.

Treatment of respiratory depression involves the following:

1. Stir-up regimen by the recovery room personnel stimulates spontaneous respiration and is often sufficient. This involves verbal and tactile stimulation.
2. Naloxone (Narcan) may be used to reverse narcotic-induced respiratory depression. It is a pure narcotic antagonist, which acts by competitive inhibition. Its duration of action is short-lived (30–60 minutes) and, hence, respiratory depression may recur. Thus, patients must be observed closely, or an intravenous dose of naloxone must be followed by an intramuscular dose to provide long-lasting effect.
3. Residual muscle relaxant may be reversed with an anticholinesterase and anticholinergic combination.
4. Controlled ventilation may be indicated to maintain a normal $PaCO_2$ and to enhance the excretion of inhalational anesthetics by increasing alveolar ventilation.

Pulmonary Aspiration

Factors which make the infant more vulnerable to regurgitation and aspiration include:

1. The resting intragastric pressure may be higher in infants than in adults due to: (a) the relatively small size of the stomach; (b) excessive air swallowing during crying; (c) encroachment of other abdominal organs; and (d) strenuous diaphragmatic breathing.
2. Short esophagus.
3. Relaxation of the gastroesophageal vestibule; regurgitation following feeding is considered a normal occurrence during the first 6 months of life.

4. Cough reflex may not be well developed.
5. Incoordination of breathing and swallowing mechanisms may occur in premature and dyspneic infants.

Anesthetic deaths for the pediatric age group are 2 to 3.3 per 10,000 anesthetics. Of these deaths 26 percent are due to aspiration of vomitus and blood.

Acid aspiration produces a chemical burn of the lungs. The critical gastric pH and volume necessary for the development of this lesion are a pH of less than 2.5, and a volume of 0.4 ml/kg (25 ml for the average adult patient). Particular food stuff aspiration or a high bacterial count of the aspirated material, such as from bowel obstruction, may produce lethal results, regardless of the pH.

The diagnosis is made on the basis of tachypnea, dyspnea, bronchospasm, cyanosis, shock, and pulmonary edema. Arterial blood gases reveal hypoxemia, initial hypocapnia secondary to tachypnea, and later hypercapnia due to increased work of breathing. The arterial pH may be decreased due to respiratory or metabolic acidosis. Chest X ray reveals irregular mottled densities, but changes may not be apparent until at least 8 hours later, typically involving the apical segment of the right lower lobe, when aspiration occurs in the supine position.

Treatment is as follows:

1. Position the patient with a head-down tilt, with the head turned to one side to aid drainage of gastric contents.
2. Suction the mouth and oropharynx to remove residual material.
3. Administer 100 percent oxygen by face mask.
4. Intubate the trachea, if the patient is not alert and cooperative.
5. Perform arterial blood gas analysis and obtain a chest X ray.
6. Apply continuous positive airway pressure (CPAP), to increase FRC (functional residual capacity) and improve ventilation-perfusion ratios.
7. Support the cardiovascular system and the acid-base imbalance as necessary.
8. Steroids are no longer recommended because studies have not indicated improvement in survival.
9. Prophylactic antibiotics are not advocated.

Acute Respiratory Failure

Acute respiratory failure is defined as an impairment of alveolar ventilation and pulmonary gas exchange sufficient to pose an immediate threat to life. Etiology is as follows:

1. Lung disease (bronchiolitis; status asthmaticus, viral pneumonia)
2. Central nervous system dysfunction (encephalitis, drug overdosage, Reye's syndrome)
3. Circulatory failure (congestive heart failure)

Clinical criteria for diagnosis of acute respiratory failure in infants and children include:

1. Severe inspiratory retractions and use of accessory muscles of respiration
2. Irregular respiration or apneic spells
3. Diminished or absent breath sounds on auscultation
4. Decreased or absent blood pressure
5. Poor skeletal muscle tone
6. Decreased level of consciousness and response to painful stimuli

Physiologic criteria include:

1. Hypercapnia ($PaCO_2$ 60 mm Hg)
2. Hypoxemia (PaO_2 100 mm Hg with $FiO_2 = 1.0$)
3. Persistent and severe metabolic acidosis

The diagnosis of acute respiratory failure is made based on the finding of any three clinical and one physiologic criteria.

Treatment aims are to improve pulmonary gas exchange by administration of 100 percent oxygen by positive pressure ventilation and suctioning of upper airway secretions. Administration of sodium bicarbonate is necessary to increase arterial pH to 7.20 or higher. Insertion of an artificial airway is essential unless there is dramatic improvement with the above measures.

SPECIAL CIRCUMSTANCES

A clinical report from the Children's Hospital in Toronto reported on the complications following minor surgery in infants. The incidence of complications in the group of infants born prematurely was significantly higher than in the group of full-term infants. All the complications seen involved the respiratory system and included:

1. Apnea
2. Postoperative atelectasis
3. Aspiration pneumonia

4. Extubation stridor
5. Excessive secretions
6. Coughing and cyanosis

Apnea was the most frequent complication. Only 36 percent of these infants had a preoperative history of apnea. It occurred up to 12 hours postoperatively and was treated by manual stimulation and/or by administration of 100 percent oxygen by bag or mask. None of the patients were hypothermic postoperatively. The cause of the apnea is uncertain and may be related to the depressant effect of halothane or the chemoreceptor response to hypoxia. Apnea occurring several hours following the anesthetic may be secondary to ventilatory muscle fatigue. Thus preterm infants should be carefully and closely observed for 24 hours postoperatively with an apnea monitor, if necessary.

RESPIRATORY SUPPORT

Endotracheal Intubation in Children

Size

The optimal size is one which passes easily through the glottic and subglottic regions and produces a small leak of gas around the tube at 15-20 cm of water peak inspiratory pressure. The formula for calculation of size of endotracheal tube is

$$\text{Internal diameter (mm)} = \frac{\text{age (years)} + 18}{4}$$

This formula is for uncuffed endotracheal tubes and is applicable for children over 2 years of age. A few patients will require an endotracheal tube that is smaller or larger than the one predicted by the above formula; therefore, tubes one size smaller and larger should also be available.

Cuffed endotracheal tubes should not be used in children less than 7 to 8 years of age, since they reduce the size of the lumen thereby increasing airway resistance and putting pressure on the delicate tracheal mucosa, thus increasing the incidence of subglottic damage. The correct size of a cuffed endotracheal tube is 0.5 mm internal diameter less than that calculated by the above formula.

Composition

The composition of endotracheal tubes is important. Toxic substances form on gamma ray sterilized PVC (polyvinyl chloride) tubes after resterilization with ethylene oxide. The clear, polyvinyl, disposable tubes that have been tissue implant-tested (Z 79) are the most satisfactory ones for general use.

Laryngoscope

Miller zero blade (straight) is used for infants up to 2.5 kg in weight and Miller one blade for larger infants. For older children, a Wis Foregger blade is preferable because the flange is wide, improving visibility. Macintosh curved blades are suitable for children over 3 years of age.

PAIN AND AGITATION

Pain

Postoperative pain is a very common problem, the consequences of which are:

1. Agitation
2. Hypertension
3. Hypoventilation due to splinting of abdominal muscles
4. Hypoxemia secondary to hypoventilation and atelectasis

Factors that influence the incidence and severity of pain are

1. Age. Pain appreciation is less at extremes of age.
2. Psychological factors, including the personality traits of the patient and the degree of anxiety and apprehension prior to the operation. Adequate preoperative preparation of the patient about postoperative pain has been shown to decrease significantly the requirement for morphine in the postoperative period.
3. Site of operation. In children pain is more severe following perineal and orthopedic operations.
4. Anesthetic techniques. If no narcotics have been administered preoperatively or intraoperatively, earlier use of narcotics in the postoperative period is necessary. The use of a narcotic as a premedicant delays the first postoperative request for pain medication, whereas preoperative medication with barbiturates appears to worsen postoperative pain.

Both pain and anxiety are more easily prevented by medication than controlled after their onset. Thus it is recommended that narcotics should be given preoperatively or intraoperatively to ease the early pain and anxiety on awakening.

Narcotics provide excellent analgesia and control excitement. It is preferable to use the intravenous route as this provides more rapid and effective pain relief, enables titration of smaller doses of the drug, and is painless compared to intramuscular administration. The first postoperative dose should be reduced by one-half the regular dose and the drug should be readministered only if needed, rather than being ordered on a regular dosage schedule. Patients should be carefully observed for the side effects of narcotics, including dose-dependent respiratory depression, excessive sedation, nausea, and vomiting. The presence of pain does not prevent narcotic-induced respiratory depression. It is prudent to avoid narcotics in patients less than 10 kg in weight for fear of profound depression.

Caudal analgesia is one of the most frequently performed blocks to reduce the postoperative pain of circumcision, hypospadias repair, and orchidopexy. It is relatively simple to perform and provides good analgesia, without delaying discharge from the ambulatory surgery unit.

Agitation

Postoperative excitement is a fairly common problem in pediatric patients, especially in those 3 to 9 years of age. The patient may awaken from anesthesia in a violent and agitated state. Etiology is as follows:

1. Drug response. This is a frequent cause of excitement. Barbiturates may lead to postoperative restlessness and may make some children wild and uncontrollable, especially in response to pain. This reaction is seen more commonly in the recovery room, if the patient has not been given narcotics at the end of the operation. Anticholinergics also increase the incidence of postoperative excitement and may lead to emergence delirium, an effect seen more with scopolamine than with atropine. Following ketamine anesthesia, hyperactivity may be prolonged. Halogenated agents have also been related to awakening delirium, with significantly greater excitement following enflurane than halothane anesthesia.
2. Pain.
3. Hypoxemia.
4. Hypercarbia.
5. Gastric distension.
6. Urinary retention with bladder distension.
7. Separation anxiety from parents and waking up in a strange room puts an appreciable emotional strain on a child.

Treatment involves the following:

1. Before giving narcotics, ascertain the adequacy of ventilation and exclude hypoxemia.
2. Relieve gastric or urinary distension.
3. Relieve pain with analgesics (see below).
4. Control continued excitement by simple measures such as the parent's presence by the patient.
5. Physostigmine (1-3 mg intravenously) crosses the blood-brain barrier rapidly and produces a nonspecific reversal of the central nervous system effects of scopolamine, major tranquilizers (droperidol, haloperidol), and diazepam.

TEMPERATURE REGULATION

Hypothermia

Infants are more likely than adults to develop hypothermia for reasons mentioned earlier. The effects of hypothermia (35°C) include

1. Increased oxygen consumption (1F° decrease in temperature increases the metabolic rate by 10 percent).
2. Hypoxemia may develop due to the increased oxygen consumption, if supplemental oxygen is not given.
3. Anaerobic glycolysis occurs secondary to hypoxia, which dissipates glycogen 20 times faster than aerobic glycolysis. Thus hypoglycemia may develop.
4. Increased lactic acid production and metabolic acidosis may develop due to the anaerobic glycolysis and to poor tissue perfusion, secondary to the vasoconstriction produced by cold.
5. Dysrhythmias.
6. Irregularity of respiration and apnea.
7. Pulmonary vasoconstriction, leading to right-to-left shunting of blood through the foramen ovale and ductus arteriosus.
8. Increased viscosity of blood.
9. Hypocalcemia.
10. Delayed anesthetic arousal.
11. Increased morbidity and mortality in the postoperative period.

To treat hypothermia:

1. Monitor body temperature.
2. Provide supplemental oxygen.

3. Cover the patient with warmed blankets, wrap the extremities with cotton, and cover the head with a stockinette cap.
4. Use a warming mattress for children weighing less than 10 kg.
5. Use overhead infrared lamps.
6. Warm intravenous fluids before administration.

Hyperthermia

Etiology of hyperthermia is as follows:

1. Elevated ambient temperature.
2. Dehydration.
3. Carbon dioxide retention.
4. Preexisting infection and fever.
5. Bacteremia, especially following urinary tract operations.
6. Transfusion reaction.
7. Atropine. Temperature elevation secondary to atropine has been difficult to document.
8. Malignant hyperthermia.

Fever increases oxygen consumption and carbon dioxide production, stimulates the cardiorespiratory system, and causes metabolic and respiratory acidosis. If uncorrected, convulsions, hypoxic brain damage, arterial hypotension, and cardiac arrest may occur. To treat the patient:

1. Cool the room.
2. Uncover the patient as much as possible.
3. Apply ice bags to the neck, groin, and axillae.
4. Infuse cold intravenous fluids.
5. Administer antipyretic agents such as aspirin, acetaminophen, or chlorpromazine.

Malignant Hyperthermia

Malignant hyperthermia is a syndrome of hypermetabolism, both aerobic and anaerobic, resulting in an intense production of heat, carbon dioxide, and lactate, and generally accompanied by tachycardia and other signs of circulatory and metabolic stress.

The defect in malignant hyperthermia appears to be an abrupt loss of control of intracellular calcium levels, resulting in a rise of sarcoplasmic calcium. The consequences of the increased calcium levels are:

1. Glycolysis secondary to activation of phosphorylase kinase
2. Hydrolysis of adenosine triphosphate (ATP) to adenosine diphosphate (ADP) due to activation of myosin adenosine triphosphatase (ATPase)
3. Troponin inhibition, leading to muscle contraction
4. Membrane instability
5. Possible uncoupling of oxidative phosphorylation

The incidence of malignant hyperthermia is 1 per 15,000 anesthetics in children and 1 per 50,000 anesthetics in adults.

Diagnosis is based on unexplained tachycardia; dysrhythmias; generalized rigidity and masseter spasm; hyperventilation; flushing, sweating, and skin mottling; cyanosis; unstable blood pressure; hyperthermia; and cardiac arrest.

To treat malignant hyperthermia:

1. Call for help.
2. Change the breathing tubing from the oxygen supply.
3. Hyperventilate with 100 percent oxygen at three times the normal minute ventilation.
4. Apply external and internal cooling measures.
5. Give sodium bicarbonate, 2 to 4 mEq/kg, titrated by monitoring of arterial blood gases and pH.
6. Maintain intravascular volume; administer iced saline at 2 to 8 ml/kg per hour.
7. Maintain urinary output at 2 ml/kg per hour with fluid infusion, furosemide (mg/kg), and mannitol (1 gm/kg).
8. To treat dysrhythmias occurring during the acute episode, give procainamide.
9. Give dantrolene sodium 1 to 10 mg/kg, up to a maximum total dose of 300 mg. The average recommended dose is 3 mg/kg, which may be repeated every 5 to 10 minutes.
10. Monitor vital signs, electrocardiogram, temperature, arterial blood gases, urinary output, and central venous pressure.
11. Send blood and urine specimens for serum electrolytes, enzymes (CPK, LDH, SGOT, aldolase), blood sugar, urea, creatinine, lactate, pyruvate, clotting studies, and urinary hemoglobin and myoglobin.
12. Avoid calcium salts, cardiac glycosides, vasopressors, and lidocaine.

FLUID REPLACEMENT

The physiologic differences in body fluid compartments, limited renal function, and a higher metabolic rate influence fluid therapy in infants and children. Fluid management falls into three categories:

1. Maintenance fluid requirement: estimated fluid requirement (EFR) and estimated fluid deficit (EFD).
2. Replacement fluid therapy (third-space loss)
3. Blood replacement

Maintenance Fluid Requirement

The aim is to provide replacement of insensible fluid losses, which includes evaporative losses through the respiratory tract to humidify the inspired gas, insensible cutaneous loss, and the minimal urine volume necessary to excrete the normal solute load of the kidney.

Type of Fluids

Because these losses are essentially sodium-free, maintenance fluids should be hypotonic with respect to their sodium concentration. Five percent dextrose in one-quarter strength saline is a suitable maintenance fluid. The solution should contain glucose to provide energy, prevent depletion of glycogen in the liver, prevent ketosis, and spare endogenous proteins. Five grams of glucose per 100 calories expended is the standard amount of glucose given for intravenous support.

Amount

EFR may be calculated on the basis of:

1. Body weight
2. Body surface area
3. Estimated metabolic rate or caloric expenditure (the most accurate method)

The following is a formula for pediatric fluid therapy based on caloric expenditure, arrived at indirectly by relating weight to caloric expenditure.

Body weight	Amount and Rate
0 to 10 kg	4 ml/kg/hour
10 to 20 kg	40 ml + 2 ml/kg/hour for each kg over 10 kg
Over 20 kg	60 ml + 1 ml/kg/hour for each kg over 20 kg

EFD

EFD = EFR × number of hours fasted. Information in the chart should indicate the number of fasting hours; one-half of this deficit is replaced in the first hour with a maintenance type of fluid. The other half is replaced as a quarter each in the second and third hours after the intravenous infusion is started. Much of this replacement should have been completed intraoperatively.

Replacement Fluid Therapy

The purpose of replacement fluids as opposed to maintenance fluids is to correct body fluid deficits caused by external losses (vomiting, nasogastric suction) or internal sequestration (burns, loss into the bowel wall and lumen in intestinal obstruction). These losses usually cease 3 to 5 days after injury.

Type of Fluids

Third-space fluid is derived initially from the plasma volume, which, in turn, is replenished from the interstitial fluid. Thus this fluid loss is nearly isotonic and suitable replacement fluids include lactated Ringer's solution, normal saline, and normosol.

Amount

The amount of third-space loss and, therefore, the amount of replacement required depends upon the severity of trauma.

Minimal surgical trauma (hernia repair)	=	1–2 ml/kg/hour
Moderate surgical trauma (pyloromyotomy)	=	2–4 ml/kg/hour
Major surgical trauma (bowel resection)	=	4–6 ml/kg/hour

Blood Replacement

The allowable whole blood loss in pediatric surgical patients is calculated to attain a final postoperative hematocrit of not less than 30 percent.

$EBV = wt$ in $kg \times y$ ml/kg

where: $y = 85$ for newborn, 80 if 6 months, 75 if 12 years.

$$ERCM = EBV \times \frac{Hct\ (A)}{100}$$

$$ERCM_{30} = EBV \times \frac{30\ (B)}{100}$$

$ARCL = (A) - (B)$

$$AWBL = (A) - (B) \times 3$$

where:

EBV = estimated blood volume
ERCM = estimated red cell mass (depends on patients preoperative hematocrit)
$ERCM_{30}$ = estimated red cell mass at a hematocrit at 30 percent
ARCL = Allowable red cell loss
AWBL = Allowable whole blood loss

The assumption made is that blood loss is occurring at a hematocrit of 30 percent. For practical purposes:

Amount of blood loss	Therapy
Blood loss is less than one-third of AWBL	Ringer's lactated solution
Blood loss is more than one-third but less than total AWBL	Colloid, preferably 5% albumin
Blood loss is equal to or more than AWBL	Blood

DRUG DOSAGES

Response to drugs is different in children than in adults. Some of the reasons for these observed differences are:

1. Differences in body fluid compartments (larger total body water and larger extracellular fluid volume) which affect the apparent volume of distribution of drugs.
2. Drugs administered intramuscularly may be absorbed more slowly due to a reduced muscle mass and decreased blood flow.
3. The gastric pH is higher, reaching adult levels by 2 years of age; this relatively higher pH results in a better absorption of orally administered drugs (e.g., ampicillin).
4. Gastric emptying time is longer in infancy and reaches normal adult values by 6 to 8 months of age, which may slow the absorption of drugs such as acetaminophen.
5. Infants have a decreased plasma protein concentration, resulting in a higher serum concentration of drugs and a narrower therapeutic range. The protein binding of drugs reaches adult levels by 1 year of age.
6. The increased permeability of the blood-brain barrier and the lack of myelination in neonates allows drugs such as phenobarbital to accumulate in the central nervous system in concentrations 20 to 100 percent higher than in adults.

7. Pathways for drug biotransformation are immature in infants less than 3 months of age, prolonging the half-life of drugs and increasing their sensitivity to drugs such as morphine.
8. Reduction in renal clearance may also lead to an altered response to drugs in infants (e.g., increased susceptibility to ampicillin toxicity).
9. Larger doses of sedatives are required during childhood due to the higher metabolic rate.

Barbiturates and narcotics are more potent in neonates than in adults because not only does more drug enter the central nervous system but there is an increased sensitivity to the drugs themselves and decreased metabolism and excretion.

Formulas for Pediatric Drug Dosages

Formulas have been derived on the basis of age, weight, and body surface area. Clark formula:

$$\text{child dose} = \frac{\text{child's weight (pounds)} \times \text{adult dose}}{150}$$

Body surface area rule:

$$\text{child dose} = \frac{\text{body surface area (sq m)} \times \text{adult dose}}{1.7}$$

Common Drug Dosages

Analgesics	*Dosage*
Morphine sulfate	0.05 to 0.1 mg/kg IM (maximum = 10 mg)
Meperidine hydrochloride (Demerol)	1.0 to 1.5 mg/kg IM (maximum = 100 mg)
Codeine phosphate	1.0 to 1.5 mg/kg IM (maximum = 60 mg)
Acetaminophen (Tylenol)	5 to 10 mg/kg
Acetylsalicylic acid (Aspirin)	60 mg/year of age orally or rectally
Sedatives	
Diazepam (Valium)	0.1 to 0.2 mg/kg IV or orally
Droperidol	0.1 mg/kg IM or IV
Pentobarbital (Nembutal)	2 to 4 mg/kg orally, or IM

Secobarbital (Seconal)	2 to 4 mg/kg orally, or IM
Others	
Atropine	0.02 mg/kg (maximum = 0.6 mg)
Lidocaine	1 mg/kg
Epinephrine	10 µg/kg or 0.1 ml/kg of 1:10,000 solution
Dopamine infusion	1 to 10 µg/kg/minute
Isoproterenol (Isuprel) infusion	1 µg/kg/minute
Propranolol (Inderal)	0.05 to 0.1 mg/kg
Calcium chloride	10 to 20 mg/kg
Sodium bicarbonate	1 to 2 mEq/kg
Furosemide (Lasix)	0.5 to 1.0 mg/kg
Naloxone hydrochloride (Narcan)	5 µg/kg

Although not a drug, it is important to note that the defibrillation dose in a child should be calculated at 2 watt-sec/kg.

SPECIAL SITUATIONS

Plastic Surgery

Children undergo plastic surgery to correct congenital anomalies and acquired lesions such as burn scars and contractures. The points to be remembered are:

1. Other defects should be suspected in the presence of one congenital anomaly.
2. If the child has congenital heart disease, antibiotics should be given in the perioperative period for prophylaxis against infective endocarditis.
3. The potential for preexisting airway problems in these patients is high. In addition, the head and neck are common sites for reconstructive surgery, which impose further problems of airway management.
4. It is essential that emergence from anesthesia be quiet and smooth to lessen the risk of damage to grafted areas and delicately sutured repairs.

Cleft Lip and Palate

The incidence is 1 per 1,000 live births. Associated anomalies are as follows:

1. Congenital heart disease
2. Subglottic stenosis
3. Pierre Robin's syndrome (micrognathia, glossoptosis, high arched palate, congenital heart disease).
4. Treacher Collin's syndrome (malar and mandibular hypoplasia, microstomia, choanal atresia, congenital heart disease).

Cleft lip repair is usually performed at 10 to 12 weeks of age. The recovery phase is the most critical period and involves several potential problems.

1. Airway obstruction is the primary problem postoperatively. The patient should be extubated awake. At the end of the operation, a long silk stitch is placed deep in the tissue of the tongue. Pulling on this traction suture is a very effective means of maintaining an adequate airway after extubation; additionally, it provides a stimulus for the patient to breathe.
2. Restlessness is common. To prevent damage to the repaired area, the infant should be restrained. The use of jackets with sleeves splinted to prevent elbow flexion is helpful in keeping the patient's hands away from his face. The Logan bow is used by some plastic surgeons for protection and relief of tension.
3. Hypothermia is observed.

Cleft palate repair is usually performed at 18 to 24 months of age. This repair is more tedious than repair of a cleft lip and involves more blood loss during and after surgery. Blood pools in dependent areas such as the hypopharynx and trachea. Postoperatively, the patient should be nursed in a croup tent and in the prone position to prevent aspiration of blood. The child should be restrained and observed closely for blood loss. The tongue suture is more critical here than following cleft lip repair.

Burns

We depend on the skin for thermal regulation, fluid and electrolyte hemostasis, protection against bacterial infection, as well as our own recognition as individuals. A peculiar aspect of burns is that no matter how small the area involved, there are systemic ramifications.

Estimating the percent of surface burns is done by the rule of nines: head = 9 percent; neck = 1 percent; upper extremity = 9 percent each; lower extremity = 18 percent each; anterior trunk = 18 percent; and posterior trunk = 18 percent. However, this rule is modified for children because a small child has a proportionately larger head (head = 18 percent in infants) and less surface area on the extremities, particularly the lower extremities, than an adult. This larger head and neck area, when burned, is more susceptible to edema formation, leading to airway obstruction. Prognosis and fluid therapy are based on knowledge of the area burned.

Anesthesia may be required for initial debridement and excharotomy, followed by skin grafts and plastic repair of burn scars and contractures. Special problems related to burned patients are given below.

Fluid Therapy

Fluid requirement is increased in burned patients due to: (1) fluid shifts secondary to changes in vascular integrity remote from the injured area; (2) evaporative fluid losses; (3) higher metabolic rate. Depending upon the magnitude of the injury, the metabolic rate doubles or triples at the time of injury and remains elevated for weeks or months until the burn is healed.

A burned child may lose up to 20 to 30 percent of his lean body mass; calories are lost due to evaporative and radiation losses. Thus the potential for hypovolemia and hypotension exists.

The Parkland formula for fluid resuscitation in burns is 4 ml/kg per 1 percent body surface area burn, up to a maximum of 50 percent burns. One-half to two-thirds of this requirement of crystalloids is given in the first 8 hours and the remainder over the rest of the first day. The aim is to give Ringer's lactate solution in sufficient quantity to maintain urinary output with a specific gravity of 1.010 to 1.020. By the second day after the burn, fluid requirement decreases as capillary integrity improves. Albumin (1 gm/kg per day) should be administered to attain a serum albumin level of at least 2 gm per 100 ml. Vital signs, urinary output, and central venous pressure should be monitored along with serial weights and laboratory tests (hematocrit, serum electrolytes, and albumin levels).

Airway Problems

Head and neck burns may be associated with edema of lips, tongue, and the airway. Airway burns produce laryngeal and tracheal edema, the major portion of which forms within 8 hours of injury but may continue to accumulate slowly for 12 to 24 hours. Such an airway should be protected immediately, if only for prophylactic reasons. Increasing edema in the first few hours may make intubation hazardous, if not impossible.

Pulmonary Problems

Hypoxemia may occur due to: (1) increased metabolic rate and oxygen consumption; (2) bronchospasm, due to inhalation of smoke, copious secretions, desquamation of the epithelium of the airways; (3) pulmonary edema due to increased pulmonary capillary permeability; (4) atelectasis and pneumonia; (5) carboxyhemoglobin formation, which shifts the oxyhemoglobin dissociation curve to the left and, therefore, decreases oxygen availability.

Psychological Problems

These problems stem from both the disfiguring nature of the injury and the need for repeated anesthetics and surgery during the prolonged phase of therapy.

Pain

The pain resulting from a second-degree burn is more severe and longer lasting than pain from a full-thickness third-degree burn.

Technical Problems

Intravenous sites may be difficult to secure, and a surgical cut-down may be necessary. Monitoring may also be difficult because of lack of intact sites. Blood pressure reading will usually be 20 to 30 mm Hg higher in the lower extremity than in the upper extremity.

Temperature Regulation

It is impaired and, hence, measures should be undertaken to maintain body temperature and prevent hypothermia (radiant lamps, warm fluids, etc.).

Infection

Aseptic techniques should be employed even for insertion of an intravenous cannula because of the increased susceptibility to infection.

Outpatient Surgery

Outpatient surgery has become popular in the pediatric population because it minimizes emotional disturbances, reduces the cost of treatment, and decreases the risk of nosocomial infection. Hospital-acquired upper respiratory and gastrointestinal infection may be reduced by 50 to 70 percent in children when operations are performed on a 1-day-stay ambulatory basis.

Factors influencing selection of patients for outpatient surgery are as follows:

1. Physical status of the patient. Healthy patients or patients with well-controlled systemic disease (e.g., bronchial asthma, epilepsy) are considered suitable candidates.

2. Age of the patient. All age groups may be considered suitable for outpatient surgery, except the ex-premature infant (less than 37 weeks gestation at birth) because of his potential immaturity of temperature control, respiration, and gag reflex. This restriction should be imposed up to 1 year of age in this group.
3. Parents. The parents should be willing and capable of caring for the child after the operation. They should live within a reasonable distance from the hospital, that is, a 1-hour driving radius. They should be informed about the possibility of overnight hospitalization of the patient.
4. Type of operation. A variety of surgical procedures are performed on an outpatient basis and include those associated with minimal bleeding and minimal physiologic derangements.
5. Duration of operation. Four hours is generally considered the upper limit for outpatient surgery.

Premedication should be minimal, using short-acting drugs. Atropine should be given to decrease secretions and to avoid adverse vagal responses.

Postoperative Care

Before discharge from the outpatient unit, the patient should be awake, alert, with stable vital signs and without anesthetic or surgical complications. Various scoring systems and discharge criteria have been set up for evaluating postanesthetic recovery in ambulatory surgical units. Those for children place greater emphasis on the adequacy of motor strength and physiologic functions, whereas evaluation of adults emphasizes mental acuity and driving fitness. The patient should be examined by a physician, preferably the anesthesiologist, before he is sent home in the care of an adult. The parents must be provided with written instructions for the care of the patient at home. Patients are usually detained for 4 hours when endotracheal anesthesia has been administered.

Complications following outpatient surgery are as follows:

1. Nausea and vomiting is commoner in children than in adults. The incidence is higher following halothane than enflurane anesthesia. While barbiturates are associated with minimal postoperative vomiting, narcotic premedication increases the incidence, which also appears to be directly related to the duration of anesthesia. Low-dose droperidol (0.05 mg/kg) may be useful in reducing postoperative vomiting. If oral intake of fluids becomes a problem, an antiemetic should be prescribed, such as dimenhydrinate (Dramamine) (2 mg/kg intramuscularly or rectally).

2. Postoperative headache occurs in 10 to 20 percent of patients. It occurs more commonly following use of inhalational than intravenous anesthetic agents.
3. Croup.
4. Sore throat is common even without endotracheal intubation.
5. Loss of appetite.
6. Muscle pain.
7. Dizziness.
8. Behavioral changes and bad dreams occur in 15 to 20 percent of young children hospitalized for surgery.
9. Postoperative surgical bleeding.

Although these complications may seem to contribute a formidable list, they have all been identified and may be minimized by careful attention to fluid replacement and careful surgical and anesthetic technique. The overall hospitalization rate secondary to these complications is less than 2 percent.

SUGGESTIONS FOR FURTHER READING

Berry FA Jr. Pediatric fluid and electrolyte therapy. Refr Cours Anesth 1975; 3:1–10.
Cullen DJ. Recovery room care of the surgical patient. Refr Cours Anesth 1980; 8:13–27.
Eckenhoff JE. Some anatomical considerations of the infant airway influencing endotracheal anesthesia. Anesthesiology 1951; 12:401–410.
Fink BR. The etiology and treatment of laryngeal spasm. Anesthesiology (July-August) 1956; 17:569–577.
Jaffe BR. Postoperative hoarseness. Am J Surg 1972; 123:432–437.
Miller RD. Anesthesia. Vol 2. New York: Churchill Livingstone, 1981.
Raphaely R. Pediatric intensive care, acute. ASA Annual Refresher Course Lectures. 1981; 232-A.
Smith RM. Anesthesia for infants and children. 4th ed. St. Louis: CV Mosby, 1980.
Steward DJ. Preterm infants are more prone to complications following minor surgery than term infants. Anesthesiology 1982; 56:304–306.

9

Postoperative Care of Neurosurgical Patients

Somasundaram Thiagarajah

Commonly performed neurosurgical procedures include (1) craniotomy for removal of intracranial tumors, clipping of cerebral aneurysm or arteriovenous fistula, and evacuation of a blood clot or an abscess; (2) cranioplasty for correction of deformed or defective skull; (3) surgery on vertebral column, including cervical or lumbar laminectomy, cervical osteophytes or fractures, and thoracic arteriovenous malformation and scoliosis; and (4) ventriculoperitoneal shunt, lumbar-peritoneal shunt, and placement of Omaya reservoir.

Following any surgery, swelling of tissues in and around the surgical site due to edema formation and minimal bleeding is usual and normally has no serious sequalae. If bleeding is excessive it is usually easily detected by observing the wound dressings or drainage tubes. But following neurosurgery, because the operative field is covered beneath a rigid cranium, not only is detection of bleeding difficult, but the increasing volume due to tissue swelling or bleeding will raise the intracranial pressure and thus decrease the blood flow to the brain, compress vital centers, or even causing herniation of the brain tissue. All of these effects adversely affect the neurological function of the patient. Furthermore, following general anesthesia, if cardiovascular and respiratory function are unstable, any hypotension, hypoxemia, or hypercapnia may decrease intracranial compliance and neurological function.

These complications in the postoperative period are amenable to therapy if detected and treated early. Therefore, vigilant care by trained staff in a well-equipped area is important. The quality of the outcome from the surgery depends on the care of these patients in the immediate postoperative period.

150   PATIENTS WHO REQUIRE SPECIAL CONSIDERATION

During transportation of the patient from the operating room to the recovery room area, he should be positioned 30° head up (unless contraindicated, e.g., following shunt procedures, lumbar laminectomy) (Figure 9-1). Breathing should be supplemented with oxygen and vital signs constantly monitored.

On arrival in the recovery room, continue oxygen administration and assessment of respiration; measure and record the baseline vital signs; determine serum electrolytes, hemoglobin, and arterial blood gases (ABG); perform skull X rays; assess neurological function. The important factors to monitor in these patients are:

1. Neurological status
2. Intracranial pressure (ICP)
3. Respiratory system: rate, tidal volume, ABG
4. Cardiovascular system: blood pressure (BP), electrocardiogram (ECG), and pulse

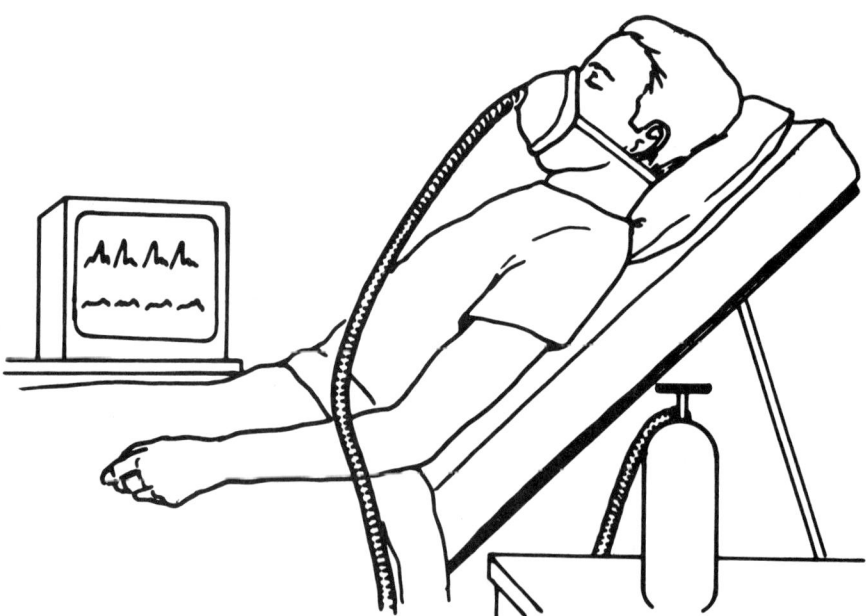

Figure 9-1. Transportation of patients following craniotomy. Note the head up position, monitoring of vital signs and oxygen supplementation.

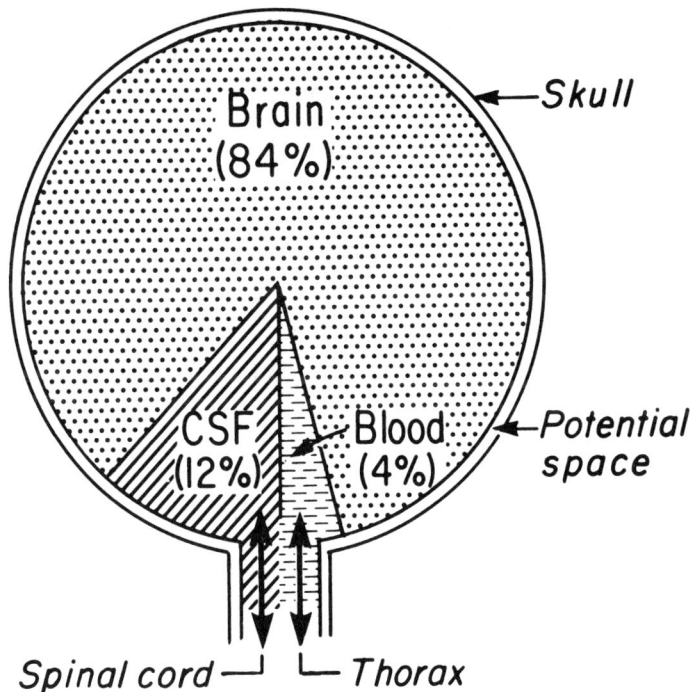

Figure 9-2. Intracranial contents: brain (84 percent), CSF (12 percent), and blood (4 percent). Communication is with spinal CSF and blood in the thorax.

PATHOPHYSIOLOGY

Within the rigid cranium are: (see Figure 9-2)

1. Brain tissue 84 percent
2. Cerebrospinal fluid (CSF) 12 percent
3. Arterial and venous blood 4 percent
4. A small potential space
5. Communication with the spinal column via spinal canal and with the thorax via the venous system

The normal ICP is less than 15 mm Hg. Uncompensated increase in the volumes of any of the above components will raise the ICP. Maintenance of the flow of oxygenated blood to the brain tissue is the most important factor in the care of these patients. It depends on:

Cerebral perfusion pressure (CPP) = mean BP-ICP

where the normal range of CPP is 70–100 mm Hg. The CPP will decrease with hypotension, increased ICP, or cerebral vessel spasm.

Several pathophysiologic changes may occur in the recovery room and cause increased ICP (Figure 9-3). These include:

1. Surgical dissection in brain substance → edema
2. Bleeding at the operative site → intracranial hematoma
3. Obstruction to CSF drainage (tumor, surgical dissection, bleeding, edema)
4. Infection (intracranial or systemic)
5. Increase in cerebral blood due to hypertension, hypercapnia, hypoxia, or cerebral vasodilation (drugs)
6. Obstruction to cerebral-venous drainage due to increased intrathoracic pressure, coughing, suctioning, positive pressure ventilation (PEEP), head low position (Figure 9-4).

MONITORING

On admission to the recovery room, baseline neurological function should be assessed, recorded, and retested at 15-minute intervals. In assessing neurological function, level of consciousness, motor activity, response to commands, and pupillary size, equality, and reaction to light are the usual parameters to observe. Immediately following anesthesia, pupillary size and its reaction to light may be the only parameters available. The Glasgow coma scale is used both as a prognostic indicator and as a monitor of neurological status (Table 9-1) following head trauma and in the postoperative period following craniotomy.

Deterioration in neurological function usually indicates that perfusion and oxygenation is decreasing to the brain and is either due to decrease in BP, increase in ICP, or spasm of cerebral vessels. A common cause of postoperative deterioration is hematoma, a formation which compresses the brain tissues and increases ICP. Less common causes are cerebral edema or pneumocephalus (Figure 9-3).

INTRACRANIAL PRESSURE

Direct monitoring of ICP in the postoperative period enables early detection of any changes in ICP before clinical manifestations on pupils, sen-

CAUSES OF ↑ICP

SURGICAL:

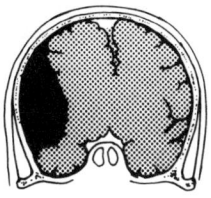
Blood clot

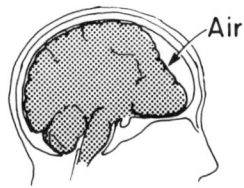
Pneumocephalus

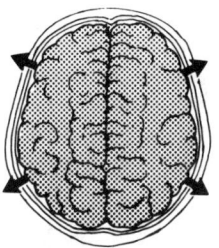
Edema

↑CEREBRAL BLOOD FLOW

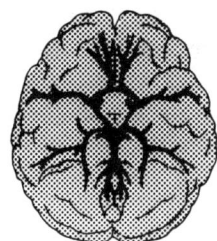

- ↑ BP
- ↑ $PaCO_2$
- ↓ PaO_2
- Vasodilators
  - Nitroprusside
  - Nitroglycerine

↑ INTRATHORACIC PRESSURE

Coughing
Straining
Suctioning
PEEP

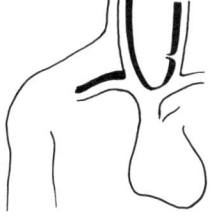

IMPAIRMENT OF CEREBRAL VENOUS DRAINAGE

Supine
Head low
Twist neck

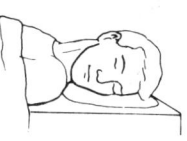

Figure 9-3. Schematic representation of the different causes of increased intracranial pressure.

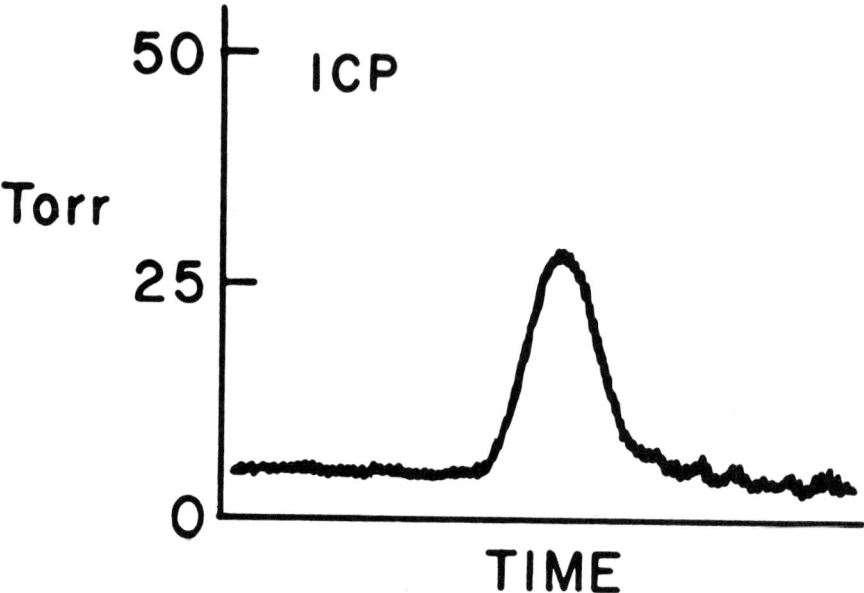

Figure 9-4. The ICP tracing shows the rise in the ICP when the head is lowered. On raising the head, the ICP returns to the baseline.

sorium, or vital signs become evident. The immediate response, if any, to therapeutic intervention is also apparent if ICP is directly monitored.

Three systems have been described to monitor ICP: intraventricular cannulation, subarachnoid bolt, and an epidural device (Figure 9-5). These systems are connected by a transducer to a graphic recorder or an oscilloscope. Advantages of the ventricular catheter include (1) withdrawal of CSF in an emergency, (2) simple calibration, and (3) easy calculation of compliance. Disadvantages include (1) liability to infection (5 percent), (2) blockage of the catheter by the choroid plexus, (3) hemorrhage, and (4) difficulty in placement within ventricles compressed by edema. The subarachnoid bolt has less chance of causing bleeding, but swollen brain or blood clots can occlude the end. Focal seizures can also occur, and CSF cannot be drained. Compliance measurements are less reliable.

All systems must be closed and aseptic conditions maintained. No heparin or external pressure is required. No more than 0.1 ml of Ringer's lactate solution should be used to clear any obstruction. For the reference point (zero point), the base of the skull or the external auditory meatus should be used. Because of the narrow range of normal values, careful calibration is important (Figure 9-5).

Table 9-1. Glasgow Coma Scale

Eyes	open	spontaneously	4
		to verbal command	3
		to pain	2
		no response	1
Best motor response	to verbal command		
		obeys	6
	to painful stimulus	localizes pain	5
		flexion-withdrawal	4
		flexion-abnormal (decorticate rigidity)	3
		extension (decerebrate rigidity)	2
		no response	1
Best verbal response			
		oriented and converses	5
		disoriented and converses	4
		inappropriate words	3
		incomprehensible sounds	2
		no response	1
Total			3-15

From Jennet B, Teasdale G. Aspects of coma after severe head injury. Lancet, April 23, 1977, pp. 878-881.

Patients who have raised ICP preoperatively or cerebral vasospasm or those in whom extensive surgical resection was required may develop cerebral edema, making ICP monitoring desirable.

The normal ICP tracing shows a pulsation with each heart beat and with respiration. Lundberg classified ICP values into four groups:

Normal	0-10 mm Hg
Slight increase	11-20 mm Hg
Moderate increase	21-40 mm Hg
Severe increase	> 40 mm Hg

As the volume in the closed intracranial system increases, ICP remains constant as long as CSF is moved from the cranium to the spinal subarachnoid space and venous blood is displaced into the chest (Figure 9-6). However, a rapidly growing lesion will quickly exhaust the compensatory buffer mechanisms. As compliance decreases, a modest increase in intracranial volume produces a rise in ICP, and when the steepest part of the

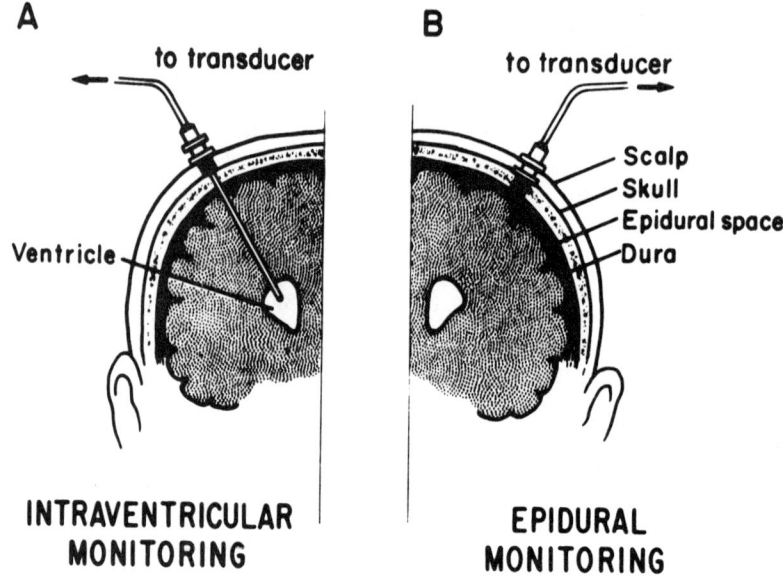

Figure 9-5. Commonly used clinical modes to measure intracranial pressure: (A) Intraventricular cannulation of the anterior horn of the right ventricle. (B) Epidural space monitor.

curve is reached, a further small increase in volume will result in a massive increase in ICP. In Figure 9-6, the flat portion of the intracranial compliance curve reflects the elastic properties of the CSF space. The steep portion represents progressive loss of CSF buffering as the elastic properties of the cerebral tissue become the main buffer. Because of this exponential curve of the pressure-volume relationship, a knowledge of ICP alone cannot define the actual tightness or decrease in reserve of the intracranial space. This can be assessed by eliciting the response to the removal or addition of 1 ml saline through the catheter. The immediate change in ICP provides an index of intracranial compliance. The amplitude of the arterial pulsations of an ICP tracing can also be used as a guide to intracranial compliance (higher peaks are associated with reduced compliance).

Sometimes neurological deterioration cannot be correlated with increasing ICP. Lesions in the medial temporal lobe and in the posterior fossa are life-threatening because of their proximity to the brain stem. In the presence of such lesions, ICP may remain normal until death.

Types of Waves

Lundberg described three types of waves, designated A, B, and C waves. A waves (plateau waves) (Figure 9-7) are associated with increased ICP up to 80 mm Hg and may persist for 15 to 20 minutes. These waves indicate

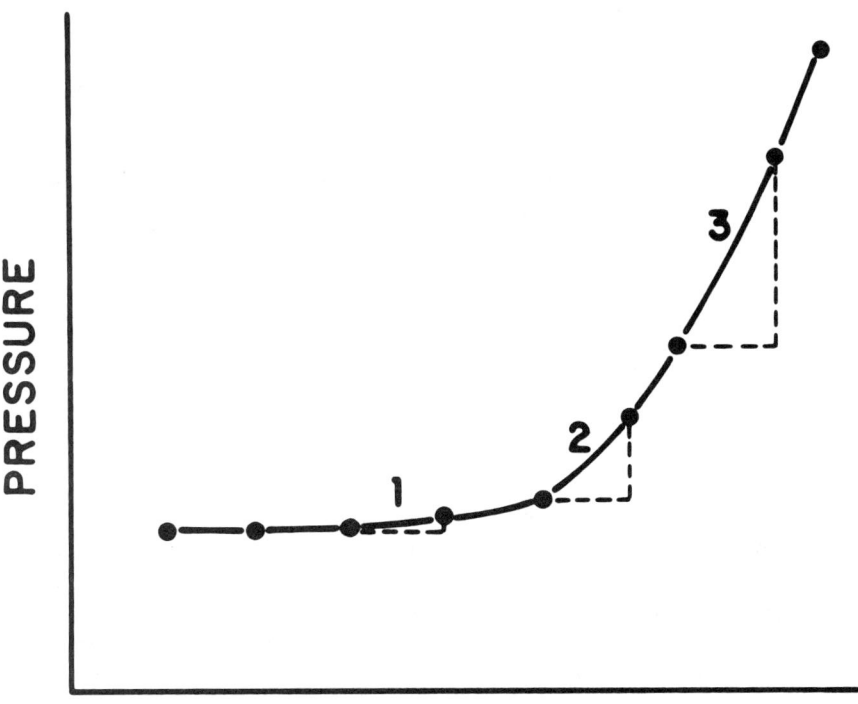

Figure 9-6. The classical intracranial pressure volume curve: (1) On the flat portion of the curve any increase in the intracranial volume hardly affects the ICP. (2) Later, a small increase in the intracranial volume produces a rise in the ICP. (3) On reaching the steeper part of the curve, any increase in volume causes a steep increase in the ICP.

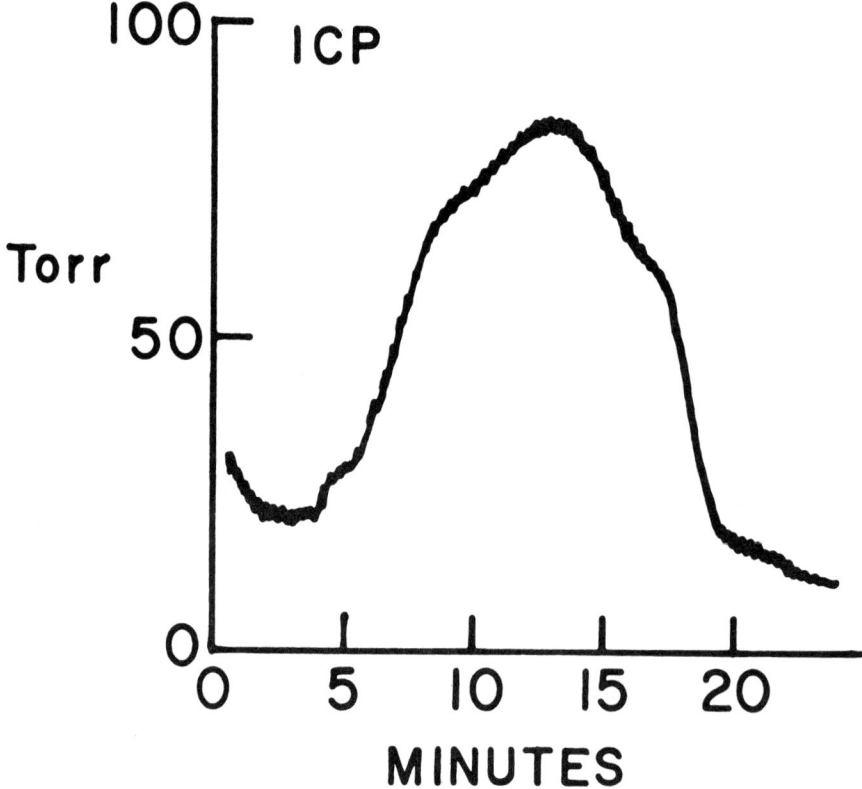

Figure 9-7. Type A (plateau wave).

that the patient is nearing the limits of the compensatory mechanism on the compliance curve. They may be associated with clinical signs of an acute increase in ICP and may be precipitated by several factors such as pain, surgical stimulation, tracheal intubation, positive-pressure ventilation, or laryngoscopic examination. B waves are smaller, 20 to 25 mm Hg, occur once per minute, and are thought to be precursors of A waves. The less-sustained C waves occur at a rate of six per minute. Their significance presently is not known, although they seem to be benign.

Effect of Rising ICP

Increasing ICP decreases blood flow to the brain, compresses vital centers, and may cause herniation of brain tissue (Figure 9-8).

Management of Increased ICP (Table 9-2)

Once an increase in ICP is suspected, the cause should be determined following skull roentgenograms, arterial blood gas estimations, and computed tomography scans. Hematomas require immediate surgical evacuation. Coagulation profiles should be recorded. Pneumocephalus can be released through a twist drill hole. Cerebral edema is treated with hyperventilation, diuretics, steroids, and barbiturates. Mannitol is administered in doses of 0.5-2 gm/kg infused over 30 minutes. The onset of action is within 20 minutes and the maximum effect is seen in 1 to 2 hours.

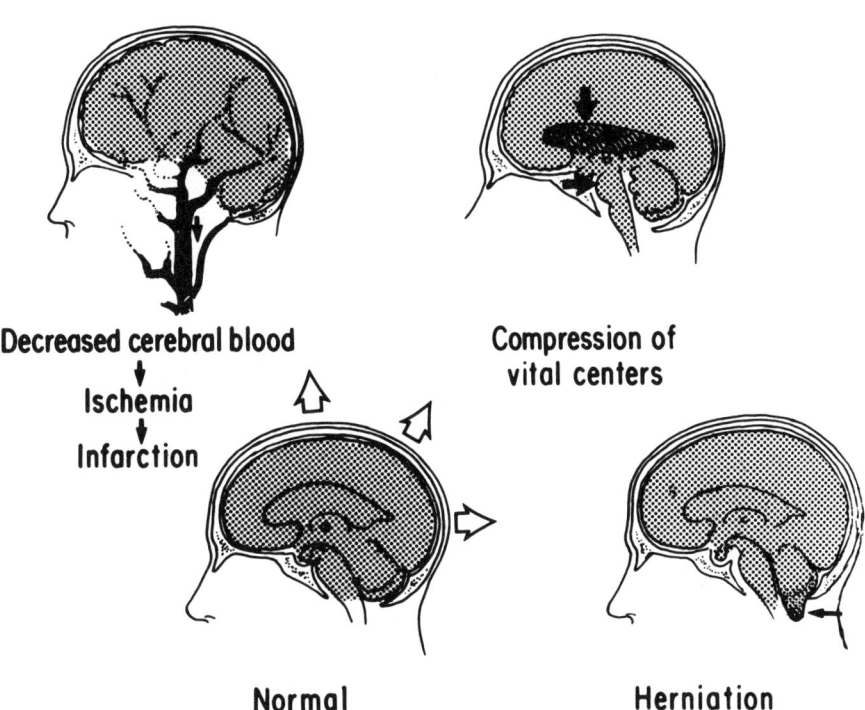

Figure 9-8. Effects of increasing ICP. Decrease in cerebral blood flow will cause ischemia or infarction of the brain tissue. Acute compression of the vital centers or herniation of the medulla are catastrophic.

RESPIRATORY SYSTEM

Respiratory inadequacy of any degree is undesirable in this group of patients because both hypoxia and hypercapnia increase cerebral blood flow and ICP and may lead to edema formation. A rise of 1 mm Hg in arterial CO_2 increases cerebral blood flow by 4 percent (Figure 9-9).

Anesthetic-related causes of respiratory insufficiency in the postoperative period include:

1. Residual effects of relaxants, anesthetics, narcotics.
2. Diffusion hypoxemia, usually a brief period related to the use of nitrous oxide.
3. Hyperventilation hypoxemia. Intraoperative hyperventilation depletes CO_2 stores which are replenished by spontaneous hypoventilation with concurrent development of hypoxemia.
4. Reduced functional residual capacity associated with general anesthetics.
5. Mechanical factors: shivering, secretion, atelectasis.

Neurological causes are as follows:

1. Damage to vital centers.
2. Damage to both carotid bodies, following bilateral carotid endarterectomy.

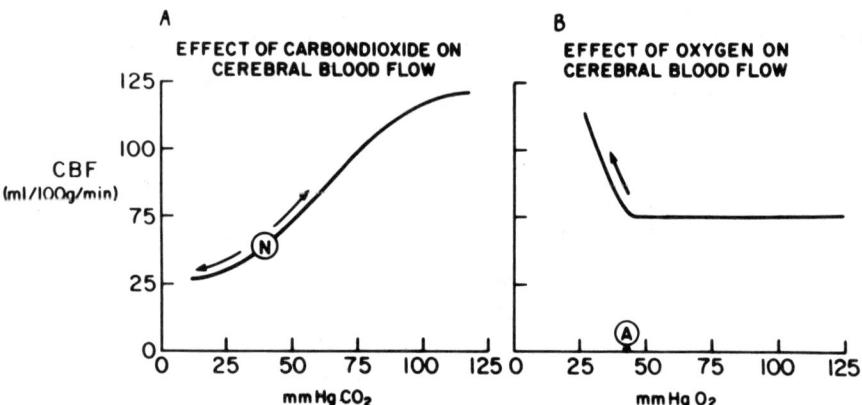

Figure 9-9. (A) Arterial CO_2 ($PaCO_2$) is a potent cerebral vasodilator. Any increase in $PaCO_2$ will increase cerebral blood flow and thus, the ICP. (B) When the arterial oxygen (PaO_2) declines below 45 mm Hg (A), there is an increase in the cerebral blood flow leading to increasing ICP.

Cardiovascular and pulmonary causes are as follows:

1. Heart failure. May be associated with infusion of hyperosmolar solutions like mannitol.
2. As postoperative sequelae of intraoperative air embolism during operations performed in the sitting position.
3. Neurogenic pulmonary edema following a variety of neurological conditions.
4. Microaggregates in pulmonary vessels after massive transfusion.

Most of these causes of hypoxemia will respond to oxygen therapy (supplemental oxygen 30-50 percent by face mask), tracheobronchial toilet, and chest physiotherapy.

Management of respiratory insufficiency involves the monitoring of respiratory rate, tidal volume, inspiratory force, chest X ray, and arterial blood gases.

Patients with airway edema, gross obesity, or preoperative pulmonary problems may require positive pressure ventilation to achieve normocapnia and adequate oxygenation.

CARDIOVASCULAR SYSTEM

Cardiovascular instability leading to hypotension, hypertension, or arrhythmias is a common complication in the postoperative period and therefore monitoring of BP and ECG is imperative.

Autoregulation

Over a wide range of systemic blood pressures, blood flow to the brain is maintained constant because of the ability of the cerebral blood vessels to change their caliber (Figure 9-10). Autoregulation in normotensive patients is limited to a range from 50 to 150 mm Hg of mean blood pressure. Above and below this range, cerebral blood flow passively follows changes in systemic blood pressure. Autoregulation is impaired by:

Surgical intervention
Head trauma
General anesthesia
Drug therapy
Diabetes mellitus
Hypertension

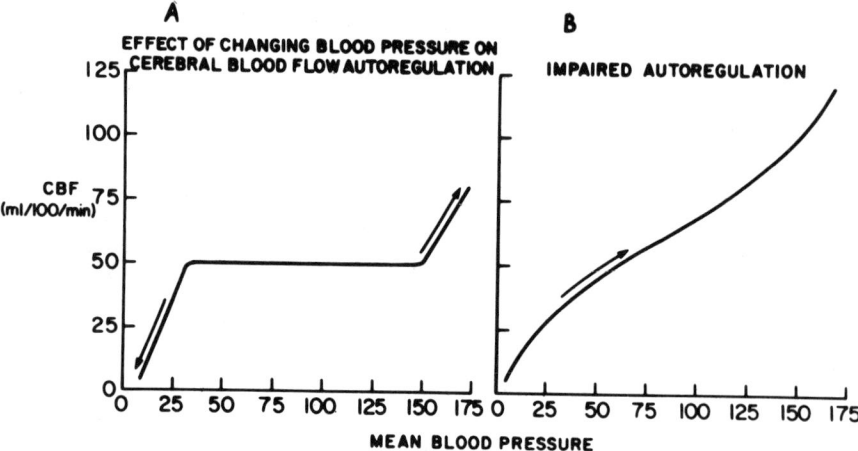

Figure 9-10. Blood flow to the brain is maintained constant during changes in the mean blood pressure from 50 to 150 mm Hg (A). After surgery, general anesthetics, or medications, the autoregulation is impaired (B).

Hypotension

Hypotension decreases CPP. Causes must be identified by assessing the fluid intake, urine output, urine osmolarity, central venous pressure, pulmonary capillary wedge pressure, or cardiac output and the appropriate therapy instituted. Causes of hypotension include:

1. Inadequate blood replacement
2. Fluid restriction compounded by diuresis
3. Hypovolemia associated with intracranial aneurysm and prolonged diuretic administration
4. Myocardial failure, arrhythmias
5. Hypoxemia
6. Brain stem damage

Hypertension

Hypertension is claimed to be the most common nonneurological complication in the postoperative period. Several causes have been identified:

1. Vasoconstriction due to hypothermia
2. Fluid overload
3. Emergence from anesthesia, pain, and shivering
4. Hypercapnia and early stages of hypoxia

5. Cushing's reflex due to intracranial hypoxia
6. Medications, e.g., dextran, naloxone, or rebound effect following nitroprusside infusion or withdrawal of antihypertensive medication
7. Revascularization techniques
8. Preexisting disease

An increase in blood pressure of more than 20 percent, if not treated, will lead to cerebral hemorrhage, myocardial failure, or myocardial infarction and can also increase ICP by increasing the tendency to bleed at the operative site, increasing cerebral blood volume, and edema formation (vasogenic edema).

Because of the serious consequences of hypertension, it should be treated aggressively. However, one cause of hypertension, Cushing's reflex, is a protective mechanism to improve cerebral perfusion. Therefore, identification of the cause is important prior to treatment (Table 9-2). Therapy includes:

1. Hydralazine 5-10 mg intravenously, repeated as necessary to control BP < 160/100 unless pulse rate is < 60/min
2. Propranolol 1 mg intravenously
3. Reinstitution of previous medications as soon as possible
4. Correction of fluid imbalance
5. Nitroprusside infusion in extreme cases

Cardiac Arrhythmias and Electrocardiogram Change

Cardiac arrhythmias and acute ECG changes (T wave inversion, ST segment elevation) are not uncommon. Hyperventilation and diuresis are common modes of therapy in neurosurgical patients, and both can lead to hypokalemia and associated supraventricular arrhythmias.

Table 9-2. Increase in ICP

Cause	Diagnosis	Treatment
Hematoma	CT scan, coagulation profile	surgery
Pneumocephalus	skull X ray	twistdrill
Edema	CT scan, ICP monitoring	hyperventilation, steroids, diuretics
Hypoxia and hypercapnia	arterial blood gas	respiratory support
Spasm of cerebral vessels	clinical deterioration angiogram	hydration, maintain BP, ? vasodilators

In these patients, particularly following head trauma and ruptured cerebral aneurysm, acute ECG changes similar to myocardial ischemia have been observed. The need for ECG monitoring and electrolyte measurements are underscored.

TEMPERATURE

During anesthesia, heat loss due to convection, conduction, and radiation (cold room, infusion of refrigerated blood or cool fluids) decreases body temperature. In the immediate postoperative period when the hypothalamus regains its function, patients begin to rebuild the lost heat by shivering. This shivering is associated with an increase in oxygen consumption (400-700 percent of the basal metabolic rate) and if respiratory and cardiac reserves are borderline, hypoxia and heart failure may follow. In anticipation of this impingement on the reserves of the vital functions, temperature should be monitored and external sources of heat made available.

FLUID AND ELECTROLYTES

Disturbances in fluid and electrolyte balance are common following neurosurgical procedures and are associated with surgery in and around the hypothalamus and pituitary areas, or hypokalemia resulting from hyperventilation, diuretics, and steroid therapy.

Monitoring the intake of fluids, urine output, and electrolytes is important. Diabetes insipidus is diagnosed by hypernatremia, extreme polyuria, and low urinary specific gravity. Therapy involves replacement of urinary losses with 0.25 normal saline and administration of pitressin (either as DDAVP nasal insufflation or injection of pitressin tannate).

SEIZURES

Approximately 20 percent of untreated patients develop seizures within the 24-hour period following intracranial surgery. Seizures cause hypoxia and may result in aspiration. Intravenous phenytoin, with careful ECG monitoring, is the drug of choice. Phenytoin must not be given faster than a rate of 50 mg per minute to minimize cardiovascular depression.

RESTLESSNESS AND PAIN

Restlessness of neurosurgical patients in the postoperative period needs careful evaluation to exclude cerebral hypoxia. Other causes include cardiac or respiratory dysfunction. Postoperative pain in this group of patients is not a major problem, and pharmacologic pain relief is generally not required. However, if necessary, mild analgesics ranging from acetaminophen to codein phosphate are adequate. Use of narcotics should be avoided in view of the depressing effect on the central nervous system and pupillary constriction. Both effects mask the changes of rising intracranial pressure. In addition, rising CO_2 due to respiratory depression caused by narcotics increases ICP.

SPINAL COLUMN SURGERY

Spinal column surgery is performed in the cervical, thoracic, and lumbar regions. The problems related to this type of surgery are shown in Table 9-3.

Pain

These operations cause muscle spasm and pain in the immediate postoperative period requiring analgesics. Unlike patients following craniotomy with compromised intracranial compliance, narcotics can be given for pain relief.

Position

In the immediate recovery period, the head-elevated position increases the functional residual capacity and thereby improves oxygenation and cerebral venous drainage. In patients who had surgery in the lower thoracic or lumbar spine area, keeping the head elevated leaves the operated site at the most dependent level. This impairs drainage of venous blood from the wound, leading to edema formation, bleeding, and poor healing. Therefore, the supine position is more appropriate.

Table 9-3.   Spinal Column Surgery

Pain: narcotics
Position: supine (lumbar laminectomy)
Respiratory function
    Phrenic nerve palsy
    Auxiliary muscle spasm
    Infection
    Bronchospasm
Hallucinations
Cardiovascular
    Bradycardia
    Pulmonary edema
    Autonomic hyperreflexia

Respiratory Function

Respiratory distress can occur due to a number of reasons.

1. Phrenic nerve damage. The diaphragm is the primary respiratory muscle and derives its nerve supply from cervical segments C3–C5. Patients are liable to experience respiratory distress either due to structural damage, or if ascending edema following surgery encroaches on these segments. Therefore, careful assessment and monitoring of respiration is necessary prior to extubation. If worsening of respiratory function is anticipated, as in surgery on the cervical vertebrae particularly following an anterior approach, extubation of the trachea should be delayed.
2. Auxiliary muscle spasm. Preoperatively if the patients had compromised respiratory function and depended on auxiliary muscles to maintain adequate ventilation, then, in the immediate postoperative period, spasm, edema, and pain in these areas may further decrease this marginal reserve. Respiratory distress should be anticipated, and supportive measures made available for several hours or days postoperatively.
3. Respiratory infections. Accumulation of secretions and regurgitation of gastric contents into the tracheobronchial tree will lead to pulmonary infection. Effective coughing can prevent both complications. However, neurologic deficits decrease abdominal and chest wall muscle action, and active physiotherapy is necessary.
4. Bronchoconstriction. Following sympathetic denervation caused by high spinal cord injury, patients tend to develop bronchoconstriction. Bronchodilators and respiratory support may be necessary.

Central Nervous System

Patients with spinal cord damage develop hallucinations and psychiatric problems because of decreased sensory input. Music, a clock, and a window in their surrounding environment increase sensory input and probably decrease psychological complications.

Cardiovascular System

Patients sympathectomized due to high spinal cord injury are liable to develop severe bradycardia, and even minimal vagal stimulation (e.g., suctioning the trachea or distended stomach) may lead to cardiac arrest, especially if some degree of hypoxia exists. Prior administration of atropine and limiting the period of suctioning to 10 seconds will eliminate this catastrophic event.

Table 9-4. Autonomic Hyperreflexia

Complete transection of spinal cord
Below T5 segment
Hyperreflexia
    Initiated by viscous distension
    Anogenital stimuli
Manifestation
    Hypertension, bradycardia
    Flushing above the level of lesion
    Pallor below the level of lesion
Complications
    Cerebral hemorrhage
    Retinal hemorrhage
    Myocardial failure and infarction

Patients are liable to develop pulmonary edema easily, and therefore, fluid management should be carefully guided, if necessary, with central venous pressure monitoring.

Patients with complete transection of the spinal cord below T5 are liable to develop autonomic hyperreflexia some weeks after the injury. Slight discomfort due to visceral distension (e.g., bladder) may cause severe hypertension and reflex bradycardia requiring immediate hypotensive therapy and sedation to prevent cerebral hemorrhage or myocardial infarction (Table 9-4).

SUGGESTIONS FOR FURTHER READING

Frost EAM. Control of intracranial pressure. Curr Rev Clin Anesth 1981; 1:16.
Lappas DG, Powell WM Jr, Dagett WM. Cardiac dysfunction in the perioperative period: Pathophysiology, diagnosis and treatment. Anesthesiology 1979; 47:117.
Lundberg N. Continuous recording and control of ventricular fluid pressure in neurosurgical practice. Acta Psychiatr Neurol Scand 1960; 36:149.
Lundberg N. Monitoring of the intracranial pressure. In: Scientific foundation of neurology. M Critchley, JL O'Leary, eds. Philadelphia: Davis, 1972.
Marshall BE, Wyche MQ Jr. Hypoxemia during and after anesthesia. Anesthesiology 1972; 37:178.
Miller JD. Intracranial pressure monitoring. Br J Hosp Med 1978; 19(50):497.
Miller JD, Garibi J. Intracranial volume pressure relationship during continuous monitoring of ventricular fluid pressure. In: Intracranial pressure, IM Brock, H Dietz, eds. Berlin: Springer, 1972.
Thiagarajah S. Postoperative care of neurosurical patients. In: International anesthesiology clinics. Recovery Room Care. EAM Frost, IC Andrews, eds. Boston: Little, Brown, 1983; 21(1):139-156.

10
Recovery from Regional Anesthetic Techniques
Richard B. Lilly, Jr.

Patients who have received regional anesthesia are sometimes felt not to need as much care in the recovery room as those who have had general anesthesia. While this is often the case, there are several problems unique to regional anesthesia that the recovery room nurse must recognize. This chapter covers: (1) general considerations after regional anesthesia, (2) local anesthetic toxicity, (3) sympathetic nervous system block, and (4) pneumothorax. Then there is a discussion in more detail of spinal and epidural anesthesia, since these have the greatest systemic effect on the patient.

GENERAL CONSIDERATIONS AFTER REGIONAL ANESTHESIA

It is not necessary for all patients who have had a regional anesthetic to go to the recovery room. At the discretion of the anesthesiologist the patient may bypass the recovery room and return directly to the ward after many types of nerve blocks. All patients who have had a spinal anesthetic should go to the recovery room. Also, patients who have had regional blocks may need recovery room care for other reasons. For example, excessive use of sedatives and narcotics to supplement an inadequate block may depress a patient as much as general anesthesia. Such a patient may need as close observation and airway support as any patient after general anesthesia.

Loss of control of an extremity is a common problem after a regional anesthetic. The patient will not be able to move his arm after a brachial plexus block and may injure himself unless the extremity is protected for him.

A nice advantage of regional techniques is that the patient will be free of pain while the residual block wears off. With the use of long-acting local anesthetics, the analgesia may last 8 to 12 hours. It certainly is not always necessary for the patient to stay in the recovery room until all the block has worn off.

A special problem of airway protection exists in patients who have had superior laryngeal nerve blocks or topical anesthesia of the larynx and pharynx. Even though these patients are awake, their protective airway reflexes will be blocked. Therefore they are not able to deal with secretions or bleeding around the airway, and they should be kept fasting for several hours until the block is well reversed.

LOCAL ANESTHETIC TOXICITY (TABLE 10-1)

High levels of local anesthetic drugs in the circulation can cause central nervous system (CNS) stimulation leading to seizures or cardiovascular depression. Excessively high levels of local anesthetic enter the circulation in two ways. The first is intravascular injection when the block is being performed. In this case the toxic effects are seen immediately. Second, there may be rapid systemic absorption of the drug from the block site, especially if the area is very vascular. Here the toxicity is usually seen within 20 minutes of injection, but may occur later if multiple doses have been given.

What Type of Block May Cause Local Anesthetic Toxicity?

Local anesthetic toxicity can occur any time a large volume of drug containing a dose close to the maximum safe dose is used (Table 10-2). Examples of common high volume, high-dose blocks are: epidural, caudal, axillary,

Table 10-1. Local Anesthetic Toxicity

	Signs and Symptoms	*Treatment*
Central nervous system	lightheaded, dysarthric, twitchy, drowsy, circum-oral parasthesia, grand mal seizures, coma	diazepam, barbiturates, airway support, and hyperventilation
Cardiovascular system	vasodilation, myocardial depression, hypotension, heart block	Trendelenberg position, O_2, fluids, ionotropic drugs dopamine, ephedrine), airway support
Epinephrine effects	tachycardia, palpitations, anxiety	reassurance, sedation, beta blockers, rarely vasodilators

Table 10-2. Local Anesthetic Drugs in Common Use

Drug	Max. Safe Adult Dose	Average Duration	Metabolism	Use/Comments
Cocaine	200 mg		plasma	topical anes. of nasopharynx only, excellent vasoconstrictor
Procaine (Novocaine)	1000 mg	50 min	plasma	infiltration, spinal
Chloroprocaine (Nesacaine)	1000 mg	30 min	plasma	epidurals, for very short duration
Tetracaine (Pontocaine)	80–100 mg	2–3 hr	plasma	topical, spinal
Lidocaine (Xylocaine)	300 mg plain 500 mg, epin.	1.5 hr	liver	infiltration, topical, nerve blocks, spinal, epidural
Mepivicaine (Carbocaine)		very similar to Xylocaine		
Bupivicaine (Marcaine)	controversial 175–225 mg	4–10 hr	liver	nerve blocks, epidural; very long duration
Etidocaine	500 mg	3–5 hr	liver	epidural, motor block may be more profound than sensory

interscalene, or multiple intercostal blocks. Topical blocks of the pharynx are among the most frequent causes of local anesthetic toxicity because tetracaine (a very toxic drug) is frequently used as the agent. Also, absorption of the drug from the mucous membranes of the pharynx is extremely rapid. While not a regional anesthetic per se, lidocaine infusions for arrhythmias are a potential cause of local anesthetic toxicity if administered too quickly.

Symptoms and Signs of Local Anesthetic Toxicity

The CNS is more sensitive to local anesthetic toxicity than the cardiovascular system, but either or both may be affected. The CNS symptoms are drowsiness, irrational behavior, or twitching and possibly some perioral paresthesia or tinnitus — all of which may progress to grand mal seizures and ultimately coma.

Diazepam raises the seizure threshold for local anesthetics and therefore is good for prophylaxis and treatment of local anesthetic-induced convulsions. Diazepam 5-10 mg intravenously is an appropriate prophylactic dose to a patient who shows early signs of twitching or convulsive movements. Patients having seizures also need oxygen and airway and ventilation control.

Symptoms of cardiovascular effects are hypotension, gray, clammy skin, a shocky appearance, and possibly, varying degrees of heart block or even cardiac arrest.

Hypotension develops because of both myocardial depression and vasodilation. Circulatory support, therefore, in the form of intravenous fluids, Trendelenberg position, and an ionotropic agent like dopamine is the treatment of choice.

Epinephrine Effects

A common side effect of local anesthesia is not related to the local anesthetic itself, but to epinephrine (adrenalin) which is added to it. Epinephrine in concentration of 1/100,000-1/200,000 is frequently combined with local anesthetics to cause vasoconstriction in the area of injection and slow the vascular absorption of the drug, thus prolonging its effect. Chances of development of toxicity are reduced by delaying the rise of systemic blood levels of the local anesthetic. But epinephrine may cause anxiety, hypertension, tachycardia, and arrhythmias. Often these symptoms are mild and need little treatment other than reassurance or mild sedation. However, severe hypertension or tachycardia in patients with coronary or vascular disease is dangerous and must be treated with beta blockers like propranolol and, if necessary, vasodilators to reduce the blood pressure. Gross overdose of epinephrine may cause hypotension, bradycardia, and ST-T wave changes. Therapy requires cardiorespiratory support including fluid replacement, vasopressor administration, intubation and assisted ventilation.

PNEUMOTHORAX

Pneumothorax may occur after any of the following blocks in which needles are placed near the pleural cavity:

1. Intercostal blocks
2. Supraclavicular brachial plexus blocks
3. Subclavian placement of central venous pressure catheter
4. Interscalene block (less common)
5. Stellate ganglion block (less common)

It is most likely to occur with intercostal blocks and supraclavicular brachial plexus blocks because the pleura lies directly under the bony landmarks toward which the needle is directed. It may also happen with some approaches to the stellate ganglion. While not a regional anesthetic technique, subclavian placement of a central venous pressure catheter is a more common cause of pneumothorax than any of the nerve blocks.

It is important to remember that the hole the needle makes in the lung is very small, so the air leak is slow. Thus the pneumothorax may not become symptomatic for several hours. Often the anesthesiologist will be suspicious that the pleura is entered, because the patient coughs, or complains of pain, or air is aspirated. However, none of these signs may occur. The nurse caring for the patient several hours later may be the first to recognize the early signs of pneumothorax. The patient will be slightly short of breath and complain of chest pain. Examination of the chest is unreliable because the pneumothorax is usually small. The diagnosis is made most reliably by chest X ray.

Important Points about Pneumothorax

The important things for the recovery room nurse to remember are:

1. Any nerve block around the chest may cause a pneumothorax.
2. The onset of the pneumothorax may be very slow and may not become symptomatic for hours.

3. A high index of suspicion is important, even though this is a rare complication.

SYMPATHETIC NERVOUS SYSTEM BLOCKADE

The sympathetic nervous system is the division of the autonomic nervous system that (among other things) causes vasoconstriction in most vascular beds. Sympathetic nerves leave the spinal cord in the thoracic and lumbar areas, synapse in the sympathetic chain ganglia, which lie alongside the vertebral column, and then supply the vascular beds of the body in a segmental distribution which coincides with the dermatomes.

Large segments of the sympathetic system are blocked by spinal and epidural anesthesia. Specific blocks of the sympathetic system may be done for vascular disease. Examples of the latter are stellate ganglion block and lumbar paravertebral sympathetic blocks. With higher levels of anesthesia, more sympathetic nerves are blocked, until a T3 sensory level is reached when all the sympathetic supply is interrupted.

What Effect Does Sympathetic Block Have?

When vasoconstrictor impulses are interrupted, arterioles dilate and blood pressure decreases. Also venodilation causes venous pooling of blood and decreased venous return to the heart. Blood pressure falls, both because vessels dilate and because cardiac output decreases (Figure 10-1).

Orthostatic Hypotension

Normally a person responds to rapid position changes with increased sympathetic tone. Blood vessels constrict and prevent gravity from pooling blood in the legs. In the presence of a sympathetic block, this effect is abolished. If the patient tries to sit or stand, severe hypotension may result. This is known as orthostatic hypotension.

Occasionally when a patient arrives in the recovery room after a spinal anesthesia, the blood pressure will be significantly lower than it was before leaving the operating room. This may be because the sympathetic block prevented the body from compensating for the position changes caused during transfer from the operating table to the stretcher.

Bradycardia

The sympathetic nerve supply to the heart comes from T1 to T5. Sympathetic stimulation of the heart causes tachycardia and increased force of contraction. If spinal or epidural blockade interferes with the sympathetic

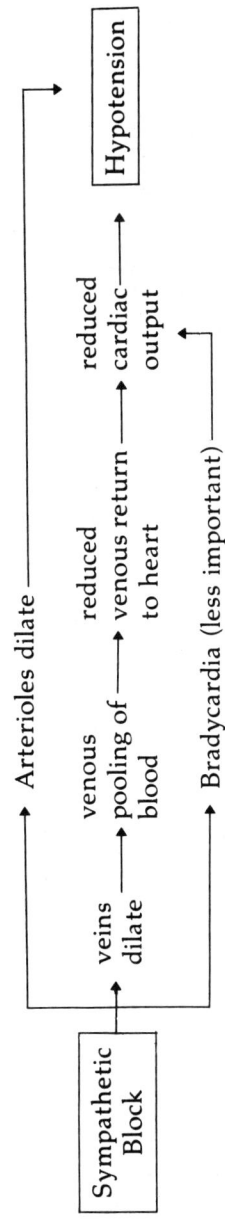

Figure 10-1. Physiology of sympathetic block.

supply to the heart, bradycardia may result. It is not uncommon to see patients with moderate bradycardia persisting for several hours after a spinal anesthetic. This is rarely symptomatic, but if it is (i.e., dizziness, nausea), it can be treated with small doses of atropine (0.4 mg intravenously).

Variability in Hypotension

The amount of hypotension caused by a given level of sympathetic block is variable and depends on the preexisting level of sympathetic tone and the adequacy of the blood volume. In patients with hypovolemia and vasoconstriction (e.g., hemorrhagic shock), profound hypotension from low levels of sympathetic block may occur, whereas healthy, relaxed, well-hydrated patients can tolerate total sympathectomy with little or no pressure change.

Treatment

Treatment of hypotension due to sympathetic block includes rapid intravenous volume expansion with an isotonic fluid (e.g., lactated Ringer's solution) and Trendelenburg position to improve venous return to the heart. If the response is inadequate, small doses of vasoconstrictor agents may be used, aiming only to bring the pressure to the low end of the patient's normal blood pressure range. Phenylepherine (40 mg per cc drip) is the most logical choice. If bradycardia is a problem, it may be treated with atropine.

SPINAL AND EPIDURAL ANESTHESIA

Spinal and epidural anesthesia are the regional techniques which usually require the most recovery room care. The greatest physiologic effect of spinal or epidural anesthesia is sympathetic nervous system block with associated hypotension, discussed in the previous section. This section covers other aspects of these major regional techniques that are pertinent to the recovery room care of the patient.

Background Physiology

In both spinal and epidural techniques, all nerves emerging from and returning to a section of the spinal cord are exposed to local anesthetic solution. The transmission of nerve impulses is thus temporarily blocked. The anesthetic solution diffuses from the injection site up and down around the cord causing a segmental spread of anesthesia. Eventually the local anesthetic is absorbed by lymph flow and blood flow around the nerves, causing gradual resolution of anesthesia. Nerve roots farther from the injection site receive less exposure to local anesthetics. Thus the anesthesia resolves gradually with the highest dermatomes recovering first and the legs and perineum regaining sensation last.

Spinal anesthesia is always injected below the level of L2 (the second lumbar vertebra). The distribution of the anesthesia is from the legs and perineum up to a given dermatome (usually below T4). Epidural anesthesia may be injected at any level of the spine. Its distribution may result in complete block below a given dermatome like a spinal, or a band of anesthesia may be obtained with nonanesthetized areas below and above.

Differential Block of Different Nerve Fibers

The size of a nerve determines how easily it is blocked by local anesthetic drugs. Sympathetic nerves are smallest and most easily blocked; sensory nerves are intermediate; and motor nerves are largest and hardest to block. This leads to a differential blockade which means that the level of sympathetic block is about 2 dermatome segments above the sensory level, which in turn is 2 dermatomes above the motor level. This effect is more pronounced after spinal than after epidural anesthesia.

Two points of practical importance relate to this phenomenon. First, the fact that a patient can move his legs must not be taken as evidence that his anesthesia has worn off. In fact, he may still have a significant level of sympathetic block. If he is allowed to sit or stand, serious orthostatic hypotension could develop. Some patients with epidural anesthesia may have no motor block, yet have significant sensory and sympathetic block, and thus are at risk for orthostatic hypotension. Second, the nerve supply to the bladder comprises very small parasympathetic fibers from the sacral plexus. Blockade in these nerves is the last to be reversed, which explains the high incidence of urinary retention after spinal or epidural anesthesia.

Spinal Headache

Spinal anesthesia is performed by placing a needle through the dura into the cerebrospinal fluid in the subarachnoid space below the end of the spinal cord. Leakage of cerebrospinal fluid (CSF) from this needle hole decreases CSF volume, which causes traction on supporting membranes of the brain and spinal headache. A typical spinal headache worsens when the patient stands and is diminished by the supine position. The onset is usually on the first postoperative day, so it is unlikely to be seen in the recovery room. However, recovery room care should include prophylactic treatment to prevent headache. The mainstay of this has always been to keep the patient flat in bed to minimize CSF leakage. The patient may have one pillow and may roll from side to side but should not sit up for 6 to 8 hours.

There is, however, contradictory evidence that recumbency prevents spinal headache. Two large studies failed to show any value of recumbency in preventing spinal headache (Jones, 1974; Carbatt and Van Crevel, 1981). Once a headache begins, however, symptoms subside when the patient lies flat. Nevertheless for cardiovascular stability and comfort, patients should be encouraged to lie "head down on one pillow" after spinal anesthesia.

Generous intravenous and oral hydration also help to prevent and treat spinal headache. Spinal headaches are more common in younger patients and especially in pregnant women. The overall incidence is less than 10 percent. The smaller the needle used, the lower the chances of developing a headache.

Respiratory Effects

Both spinal and epidural anesthesia may have significant respiratory depressant effects. The phrenic nerve (C3–5), which controls the diaphragm, is rarely blocked. However, it is quite common for a high spinal or epidural to paralyze other muscles of respiration such as intercostals and accessory muscles. In a normal patient this will have little effect on ventilation, but in a person with lung disease, serious respiratory depression can result.

Severe hypotension from a spinal or epidural anesthetic may cause central nervous system hypoxia which in turn may cause respiratory arrest. Finally, sedatives and narcotics given to patients to supplement the block may add their own respiratory depressant effects.

Shivering

Spinal and epidural anesthesia causes skin vasodilation, which causes significant heat loss as warm blood comes to the surface of the body. This effect lasts until the block resolves. All patients lose heat in the operating room because of reduced ambient temperature and use of cold irrigating and infusing solutions. Patients who have had spinal or epidural anesthesia stay hypothermic longer, as vasodilation lasts into the recovery phase. Shivering to generate heat may be violent, increasing oxygen consumption (by 500 percent) cardiac output, and ventilation. Supplemental oxygen must be given to hypothermic or shivering patients. All patients must be kept warm by generous use of blankets or infrared heaters.

Discharge Criteria

In many institutions the traditional criteria for discharge from the recovery room after spinal or epidural anesthesia is the patient's ability to move his toes. As explained above, that certainly does not mean that the block has worn off, but it does show that resolution is progressing normally.

Additional factors must be considered prior to discharge to the ward. Are his blood pressure and pulse normal? Is he breathing well? Is he awake and alert? Is his temperature normal? Although the ability of the patient to move his toes is a good indication that the block is decreasing as expected, it must not be the only criterion for discharge.

It is essential that nurses on the wards receiving patients from the recovery room understand that spinal or epidural anesthetics may not be totally worn off when the patient leaves the recovery room, and that the patient may still experience orthostatic hypotension if allowed to sit or stand rapidly. This understood, if vital signs are stable, the patient can be released from the recovery room even before regaining the ability to move his feet. Generally ambulatory care patients are not suitable candidates for spinal or epidural anesthesia. These techniques are used, however, in some Surgicenters.

Differences in Spinal and Epidural Anesthesia (Table 10-3)

Spinal anesthesia is achieved by injecting a small amount of local anesthetic into the CSF surrounding the spinal cord. Epidural anesthesia is performed by injecting a much larger volume of local anesthetic into the fat-filled, highly vascular epidural space which lies just outside the dural sac and spinal cord. There are two important differences in the two techniques. First, the very small dose of drug required for spinal anesthesia minimizes local anesthetic toxicity. During an epidural injection drug amounts approaching the maximum safe dose are often used. Thus, in addition to all the effects caused by a spinal anesthetic of comparable level, an epidural anesthetic may cause toxic reactions as the drug is absorbed. Second, in a well-conducted epidural anesthetic, the needle does not penetrate the dura into the subarachnoid space. Therefore spinal headache does not occur and maintenance of a supine position is unnecessary. However, patients should not be allowed to sit up until the sympathetic block resolves, or orthostatic hypotension may occur.

Table 10-3. Spinal and Epidural Comparison

	Spinal	Epidural
Drug dose	small	large
Local anes. toxicity	none	possible
Sympathetic block	very significant	significant, but may be of slower onset and cause fewer symptoms than spinal at same level
Distribution	from a given dermatome down to feet and perineum	may be like spinal or may be a band of anesthesia with no anesthesia above and below
Catheter used for continuous technique	rarely	commonly allows unlimited duration and postop analgesia
Drugs and approximate duration*	procaine 30–60 min lidocaine 60 min tetracaine 2–3 hr	chloroprocaine 30 min lidocaine 60 min bupivicaine 150 min
Headache	possible	no

*Epinephrine added to local prolongs these times by 25–33 percent.

Continuous Techniques

A spinal anesthetic may last 1 to 4 hours, depending on the drug used. With an epidural technique, a catheter may be left in the epidural space and repeated doses of local anesthetics may be given. In this way the duration of analgesia can be prolonged well into the postoperative period, which is one of the real advantages of epidural anesthesia. Careful monitoring for all the effects of epidural anesthesia, especially orthostatic hypotension, is essential.

Epidural Hematoma

An epidural hematoma is a rare complication of spinal or epidural anesthesia. It is caused by damage to an epidural vein by the needle in a patient with a coagulation defect. The symptoms are severe back pain and tenderness and residual neurologic deficit in the legs. This is an emergency which requires immediate surgical decompression.

Epidural Narcotics

Since the late 1970s narcotics, especially morphine, have been injected into the epidural space. Some use of epidural morphine for surgical anesthesia has been made, but more usual indicators are postoperative pain relief. Epidural morphine gives far more profound and long-lasting pain relief than parenteral morphine. However, there are several side effects. The most important is respiratory depression. Although small doses of morphine (4-10 mg) are used, some patients have had severe respiratory depression many hours after the epidural injection. The patient who receives epidural morphine, therefore, must be in an intensive care environment for 24 hours after the epidural narcotic is given. Lesser side effects are generalized pruritus and urinary retention. Naloxone (Narcan 0.4 mg intravenously) can reverse all these adverse effects, but will also reverse the analgesia (Table 10-4).

Table 10-4. Summary of Important Recovery Room Considerations after Spinal and Epidural Anesthesia

1. Sympathetic block → hypotension (especially orthostatic).
2. Spinal headache precautions after spinal, but not epidural.
3. Moving feet does not mean block is totally gone.
4. Heat loss continues as long as block is present.
5. Shivering increases oxygen consumption dramatically.
6. Urinary retention is common.
7. Delayed respiratory depression after epidural narcotics.

SUGGESTIONS FOR FURTHER READING

Bromage PR. Epidural analgesia. Philadelphia: WB Saunders, 1978.

Carbatt PAT, Van Crevel H. Lumbar puncture headache: controlled study on preventive effect of 24 hours bed rest. Lancet 1981; 2:1133-1135.

Dripps R, Eckenhoff J, Vandam L. Introduction to anesthesia, the principles of safe practice. Philadelphia: WB Saunders, 1982.

Greene NC. Physiology of spinal anesthesia. Baltimore: Williams & Williams, 1981.

Jones RJ. The role of recumbency in prevention of postspinal headache. Anesth Analg 1974; 53:788.

Miller RD. Anesthesia. New York: Churchill Livingstone, 1981.

Moore DC. Complications of regional anesthesia. Springfield, IL: Charles C Thomas, 1955.

11
Recovery Room Care of the Patient with Renal Disease
Rhoda D. Levine

This chapter deals with: (1) the laboratory evaluation, symptomatology, medications, risk factors, and proper monitoring of the patient with chronic renal disease; (2) the diagnosis and management of the patient with normal kidney function who develops acute perioperative renal failure; and (3) the special problems posed by the donor and recipient of a renal transplant.

CHRONIC RENAL DISEASE

Laboratory Evaluation

Serum Creatinine

This is the most useful single test of renal function. Normal level is approximately 1 mg/dl. It may be elevated in patients with normal renal function with severe volume depletion (postural hypotension, tachycardia, and decreased skin turgor), or who have muscle necrosis (rhabdomyolysis). Generally, renal function is estimated as 1/serum creatinine (a patient with a serum creatinine of 2 mg/dl has roughly one-half the normal renal function, while a serum creatinine of 10 mg/dl suggests that one-tenth of normal renal function remains). When rapid changes in renal function are present, creatinine clearance should be measured.

Creatinine Clearance

This simple measure of glomerular filtration rate can be obtained on any timed urine collection:

$$\text{Creatinine clearance} = \frac{\text{urine volume (ml)} \times \text{urine creatinine}}{\text{collection time (min)} \times \text{plasma creatinine}}$$

Normal creatinine clearance is about 120 ml per minute in a 70 kg person.

BUN

Blood urea nitrogen (BUN) is a less specific indicator of renal function than serum creatinine. Normal value is usually < 20 mg/dl. BUN elevations occur in many situations not associated with decreased renal function (mild volume depletion, heart failure, hypercatabolic states such as infection or burn injury, gastrointestinal hemorrhage, hyperalimentation, and urinary tract obstruction).

Urine Production

This is the easiest function of the kidney to measure and thus the one most usually recorded, but it is a poor indicator of renal function, particularly in patients with preexisting renal disease. Low urine volume (< 300 ml per hour), or oliguria, may be an appropriate response of a normally functioning kidney to volume depletion. A seemingly normal urine volume may be seen in patients with "nonoliguric" acute tubular necrosis.

Urine Specific Gravity

This is often measured to evaluate adequacy of hydration. This may be misleading in the patient with renal failure who is unable to concentrate or dilute urine and in the patient who is excreting large amounts of solute (e.g., glucose, mannitol).

Other Laboratory Tests

Complete blood count (CBC)
    Hemoglobin   normal = 14–16 g/dl ± 2
    Hematocrit   normal = 42–47 ± 5%
Serum electrolytes
    Potassium   normal = 3.5–5.0 mEq/liter
    Sodium   normal = 135–145 mEq/liter
    Bicarbonate   normal = 24–30 mEq/liter
Serum osmolality   normal = 280–300 mOsm

Clinical Symptomatology (Table 11-1)

Cardiovascular

Many problems in the patient with chronic renal failure arise from decreased ability to excrete water and sodium, or from complications of chronic hypertension. These patients respond slowly to changes in sodium intake, and urinary sodium excretion reflects chronic intake rather than acute needs. To maintain sodium balance, a nonedematous patient with renal insufficiency should receive approximately as much sodium as his chronic intake. The 24-hour urinary sodium content can be used to establish this level, although a daily intake of 2-3 gm sodium chloride (approximately 1-1.5 gm Na^+, or 35-50 mEq) is adequate in most patients. As a reference, 500 ml of 0.9 percent NaCl contains 4.5 gm Na^+. If salt intake exceeds excretory ability, circulatory overload may develop (peripheral edema, pulmonary congestion, hypertension). Treatment includes salt restriction and administration of diuretics. Caution should be used in diuresing edematous patients with hypoalbuminemia who may also have intravascular volume depletion. Measurement of central venous pressure is a useful guide in treating these patients.

A person with normal renal function rapidly decreases urinary sodium excretion almost to zero when faced with dietary sodium restriction or extrarenal sodium losses. In chronic severe renal disease, urinary sodium excretion cannot be decreased rapidly, and the kidneys continue to excrete sodium, leading to extracellular fluid volume depletion, hypotension, and a further decrease in glomerular filtration rate (GFR). Patients with severe renal disease who sustain significant unreplaced volume loss (trauma,

Table 11-1. Clinical Symptomatology Found in the Patient with Chronic Renal Disease

Cardiovascular	Neurologic
Hypertension	Confusion
Peripheral edema	Disorientation
Pulmonary congestion	Coma
	Convulsions
	Peripheral neuropathy
Hematologic	Musculoskeletal: 2° hyperparathyroidism
Anemia	
Platelet function	
Metabolic	Gastrointestinal
Acidosis	Bleeding
Hyperkalemia	Nausea and vomiting

Only those symptoms relevant to the recovery room setting are discussed in the text.

diarrhea, surgery, inadequate intake, etc.) may suffer further deterioration of renal function on a temporary or even permanent basis.

Patients with severe renal disease excrete urine which is more or less the same osmolality as plasma. They dilute and concentrate urine poorly in response to alterations in water intake. Urine volume will be 1.5-2 liters per day as long as the GFR exceeds 3-5 ml per minute. Hypothalamic osmoreceptors control water intake by alterations in thirst to maintain serum osmolality and sodium concentration.

Surgical patients with renal insufficiency may develop hyponatremia from water overload or sodium depletion. Water overload results when sodium-containing losses (urine, "third-space," i.e., edema fluid sequestered in traumatized tissue) are replaced only with water or as the result of inappropriate antidiuretic hormone (ADH) secretion (positive pressure ventilation, neurologic lesion). This is best treated by restricting the amount of free water the patient receives. If the patient is symptomatic (confused, lethargic, convulsing), hypertonic saline is administered at 50 ml per hour up to ~200 ml. In addition, the actual seizure activity is treated with anticonvulsants. Diuretics are also administered to the volume overloaded patient to speed the removal of water from the body. Sodium depletion is infrequently seen as an acute postoperative event. It is best treated with isotonic sodium chloride or, in acidotic patients, sodium bicarbonate.

Hypernatremia is most commonly the result of water depletion and thus should be treated by increasing the amount of free water administered to the patient.

Hematologic

The anemia of chronic renal insufficiency is caused by decreased erythrocyte synthesis (in part due to decreased renal erythropoietin) and shortened erythrocyte life. Patients in an unstressed situation may tolerate hemoglobin levels as low as 5 gm/dl, but blood oxygen-carrying capacity is markedly reduced and increased heart rate, intravascular volume, and cardiac output maximize oxygen delivery to tissues. Perioperative decreases in cardiac output as seen with myocardial depressant drugs (e.g., anesthetic agents) or increases in tissue oxygen requirements (shivering, hyperthermia) may decrease tissue oxygenation to dangerously low levels in such anemic patients. Administration of humidified oxygen to the postoperative anemic patient is essential.

Although transfusion is not without risks (including volume overload, hepatitis, and transfusion reaction) hemaglobin levels of 10 gm/dl are often necessary to provide an adequate oxygen-carrying capacity. The possibility of stimulating antibody formation which was thought to increase the risk of rejection of future transplants is no longer a contraindication.

Metabolic Acidosis

Metabolic acidosis is relatively benign at a bicarbonate level of 15 mEq/liter or above, although it prolongs the effect of nondepolarizing neuromuscular blocking agents (curare and pancuronium) and decreases buffer reserve. Acidosis may be treated with sodium bicarbonate (1 ampule of $NaHCO_3$ will increase the plasma HCO_3^- of a 70 kg person by about 1 mEq/liter. This treatment carries with it the risk of sodium overload.

Potassium

The ability to excrete a normal daily potassium intake is usually preserved in severe renal disease as long as urine output is maintained; however, rapid changes in potassium excretion cannot be made. Hyperkalemia is seen in the perioperative period when large potassium loads (cellular breakdown, blood transfusion) occur. A serum potassium > 5.5 mEq/liter is associated with an increased risk of life-threatening arrhythmias in the surgical patient with renal insufficiency. Electrocardiographic evidence of hyperkalemia includes T-wave peaking with modest elevations and loss of P waves with widening of QRS complexes as the hyperkalemia becomes more severe. As cardiac muscle function is impaired, cardiac output is severely compromised.

The most rapid treatment of hyperkalemic cardiac toxicity is the slow infusion of 10 to 20 ml of 10 percent calcium gluconate which should be reserved for the patient with severe hyperkalemia (> 7.5 mEq/liter). Calcium infusions do not alter serum potassium concentrations but decrease the neuromuscular irritability seen with hyperkalemia. Electrocardiogram (ECG) monitoring should be continuous, particularly in the patient who is receiving digitalis and who may respond to calcium infusion with an increase in the frequency of digitalis-related arrhythmias (e.g., premature ventricular contractions, PVCs). The effects of calcium infusions are rapid (< 5 minutes) but short-lived, and more definitive treatment should be begun immediately.

Administration of 50 ml of 50 percent glucose with 10 units of regular insulin to move potassium into cells from the extracellular fluid (ECF) is indicated for K^+ levels < 7.5 mEq/liter. If acidosis is present in addition to hyperkalemia (in the normovolemic patient), infusions of sodium bicarbonate at a rate of 1 ampule (44 mEq) per hour for 2 to 3 hours are beneficial. However, the potassium will return to ECF after several hours.

Removal of potassium from the body is accomplished by using cation exchange resins administered orally or rectally (e.g., Kayexalate) to slowly exchange sodium for potassium in the gastrointestinal tract. The use of dialysis in the hyperkalemic patient is discussed below.

Medications

Antibiotics

Many are excreted by the kidney and may accumulate to toxic levels in patients with impaired renal function. This is particularly important for the nephrotoxic aminoglycosides (e.g., kanamycin, gentamycin) and tetracyclines where excessive plasma levels can further impair renal function. Tetracyclines are best avoided in patients with decreased GFR because of their antianabolic effect (increased BUN, hyperkalemia, and acidosis) with the exception of doxycycline which is excreted by the liver. Aminoglycosides should be carefully monitored with plasma levels. As a rule of thumb, the physician increases dosage intervals in proportion to the fall of GFR (i.e., a patient with a GFR one-third normal should be given aminoglycosides one-third as often as normal). A detailed description of drug dosage may be found in the review by Anderson et al (1981).

Antihypertensive Agents

These alter the responsiveness of the autonomic nervous system both to normal homeostatic stimuli and to exogenously administered drugs. Morbidity is increased in the patient whose hypertension is poorly controlled (diastolic blood pressure greater than 110 mm Hg). Antihypertensive therapy should not be discontinued in the perioperative period.

Reserpine and guanethidine deplete peripheral catecholamine stores and reduce the response to indirect-acting vasopressors (e.g., ephedrine) but increase sensitivity to exogenously administered norepinephrine. Clonidine and alpha methyldopa are centrally acting alpha agonists, and their abrupt discontinuation may cause rebound hypertension especially in the recovery room.

Beta-adrenergic blocking agents (e.g., propranolol, metoprolol) decrease blood pressure by decreasing myocardial contractility, decreasing plasma renin levels, and also acting in the central nervous system. Patients chronically maintained on these drugs may be unable to increase heart rate in response to volume depletion, hypoglycemia, or other sympathetic stimuli. Therefore, a slow, stable heart rate cannot always be regarded as a reassuring sign.

Postoperative hypertension is frequently seen in patients with chronic renal disease. The differential diagnosis includes hypoxia, hypercapnia, pain, volume overload, and "inadequately" treated preexisting hypertension. Therapy should be directed at the etiology: improvements in oxygenation and ventilation, administration of analgesics or diuretics, institution of dialysis. In the acute setting, vasodilators such as hydralazine or nitroglycerine may be used. Sodium nitroprusside should be avoided in these patients because thiocyanate, a metabolite of nitroprusside, is excreted by the kidney and can accumulate to toxic levels.

Corticosteroids

These are frequently prescribed either as a treatment for glomerulonephritis or as immunosuppression after renal transplantation. Because of chronic suppression of adrenal steroid synthesis, these patients may not be able to respond to the stresses of the perioperative period with a release of endogenous glucocorticoids. Supplementation using a total parenteral steroid dose of 300 mg hydrocortisone per day (which is equivalent to the amount of endogenous steroid normally released in response to stress) in divided doses is recommended in the immediate perioperative period.

Digitalis Preparations

Digoxin is excreted largely by the kidney, and its dosage should be decreased to prevent toxicity in the form of cardiac dysrhythmias. Serum digoxin levels can be monitored to ensure a proper therapeutic effect. Digitoxin is metabolized by the liver and its dose need not be altered in renal insufficiency.

Diuretics

Diuretics such as furosemide and hydrochlorothiazide are used to treat both volume overload and hypertension. Excessive volume depletion may occur, further decreasing renal function and causing hypokalemia which can precipitate digitalis toxicity.

Fluids

Fluid therapy is directed at replacement of losses. Insensible loss (sweat, respiratory) is replaced by free water as 5 percent dextrose in water (D5W); ~500 ml/day is required for the 70 kg adult with no renal function. If the patient has a urine output, enough fluid should be given on a daily basis (as one-third or one-half normal saline) to provide for the anticipated urine output.

Blood loss must be replaced with blood. The use of triple-washed red blood cells allows the replacement of oxygen-carrying capacity without addition of excess volume or potassium. The amount of blood that may be lost before replacement is begun depends upon the type of surgery and the individual patient.

Third-space losses should be replaced with a sodium-containing solution, preferably normal saline. If D5W is given alone for replacement of third-space losses, hyponatremia may result. Colloid (5 percent albumin) may be given as part of the third-space replacement when the surgery involves viscera or moderate blood loss. Third-space losses in the anephric patient are replaced at the rate of 1-5 ml/kg per hour depending on the extent of tissue trauma. Corresponding replacement rates in the patient with normal renal function and these losses are: up to 5 ml/kg per hour for surgery involving minimal trauma (hernia repair, D&C), 5-10 ml/kg per hour for moderate trauma (cholycystectomy), and 10-15 ml/kg per hour for major trauma (bowel resection, burns). These numbers are only guidelines; volumes actually administered will be altered based on measurement of vital signs and central venous pressure (CVP). As mentioned previously, urine output may not readily reflect rapid changes in volume status in the patient with chronic renal disease.

Exogenous potassium should not be given to the patient with chronic renal disease unless the renal disease is mild or the patient has a specific K^+ losing renal defect. Preoperative or intraoperative tissue trauma and blood transfusions increase serum K^+ levels.

Monitoring

Monitoring of the patient with renal disease should include routine parameters such as blood pressure, pulse, ECG, fluid intake and output, level of consciousness, and temperature. Where major blood loss or fluid shifts have occurred, a CVP or pulmonary artery catheter is useful. The need for an indwelling urinary catheter is controversial as urine output may not reflect acute changes in volume status or renal function and the risk of urinary tract infection is high.

A postoperative hemoglobin determination should be made and blood obtained for serum K^+, Na^+, and HCO_3^-. (An ECG may be useful here when looking for signs of hyperkalemia.)

Nondepolarizing muscle relaxants (d-tubocurarine, pancuronium) are excreted primarily via the kidney. Although biliary pathways are available for excretion of these drugs, half-lives will be prolonged and the patient may need postoperative ventilatory assistance. The degree of residual neuromuscular blockade can be evaluated using a nerve stimulator.

Dialysis

Perioperative management of the chronically dialyzed patient is often less complex than management of the nondialyzed patient with severe renal insufficiency because dialysis provides a means to control body fluid and electrolyte content, decrease acidosis, improve hematocrit, and decrease most symptoms of uremia.

The dialysis site in the arm or leg must be protected at all times. Peritoneal dialysis catheters should be handled with aseptic technique. Hemodialysis access sites (either an external shunt or, more commonly, a subcutaneous fistula) should not be used for blood sampling. Blood pressure cuffs and tourniquets should not be placed on those extremities. Volume depletion or hypotension may result in shunt or fistula clotting. Presence of a bruit or thrill should be confirmed frequently by palpation or with a stethoscope. Any changes should be reported immediately to the physician.

Indications for acute postoperative dialysis in the patient with chronic renal failure (a very rare event) include volume overload with congestive heart failure and symptomatic hyperkalemia.

RENAL FAILURE IN THE PATIENT WITH PREVIOUSLY NORMAL RENAL FUNCTION

Acute renal failure refers to a rapid decrease in GFR and a concomitant increase in serum creatinine concentration. It is frequently accompanied by oliguria (urine volumes of less than 20 ml per hour or 400 ml per day), but may at times be observed with a normal urine output ("nonoliguric" renal failure). An outline of causes of acute renal failure is presented in Table 11-2. There appears to be a wide range of variability in degree of insult and the number of factors necessary to produce acute tubular necrosis (ATN) in any individual patient. Some patients develop ATN after only transient hypotension, while others do not do so even after prolonged

Table 11-2. Etiology of Acute Renal Failure

1. Structural Lesions
    Arterial (thrombus, embolus)
    Venous (kinking, ligation)
    Renal tubular occlusion
    Renal pelvis, ureter, bladder
	3. Prerenal failure
	    True hypovolemia
	    Other low cardiac output states

2. Acute renal disease
    Vasculitis
    Glomerulonephritis
    Malignant hypertension
    Pregnancy-related
	4. Acute tubular necrosis 2° to 1 or a combination of the following:
	    Any prerenal cause
	    Nephrotoxins
	    Heme pigments
	    Sepsis

sepsis and shock. The reasons for this are unclear but suggest multifactorial causes. Incipient ATN may be reversed with vigorous treatment of volume depletion, low cardiac output states, and sepsis, together with discontinuation of nephrotoxic agents; therefore, early diagnosis and prompt and aggressive treatment of these conditions should be undertaken.

Diagnosis

Renal dysfunction usually presents as a decreased or absent urine output. There are many situations in which the kidney is predictably at risk, when urine output should be closely monitored with an indwelling catheter. Perioperative situations with a high risk for acute renal failure include:

1. Major trauma
2. Cardiopulmonary bypass
3. Surgery of the aorta or renal vessels
4. Massive blood transfusion
5. Major biliary surgery or obstructive jaundice
6. Hypovolemic hypotension
7. Long or extensive surgery in the elderly patient
8. Surgery in the patient with preexisting renal disease
9. Sepsis
10. Nephrotoxic antibiotics
11. Obstetric complications (abruptio placenta)

Surgical intervention in any of these situations may result in postoperative acute renal failure.

If urine output ceases entirely, the system should be checked first for any obstruction (kinks, clots, etc.). Complete anuria is rare in the perioperative period and is caused only by vascular occlusion or the disruption of the continuity of the urethra or both ureters.

Distinguishing prerenal from acute renal disease is best accomplished by using a combination of clinical and laboratory evaluations. Clinical parameters for hypovolemia or cardiovascular failure can be rapidly evaluated and the problem(s) corrected even before results of laboratory tests are obtained. Oliguria in most surgical patients is the result of volume depletion, and unless signs of fluid overload are present, infusion of balanced salt solution should be tried.

The patient with cardiac failure (with or without volume overload) may also be oliguric. This diagnosis should be apparent after demonstration of an elevated CVP or pulmonary capillary wedge pressure (PCWP). The exact level depends on the particular patient, but a CVP >10 cm H_2O or PCWP >18 mm Hg is suggestive of cardiac failure.

On the other hand, in many patients a diagnosis is not readily apparent from clinical evaluation alone. Simple laboratory tests which assume that in prerenal states the kidney concentrates urine better and reabsorbs sodium and water more effectively than if ATN is present can establish the diagnosis.

Usually, urine specific gravity and osmolality (a measure of renal concentrating ability) tend to be fairly high in prerenal states, while urine and plasma osmolalities are nearly equal in ATN.

	Prerenal	ATN
Urine specific gravity	>1.015	1.010–1.015
Urine/plasma osmolality	>1.1/1	<1.1/1

Considerable overlap may exist. These parameters are useful only for distinguishing ATN from prerenal states in the acutely oliguric patient. These values are compatible with many other conditions in the nonoliguric patient. In addition, heavy solutes such as glucose or iodinated contrast media can increase urine specific gravity, even in patients with ATN.

Indices of water reabsorption by the kidney can be used to differentiate renal from prerenal oliguria. The urine/plasma (U/P) concentration ratio of a filtered, but nonreabsorbed solute such as creatinine is an accurate index of the fraction of the glomerular filtrate volume that is unreabsorbed by the kidney and appears in the urine. For example, if the U/P creatinine ratio is 3, then one-third the originally filtered water must have been reabsorbed in order to triple the creatinine concentration in the urine. Similarly, a U/P creatinine ratio of 100 means that 99 percent of the filtered water was reabsorbed, and only 1/100 or 1 percent appears in the urine. This is true regardless of the glomerular filtration rate or the serum creatinine concentration. The U/P urea ratio may be used in a similar manner, although a significant fraction of the filtered urea is reabsorbed by the tubules so that U/P urea will always be less than U/P creatinine.

	Prerenal	ATN
U/P creatinine	>40/1	<10/1
U/P urea	>20/1	<10/1

Intermediate values are consistent with either diagnosis.

Indices of sodium reabsorption also differ in prerenal states and ATN. In prerenal states, urine sodium concentration is typically low (less than 25 mEq/liter), while it is more than 10 mEq/liter in almost all patients with ATN. The range of 10 to 25 mEq/liter is consistent with either diagnosis. Since urine sodium concentration is affected both by sodium reabsorption and by water reabsorption, as more water is reabsorbed, urine sodium concentration will increase, though sodium excretion may remain unchanged.

To correct for the effect of water reabsorption, the renal fractional excretion of sodium or FE_{Na} has been used as a diagnostic tool.

$$FE_{Na} = \frac{\text{urinary sodium excretion}}{\text{sodium filtered at the glomerulus}}$$

FE_{Na} is calculated as: U/P Na divided by U/P creatinine (expressed as a percentage of filtered sodium). An untimed sample of urine is sufficient for the test. Measurement of FE_{Na} appears to give a more clear-cut separation between prerenal disease and ATN than any of the other methods mentioned so far, as little overlap has been observed between the two groups of patients using this test.

	Renal	Prerenal
FE_{Na}	< 1%	> 2%

As with specific gravity and U/P osmolality, the U/P urea, U/P creatinine, and FE_{Na} tests are of use for distinguishing ATN from prerenal disease only in the acutely oliguric patient. These tests are applicable only during acute deterioration in patients with previously normal renal function. The patient with severe chronic renal disease, even when otherwise well, excretes urine of low specific gravity which contains a large fraction of filtered salt and water which may mimic ATN. The use of potent diuretics or an acute saline infusion can increase urinary sodium excretion and produce a picture identical to that of ATN. A patient with mild urinary tract obstruction will have a picture consistent with prerenal oliguria, while one with more severe or prolonged obstruction will appear to have ATN.

Prevention

Prevention is best accomplished by prompt recognition and effective treatment of the clinical states associated with prerenal azotemia and oliguria. Fluid administration or antibiotic therapy in the volume-depleted or septic patient may prevent renal failure. Renal function should be carefully monitored when nephrotoxic agents (e.g., aminoglycosides) are used.

The role of diuretic agents such as mannitol and furosemide (Lasix) as prophylaxis and therapy for ATN is more controversial. There are several theoretical mechanisms by which mannitol and furosemide might protect the kidney from ATN, including: (1) decreasing tubular reabsorption, minimizing intratubular obstruction from cell debris, precipitated pigment and proteins; (2) perhaps reversing arteriolar vasospasm; and (3) in the case of mannitol, shrinking swollen capillary endothelium and decreasing renin secretion. Despite extensive investigation in animals and uncontrolled studies in humans, there is not yet convincing evidence to support the use of mannitol or furosemide as either prevention or treatment of acute tubular necrosis. In clinical settings in which the formation of obstructing intratubular casts or crystals appears to play a major pathogenic role (crush injury to muscle, malignant hyperthermia, mismatched transfusions, massive intravascular hemolysis and acute hyperurecosuric states), the use of mannitol or furosemide and intravenous fluids to maintain urine flow at a high level to "flush" the kidney may avert renal failure. When these conditions are present, urine flows of 2 to 4 liters per day should be maintained for 2 or 3 days.

In situations known to carry a high risk of ATN, particularly in open heart or aortic surgery, the addition of 25 to 50 gm of mannitol per day to intravenous infusions may be helpful, but it is probably more important to avoid volume deficits through careful fluid management.

The possibility that oliguric ATN may be converted to nonoliguric ATN by diuretics is also questionable. The risk of a single dose of mannitol (25 gm) or furosemide (20-40 mg) is small. Doses > 500 mg of mannitol may cause serious volume overload while a large dose of furosemide (1gm) may cause deafness. It must be remembered that any diuresis in a volume-depleted patient must be accompanied by vigorous fluid replacement in order to prevent even more severe volume depletion with further diminution of renal function.

Treatment

Established postsurgical acute tubular necrosis carries a poor prognosis. About 60 percent of patients die, usually from infection or from the illness which precipitated the renal failure. Optimal patient survival requires careful management of fluids and medications, with timely use of dialysis. Fluid intake is limited to replacement of urinary and extrarenal losses. In the afebrile patient without diarrhea, a fluid intake limited to urine volume plus 500 ml per day is a reasonable regimen. Sodium should be provided in sufficient quantity to replace losses.

Potassium should not be given to the oliguric patient (volume<400 ml per day). Kayexalate may be used to prevent or treat hyperkalemia. In the nonoliguric patient, urinary losses of potassium are replaced with careful monitoring of serum and urinary potassium.

Particular attention to detail should be paid to the postoperative monitoring and management of the patient with impaired renal function to preserve all remaining kidney function. It is important to be aware of the situations that place a patient at risk for developing acute renal failure. The early diagnosis and treatment of prerenal states may prevent acute tubular necrosis. Should acute renal failure occur, its prompt recognition and the institution of appropriate therapy will decrease morbidity and possibly mortality.

RENAL TRANSPLANTS

The Recipient

Patients who receive renal transplants usually have little if any remaining renal function. Postoperatively they present particular problems in terms of volume status and infection control.

Unlike the patient whose intravascular volume must be restricted to prevent volume overload, the transplant recipient needs an adequate circulating volume so that oliguria on the basis of volume depletion will not complicate the clinical picture. Moreover, almost all transplant recipients receive immunosuppressive drugs, and their ability to combat infection is impaired. Even greater attention than usual needs to be paid to aseptic technique.

The Donor

The recovery room is often the site where patients whose kidneys are to be used as donor organs are nursed until criteria for brain death are met. These patients must be carefully monitored (urine output, blood pressure, temperature, arterial blood gases, and if available CVP or PCWP). Strict aseptic techniques should be adhered to as sepsis in the donor or the need to use potentially nephrotoxic antibiotics might render the kidneys unsuitable for transplantation. Particulars of drug therapy for organ preservation vary from center to center. A good review of the topic is presented by Slapak. The protocol followed at the Montefiore Hospital and Medical Center is a typical example (see Figure 11-1).

SUGGESTIONS FOR FURTHER READING

Anderson RJ, Bennett WM, Gambertoglio JG, Schrier RW. Fate of drugs in renal failure. In: The kidney, 2d ed. Brenner BM, Rector FC Jr. eds. Philadelphia: WB Saunders, 1981.

Once brain death has been determined, it is imperative to maintain the donor until consents can be obtained and the organs removed.

It is important to maintain adequate circulatory volume in order to insure good organ perfusion and urinary output.

SUGGESTED M.D. ORDERS FOR DONOR MAINTENANCE

1. Vital signs q̄. 1 Hour
   Notify M.D. If: B/P ↓ 100 mmHg.
   Pulse ↑ 120/min.
   or ↓ 70/min.
2. Record hourly intake and output.
3. Central venous pressure q̄. 1 hour (if possible)
   Notify M.D. if CVP: ↓ 10 cm. H_2O
   or
   ↑ 16 cm. H_2O
   Hypovolemia insidiously develops in patients with brain death and accounts for nearly 100% of all the hemodynamic instability. A central venous catheter should be inserted either by percutaneous technique or by cutdown.
4. I.V. fluids and medications
   a. Vigorously hydrate donor with appropriate fluids. The nature and volume of I.V. fluids should vary according to changes in serum electrolytes and urinary output. The following solutions may be used at a rate equal to urinary output plus 50 cc per hour:
      1. 5% dextrose in ¼ normal saline solution
      2. 0.5% saline in 2.5% dextrose solution
      3. Lactated Ringer's solution
      Also, plasma, plasmanate or other volume expanders may be used at 500-1,000 cc.
      Please note, additional fluids may be needed to compensate for preexisting deficits, particularly in patients in whom dehydration to reduce cerebral edema has been induced.
   b. Push intravenous fluids until central venous pressure is about 10 cm. H_2O.
   c. A systolic blood pressure of 100 mmHg or greater is desirable. If necessary, Dopamine is the recommended vasopressor of choice. However, Isuprel, Levophed, or Aramine may be used but are not desirable.
   d. Attempt to maintain urinary output above 100 cc. per hour with Mannitol, 25 grams in 1,000 cc. Lactated Ringer's, Lasix 40 mg. to 1.0 grams.
   e. If diabetes insipidis occurs, use Pitressin in water (not oil) 2-5 units, initially, depending on urine volume, may repeat in four hours, etc.
5. Use hypothermia blanket to maintain temp. ↓ 100°F and ↑ 95°F.
6. CBC, SMA-12 (serum creatinine and blood urea nitrogen), daily.
7. Blood culture × 1 (daily, if indicated).
8. Urinanalysis daily.
9. Urine culture × 1 (daily, if indicated).
10. Sputum culture × 1 (daily, if indicated).
11. Blood type, VDRL and HAA (Hepatitis Associated Antigen) once during hospitalization.
12. Toxicology screen (if indicated).

Since patients with widespread systemic infections are not considered suitable donors, it is important to take care in avoiding contamination. Rigorous techniques should be employed in catheter, tracheostomy and wound care. However, patients with bacterial infections, such as pneumonia, that can be successfully treated with antibiotics, may be suitable donors if the infection is eliminated prior to the organ retrieval.

Figure 11-1.   Donor maintenance protocol.

Goldman L, Caldera DL. Risks of general anesthesia and elective operation in the hypertensive patient. Anesthesiology 1979; 50:285–292.

Mazze RI. Care of the patient with acute renal failure. Anesthesiology 1977; 47:138–148.

Slapak M. The immediate care of potential donors for cadaveric organ transplantation. Anaesthesia 1978; 33:700–709.

12
Recovery Room Care after Intrathoracic Surgery
Patricia Hartwell

Recovery room needs of patients after intrathoracic surgery depend on the preoperative condition, the nature of the operative procedure and the anesthetic management.

The cardiopulmonary system is particularly stressed by thoracic surgery. The preoperative condition of these patients must be assessed from several points.

1. How much pulmonary reserve does the patient have? This may be assessed by evaluation of excercise tolerance, smoking history, signs of emphysema (e.g., finger clubbing, increased anterior-posterior diameter of the chest, wheezing), and review of pertinent laboratory data. Preoperative evaluation includes chest X ray, arterial blood gas estimation, and particularly if lung resection is considered pulmonary function tests.

Normal values for many of the pulmonary function tests take into consideration the patient's age, sex, height, and weight. When pulmonary function tests are performed in the laboratory, the normal values, i.e., the "predicted values," are usually reported along with the patient's values. An example of normal blood gas and pulmonary function is given in Table 12-1. Within the first 18 hours following thoracic surgery, there is a 50 to 75 percent reduction of vital capacity. This improves to some degree over the next few days, but if the patient's preoperative pulmonary function is severely decreased, any superimposed reduction would not be tolerated, and the patient would require ventilatory support. Generally speaking, a patient whose vital capacity and expiratory flow rates are at least 80 percent of the predicted or normal values can be expected to have a normal postoperative course. Fifty percent reduction, however, means very severe disease and predicts the greater need of postoperative respiratory support.

Table 12-1. Normal Arterial Blood Gas and Pulmonary Function Test Values (50-year-old man, 70 kg, 180 cm, sitting position)

Arterial blood gas	pH 7.40
PCO_2 40 mm Hg	
PO_2 90 mm Hg	
Base excess 0	
Pulmonary function tests	
FVC (forced vital capacity)	4.74 liters
FEV_1 (forced expiratory volume in 1 second)	3.87 liters
FEV_3 (forced expiratory volume in 3 seconds)	4.41 liters
Expressed as a % of the FVC,	
$FEV_1 = $ 83% (i.e., 3.87 liters is 83% of 4.74 liters)	
$FEV_3 = $ 97% (i.e., 4.41 liters is 97% of 4.74 liters)	
PEFR (peak expiratory flow rate)	8.97 liters/sec
MMF (mid maximal flow rate, also called "FEF 0.25–0.75," measures the forced expiratory flow rate in middle of effort)	3.08 liters/sec
$D_{L_{CO}}$ SB (diffusion capacity for carbon monoxide measured during single breath)	32.08
ERV (expiratory reserve volume)	0.96 liters
RV (residual volume)	1.77 liters
TLC (total lung capacity)	6.51 liters
RV/TLC × 100%	27%
FRC (functional residual capacity)	2.73 liters
IC (inspiratory capacity)	3.78 liters

2. Is there a previous history of angina or congestive cardiac failure? If so, cardiac reserve is limited. Prior placement of central venous and arterial catheters may be indicated. Shivering, which increases oxygen consumption and hence cardiac output by up to 400 percent, must be prevented by careful attention to maintenance of normothermia, sedation, or administration of small doses of methylphenidate, narcotics, or (very rarely) muscle relaxants (which of course would mandate continued ventilatory support with appropriate sedation and analgesia).

3. What preoperative medication was the patient receiving? Drugs such as antibiotics, steroids, most antihypertensives, vasodilators (e.g., Isordil and nitroglycerine (Nitrobid) paste), beta-blocking agents (e.g., propranolol) and eye drops for glaucoma should be continued perioperatively. Diuretics are often withheld and given as necessary. Calcium channel blockers may or may not be maintained depending on the postoperative condition.

The anesthetic technique generally aims to allow the patient to be awake and extubated on arrival in the recovery room to minimize complications of air leaks caused by mechanical ventilation. Occasionally intraoperative problems or the complexity of surgery dictate that the patient remain intubated for a prolonged period.

The nature and extent of the operative procedure determine to some extent the type and intensity of monitoring. Some of the more commonly performed intrathoracic procedures are considered.

LOBECTOMY

Lobectomy involves resection of a lobe of the lung. Postoperative management of patients who have undergone total or partial lobectomy or wedge resection involves several considerations.

Care of Chest Tubes

Chest tubes have three functions:

Drainage of fluid and air from the pleural space
Prevention of air entering the chest through the drainage site
Application of controlled suction or negative pressure to the pleural space to aid in pulmonary reexpansion

Three chambers usually combined as one package (Pleur-evac) are connected to the chest tube (Figure 12-1). The first, or collection chamber, collects fluid drained from the chest. Calibration allows accurate measurement and recording of drainage. The second chamber is a water seal which acts as a one-way valve allowing air to leave the chest and preventing its return. The third bottle provides controlled negative suction by a predetermined height of a water column (usually 20 cm). The small port that is open to air provides a safety valve and allows room air to enter and prevents the negative pressure from exceeding the preset limits.

If the tube is patent and functioning normally, the fluid in the second chamber moves slightly with respiration. If the patient is breathing spontaneously, negative intrapleural pressure during inspiration is transmitted to the chamber, and the water level moves 1-2 cm upward, against the direction of arrow A (Figure 12-1). Conversely, when positive pressure ventilation is applied, the water level dips, moving along the direction indicated by arrow A. If fluctuation of the fluid level stops, a blocked or kinked chest tube should be suspected. Air bubbles, which represent an air leak, pass along in the direction of the arrow. If the connections to the

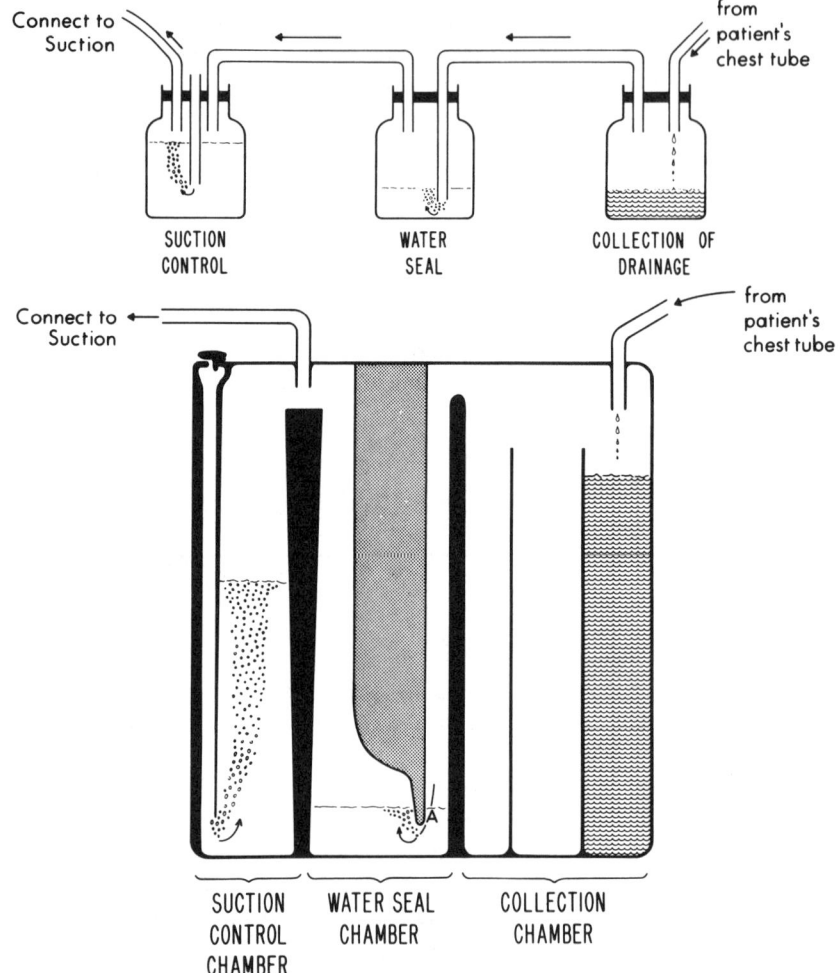

Figure 12-1. Schematic drawing of the Pleur-evac unit. If bottles are used instead, each bottle functions as the corresponding chamber in the Pleur-evac.

chest tubes are sealed and the tube securely sutured in place, the leak is from the lung. Small air leaks are common and usually close spontaneously.

Application of suction to the system causes a gentle and steady bubbling in the third chamber which results in a controlled negative pressure effect in the pleural space. If the suction is increased to excessive levels, more air is drawn in so more bubbles pass in this chamber, but the pressure applied to the lung space stays at the desired level. During transfer, or if continued negative pressure is undesirable, the tubing at the suction chamber is disconnected and left open to room air. This tube should not be clamped as it provides an escape for air from the chest passing through the water seal chamber.

Pain Relief

Postoperative pain caused by the incision, pleural irritation, and the presence of chest tubes is a major problem. Deep breathing and coughing may become ineffective, and therefore secretions can become a major problem, especially if the patient has been a heavy smoker. Pain relief is achieved by the use of parenteral narcotics (which are respiratory depressants). Alternatively, the thoracic nerves may have been blocked intraoperatively with local anesthetic solution. Analgesia is incomplete with this method as pleural pain is not relieved adequately. Thoracic epidural techniques have been used successfully in some centers but are invasive and have the potential side effects of bradycardia and hypotension.

Adequate analgesia is obtained when the patient is comfortable enough to sleep intermittently but continues to breathe at a rate at least 14 per minute and remains promptly responsive to verbal stimulation. Although slight hypercapnia may prevail ($PaCO_2$ 40–47 mm Hg), the analgesia should allow the patient to clear his own secretions and improve oxygenation. Recommended therapy is morphine 1–2 mg or meperidine 10–20 mg intravenously, repeated after 10 minutes if necessary.

Respiratory Adequacy

With adequate pain relief, coughing and deep breathing should be encouraged. In the awake, extubated patient this is achieved by turning, supporting the thorax and tubes, cupping or clapping the chest, and using postural drainage. Occasionally, gentle nasotracheal suctioning may be necessary to stimulate a cough response and clear secretions. This maneuver should only be attempted while the patient continues to breathe an enriched oxygen supply because suctioning causes hypoxia.

If the patient is still intubated, appropriate support is necessary. If the tidal volume is adequate (> 4–5 ml/kg), the endotracheal tube should be attached to an enriched oxygen supply via a T-piece. Up to 50 percent oxygen can be inspired safely by most patients indefinitely without causing lung damage. One exception to this is the premature infant in whom high oxygen concentration may lead to retrolental fibroplasia and blindness. Another exception is the patient who breathes by hypoxic drive, e.g., the emphysematous patient who is chronically hypoxemic ($PaO_2 < 60$ mm Hg) and hypercapnic ($PaCO_2 > 45$ mm Hg). In this situation hypoxemia, not

204 PATIENTS WHO REQUIRE SPECIAL CONSIDERATION

hypercapnia, is a stimulus to respiration. As supplemental oxygen increases the PaO_2 above the triggering level, respiratory depression leads to apnea and coma and ultimately cardiac arrest. The process may be accelerated by administration of narcotics. Careful observation should be combined with arterial blood gas measurement.

Gentle suctioning after three to five assisted ventilations with oxygen should be used as necessary, avoiding entering one or other bronchus and incurring the risk of irritation to the surgical site or bronchial stump. If spontaneous ventilation is inadequate, respiratory support must be available (see Chapter 3).

The patient may be extubated if the criteria listed in Table 12-2 are realized. Failure to precisely meet all the criteria does not necessarily preclude extubation, but it does mean the patient is marginal and should be watched closely for signs of respiratory failure.

Causes of Hypoxemia

One of the most common complications of lobectomy in the recovery room is inadequate oxygenation. Apart from respiratory depression caused by pain or narcotic administration, several other situations may prove hazardous.

Intrapulmonary Shunting due to Atelectasis or Endobronchial Intubation

Inadequate pulmonary toilet and low tidal volumes predispose to areas of alveolar collapse. Any change of the patient's position should be followed by auscultation of the lungs to verify that the endotracheal tube has not

Table 12-2. Criteria for Safe Extubation

Mental status
    Conscious, following commands
    Functional reflexes (swallowing, gag)
Upper airway clear
    No bleeding, foreign bodies, or vomitus
Lungs fully expanded:
    Breath sounds are equal (and clear)
    X ray is satisfactory
Oxygenation adequate
    No cyanosis (examine conjunctiva of a dark-skinned patient)
    PaO_2 is 90, when FiO_2 is 40 or less
Air exchange adequate
    Vital capacity of > 15 ml/kg
    Tidal volume of > 5 ml/kg
    Spontaneous respiratory rate < 25 per minute
    Inspiratory force of at least -25 cm H_2O

entered the right main stem bronchus. Movement of the chin toward the sternum causes the tip of the endotracheal tube to move toward the carina where it may enter the bronchus. Neck extension pulls the tube up the trachea and accidental extubation may occur, especially in children.

Pneumothorax or Hemothorax

Loss of the vacuum between the lungs and thoracic wall caused by the surgical incision allows air or blood to enter the newly created space and hamper full expansion of the lung. Chest tubes are usually inserted intraoperatively to prevent such accumulations. Pneumothorax may occur, however, due to disconnection of chest tubes, leakage of air from incision sites or a ruptured bleb, or puncture of the lung during placement of central venous pressure monitoring catheters, especially if a subclavian or internal jugular route was used. Flap valves may create a one-way system and allow a tension pneumothorax to develop quickly. A life-threatening situation occurs as the mediastinum is shifted, impairing ventilation of the other lung, and compromising cardiac output.

Signs and symptoms of pneumothorax include an initial sharp pain (masked perhaps by incisional pain or narcotics). Asymmetry and decrease of the breath sounds occur when the pneumothorax reaches 15 to 20 percent. Tachypnea and hypoxia are late developments as the pneumothorax increases in size. Hypotension and cardiovascular collapse occur as a tension pneumothorax develops. Chest X ray, preferably in an upright position, affords definitive diagnosis, but lifesaving therapy should not be delayed.

Therapy requires careful examination of the chest tube for blockage by external kinking. Intraluminal clots may be dislodged by milking the tube or passing a catheter up the tube. If these measures do not correct the situation, the chest tube should be replaced. In emergencies, a large bore needle (#14) can be inserted in the second or third interspace anteriorly and connected via intravenous tubing to an open bottle of saline below the patient. Supplemental oxygen must be given and positive pressure ventilation reduced as much as possible until another chest tube can be inserted.

Hemothorax causes hypotension and tachycardia before tachypnea develops. Breath sounds are diminished in dependent parts of the lung where there is dullness to percussion. Blood collects in the thorax if the chest tube is blocked. Otherwise it will drain into the collection chamber. Rapid accumulations usually dictate prompt surgical reexploration.

PNEUMONECTOMY

Removal of an entire lung, a radical thoracic procedure, is performed either when extensive disease involves the lung or when a resectable cancer is too close to the hilum for lobectomy.

Following pneumonectomy, chest tubes are not normally used as negative pressure would pull the mediastinum to the resected side, causing overdistension of the other lung.

The newly transected bronchus has been oversewn and is susceptible to breakdown by trauma (e.g., caused by a suction catheter) or by positive pressure. Early extubation is desirable. Suction catheters should be premeasured and care taken not to pass them below the level of the carina.

Central venous pressure must be monitored carefully. Modest fluid restriction may be necessary to prevent development of right-sided heart failure. Following resection of the entire lung, the resistance through the pulmonary vascular bed is almost doubled (i.e., same volume of blood must traverse half the blood vessels). This is usually only temporary, because the vessels can normally dilate. But if disease is present in the remaining lung, the resistance to blood flow may remain elevated. This may lead to heart failure and arrhythmias.

PERICARDIAL WINDOW

An effusion may develop in the pericardial sac and compromise hemodynamic function. If the fluid collects rapidly, cardiac tamponade may occur with as little as 250 ml fluid. A slowly increasing collection may reach a volume of 1 liter before a life-threatening situation develops. Therapy involves evacuating the fluid and removing a piece of pericardium to create a pericardial window.

Several signs are associated with cardiac compression. Tachycardia is common and pulse pressure is narrow. Arterial blood pressure decreases more than normally during inspiration. Detection of this so called "pulsus paradoxus" may be made by listening carefully to the Korotkoff sounds as the blood pressure cuff is deflated slowly. When the sounds are first heard, the cuff pressure is slightly increased until the sounds are heard only during expiration. The highest pressure at which any Korotkoff sounds are heard is noted. The cuff is slowly deflated until the sounds are heard throughout the respiratory cycle and this pressure noted. Normally the difference between the two recordings is 5 mm Hg. A difference of 10 mm Hg suggests a significant cardiac tamponade. Kussmaul's sign is a paradoxical increase in central venous pressure during inspiration. Neck veins fill as the patient takes a deep breath in the semireclining position.

Postoperatively, hemodynamic stability is usually regained. Care depends largely on the extent of the disease which caused the tamponade. A posttraumatic hemorrhagic pericardial effusion may recur and cause tamponade in the recovery room. Lung contusion may coexist and require ventilator support. If the cause of the pericardial tamponade is uremia, careful attention to fluid and electrolyte balance is essential, and potassium-containing solutions must be avoided. Other pathologic conditions associated with pericardial effusions include collagen vascular disease, infection, or tumor.

MEDIASTINOSCOPY AND BRONCHOSCOPY

Evaluation and biopsy of tumors and other lung disease are performed by mediastinoscopy and bronchoscopy. Mediastinoscopy is usually done through the suprasternal notch using an instrument like a short, straight bronchoscope through which long forceps are passed. On arrival in the recovery room, patients are usually extubated, have no chest tubes, and have only a small suprasternal incision.

Complications include bleeding and tearing of the lungs and airways. Bleeding in the mediastinum may manifest itself as progressive dyspnea and airway obstruction with deviation of the trachea. Chest X ray shows widening of the mediastinum. Perforation of the lung may cause pneumomediastinum or pneumothorax. The pneumomediastinum results from air that has leaked either from the periphery of the lung and tracked into the hilum, or from air that has escaped directly from a larger bronchus. Air in the mediastinum diffuses up into the neck and dissects into the subcutaneous tissues of the neck, upper chest, and even the face. This results in subcutaneous emphysema, which is a swelling of the tissues caused by air, and it has a feeling of crepitance on palpation. It is essential to treat any of these complications with supplemental oxygen. Adequate patency of the airway must be assured. Surgical exploration may be indicated, and a chest tube may be necessary for a pneumothorax.

THYMECTOMY

Remission of myasthenia gravis may be achieved by removal of the thymus. Myasthenia gravis is characterized by progressive weakness from impaired neuromuscular transmission. Antibodies develop to the acetylcholine receptors in muscle. Thymectomy decreases this autoimmune response. Muscles supplied by the cranial nerves are affected most. Ptosis, double vision, and difficulty in swallowing are common findings. Extreme sensitivity to nondepolarizing muscle relaxant drugs (e.g., curare, pancuronium) exists. Therapy of myasthenia gravis includes administration of anticholinesterase drugs such as pyridostigmine and neostigmine which improve muscle strength. Complications of these drugs include increased secretions and bradycardia, requiring concurrent administration of atropine.

The thymus may be approached surgically by splitting the sternum. This incision is painful and patients usually require sedation and ventilatory support for 24 to 48 hours postoperatively. Another cervical approach involves removal of the thymus through an incision in the neck. Extubation is frequently possible much earlier in the postoperative course.

If the patient requires anticholinesterase medication to maintain adequate respiratory function, the dose must be adjusted postoperatively prior to extubation. Dose is adjusted using a repeated "Tensilon test." Tensilon (edrophonium) is a short-acting anticholinesterase. When the longer acting anticholinesterase agent (e.g., pyridostigmine) is adjudged to be at peak effect, Tensilon is given. If the motor strength improves, dosage is increased. If the dosage is already excessive, greater weakness may develop. Excessive doses of anticholinesterase can progress to a cholinergic crisis (excess secretions, profound weakness, bradycardia).

Extubation is performed when the patient meets all the criteria as outlined earlier. Disproportionate bulbar weakness can result in airway obstruction following extubation because of decrease in protective pharyngeal reflexes. Difficulty in swallowing secretions make aspiration and progressive respiratory distress an ever-present hazard. Careful observation for the first signs of respiratory distress, bleeding, and pneumomediastinum is essential.

CARDIAC SURGERY

Because most hospitals have separate areas or intensive care units for patients who have undergone open heart surgery, care of these patients is not considered in this chapter. But most of the general principles given apply also to these patients. Ventilatory support with supplemental oxygen administration is necessary. Intrapleural and mediastinal tubes require routine care and careful observations. The most usual complications include arrhythmias, atelectasis, pneumothorax or hemothorax, and cardiac tamponade. Endotracheal tube displacement is a likely hazard.

SUMMARY

The patient who has undergone intrathoracic surgery represents a special challenge for the recovery room nurse. Life-threatening complications can develop rapidly. Special vigilance and preparedness are essential.

SUGGESTIONS FOR FURTHER READING

Kuddusi G, Israel RH. The pulmonary function test. In: Problems in pulmonary medicine for the primary physician. RH Pie, RH Israel, eds. Philadelphia: Lea & Febinger, 1982.

Poe RH, Dale RC. The surgical patient. In: Problems in pulmonary medicine for the primary physician. RH Poe, RH Israel, eds. Philadelphia: Lea & Febinger, 1982.

Pontoppidan H, Geffin B, Lowenstein E. Acute respiratory failure in the adult. Boston: Little, Brown, 1973.

Shapiro BA. Evaluation of respiratory function in the perioperative period. In: 31st annual refresher course lectures. American Society of Anesthesiologists, 1980.

Shapiro BA, Walton JR. Ventilatory support of the postoperative patient. In: General thoracic surgery. TW Shields, ed. Philadelphia: Lea & Febinger, 1983.

Wilkinson CJ. General principles of postoperative management. In: General thoracic surgery. TW Shields, ed. Philadelphia: Lea & Febinger, 1983.

13
The Recovery Room as an Ambulatory and Special Procedures Unit
Elizabeth A. M. Frost

Medicosocioeconomic trends are toward shorter hospital stays. An increasing number of surgical procedures are performed on a one-day stay, or ambulatory basis. Frequently, because of space restrictions, other areas in the hospital are not available for care of these patients. The recovery room, therefore, has assumed a critical role as it is here that many patients are monitored until they regain "street fitness" and may be discharged home.

Yet another role for the recovery room has developed as that of a special procedures unit. It is difficult to predict operating times and thus recovery room time on a daily basis. Periods occur in the recovery room when, although staffing is available, there are few, if any, patients. This situation is most likely to occur early in the morning before the first operative procedures are completed. In many recovery rooms it has become routine to schedule certain procedures to fill these anticipated gaps. Other advantages of using the recovery room as a special procedures unit are as follows:

1. Operating room proximity
2. Improved recovery room utilization
3. Availability of intensive care nursing staff
4. Sterile area
5. Intensive care facility
6. Accessibility to anesthesiology and surgical departments

AMBULATORY SURGERY

Although 60 percent of all surgical procedures may be performed on an outpatient basis, the actual number is determined by several factors including available supporting services, patient population, and acceptability and financial resources. Most frequently pediatric operations are suitable for ambulatory care because of short surgical duration and ready availability of family support. However, with increasing public awareness and involvement of close relatives, many other procedures may be treated safely on a one-day stay basis.

Operations most frequently performed on an ambulatory basis include:

Pediatrics	*Adults*
Hernia repair	D&C
Myringotomy and tube insertion	Breast biopsy
Circumcision	Varicose vein ligation
Cystometrics	Hernia repair
	Cystoscopy

An area should be designated in the recovery room or an adjacent room where these patients may be watched until they can be safely discharged home. Equipment requirements for such an area include:

1. Stretchers
2. Basic monitoring equipment: electrocardiogram (ECG); blood pressure
3. O_2 supply, suctioning apparatus
4. Lounge chairs
5. Closets for storage of clothes
6. Kitchen facilities to prepare light foods and beverages (e.g., warm milk, tea, soda and ice)
7. Drug cabinets
8. Bathroom facilities
9. Nearby waiting room for parents and relatives

Patients treated on an ambulatory basis should be given instructions such as those outlined in Table 13-1 prior to admission to the hospital. It is especially important to emphasize that patients must be accompanied home by a responsible adult. They should not drive within 24 hours of a general anesthetic procedure.

The criteria which must be met prior to discharge are outlined in Chapter 7. Patients should be able to tolerate fluids, dress themselves, and walk with only minimal assistance.

Table 13-1. Instructions to Be Given to Patients before Admission for Ambulatory Surgery

Do
- Bring with you an early morning urine specimen.
- Bring someone with you to drive you home. If a child is having surgery, two adults are required: one to drive the car and one to care for the child.
- Wear loose-fitting, easy-to-put-on garments or a robe.
- Bring your insurance papers or their identifying numbers.

Do not
- Eat or drink anything after midnight prior to the day of surgery. Take nothing by mouth. Bring no food to the hospital.
- Bring jewelry or other valuables. We cannot be responsible for them.
- Bring pajamas, gowns, or slippers. The hospital supplies these.
- Bring children with you since they may become apprehensive while waiting.

On discharge
- You will not be permitted to leave the hospital alone after administration of anesthesia. Please have someone drive you home.
- You will be discharged on your physicians's orders. Do not drive or drink alcoholic beverages for at least 12 hours after discharge.
- You may be dizzy or drowsy. Follow your doctor's orders regarding diet, rest, and medication.
- If you have medical problems, call your doctor (Tel. #_____) or Emergency Room (Tel. #_____), or Ambulatory Surgery Center (Tel. #_____).

SPECIAL PROCEDURES

Procedures commonly scheduled for the recovery room are as follows:

1. Electroconvulsive therapy
2. Cardioversion
3. Diagnostic nerve blocks
4. Blood patches
5. Blood transfusions
6. Monitoring placement

Staffing should be planned on a one-to-one basis. Most of these therapies, which usually do not require longer than 15 to 30 minutes, are performed by an anesthesiologist, assisted by a recovery room nurse. During electroconvulsive therapy, a psychiatrist is present; during cardioversion, a cardiologist is usually in attendance.

Although epidural saline and blood patches can be completed in about 15 minutes, frequently a catheter is left in place should further administration be necessary. Patients should be observed for 1 to 2 hours.

Blood transfusions are administered slowly, and the patient's stay in the recovery room may last several hours. After an initial observation period of about 15 minutes, critical nursing care is no longer essential and vital-sign monitoring every 15 minutes is adequate.

Emotional support of all these patients before, during, and after these procedures must be viewed as a major aspect of their care. Although infection control is the responsibility of all medical personnel, the recovery room nurse is frequently the main overseer of this essential aspect of patient care. Ideally a section of the recovery room which can be physically isolated should be used for all special procedures. Donning of operating room garb should be required before entering this area. Sterile gloves, masks, caps, and washing facilities should be readily available. Use of disposable equipment is recommended. Frequent hand washing between patient contact and a one-to-one patient-nurse ratio curtails infection transfer.

Electroconvulsive Therapy

Electroconvulsive therapy (ECT) is a form of treatment for many manic-depressive types of psychiatric illnesses. Important considerations in these patients include:

History of cardiovascular disease. Hypertension and bradycardia may result from electrically induced convulsions. Prior to therapy, medical consultation should indicate that any hypertensive state or arrhythmia is under the best possible control.
Evaluation of musculoskeletal disease. History of osteoporosis, frequent fractures, back pain, or disk disease should be noted as one of the complications of ECT is bony injury caused by muscle contraction.
Careful emotional support. A course of ECT involves usually five to 10 applications over a 3 to 5 week period. Moreover, by the nature of the illness, patients are frequently depressed or withdrawn. Special efforts should be made to communicate with the patients and to reassure them.
Oral intake. Two problematic areas may exist. Frequently patients are extremely dehydrated because of disinclination to eat. Preanesthetic preparation may require intravenous infusion of 1 liter or more of dextrose and lactated Ringer's solution. As patients on the psychiatric service are frequently unreliable, a careful check must be made that

a fasting state has been maintained for 6 hours prior to induction of general anesthesia.

Dentition. Poor attention to physical well-being is often manifest by oral sepsis. Loose teeth should be identified and, if necessary, removed as the induced seizure may cause them to break loose under anesthesia.

These patients are often treated as outpatients either from home or during a short transfer from a nearby psychiatric hospital. The usual preanesthetic checklist prevails and includes:

1. Identification.
2. Consent.
3. Nothing orally during the preceding 6 hours.
4. Securing of personal items (jewelry, clothing, etc.). Removal of dentures may not be necessary if these are tightly secured within the mouth.
5. History and physical, including careful note of all maintenance medications.
6. Basic laboratory tests: serum chemistries, Hb, white cell count, urinalysis, ECG, and chest X ray. These tests need not be repeated prior to every treatment if no new disease processes have developed. Individual local and hospital requirements vary, but laboratory findings are generally valid for 2 to 3 weeks.

ECT should be administered in a section of the recovery room which can be curtained off to provide privacy and space for treatment and recovery.

The necessary medications and equipment are listed in Table 13-2. The patient is prepared in bed by monitoring the blood pressure and electrocardiogram. A peripheral vein is cannulated. After preoxygenation, atropine (0.4 mg) and a barbiturate are given. Prior to injection of the short-acting muscle relaxant, the blood pressure cuff is inflated to prevent flow of blood to one arm. Should frequent premature ventricular contractions develop, lidocaine 1-2 mg/kg is given. As soon as the patient loses consciousness, ventilation must be supported. When muscle relaxation is complete, a bite block is inserted in the mouth. Electrodes coated with sufficient paste are applied bilaterally or unilaterally to the head. A single shock is administered. An attenuated seizure or downward toe movement may be observed which lasts 1 to 2 minutes. The seizure can usually be followed more accurately by observing the nonparalyzed arm.

Hypertension and either bradycardia or tachycardia occur almost immediately after the treatment. These effects are usually transient (lasting 1 to 15 minutes) and rarely require treatment. However, careful

Table 13-2. Equipment and Medications Necessary for ECT

Medications	Equipment
Atropine 0.4 mg	Anesthetic machine or AMBU bag
Pentothal 3-5 mg/kg	ECG
Succinylcholine 1 mg/kg	Suction apparatus
Lidocaine 1-2 mg/kg	Sphygmomanometer
O_2 supply	Electrodes delivering shock
Intravenous solutions	Conductive paste
	Artificial airways
	Equipment for endotracheal intubation
	Intravenous cannulation equipment

monitoring is essential. The patient should be responsive and awake within 10 minutes.

Record keeping of the vital signs, amounts of medication given, and the shock strength are very important as individual variation is commonly seen in these patients due to interaction with other long-acting drugs (tranquilizers, sedatives, antidepressants, etc.). Appropriate modification of drug dose can then be made during subsequent treatments.

Cardioversion

Cardioversion is a simple, safe, and usually effective means of converting cardiac arrhythmias to sinus rhythm. The main indications, atrial flutter and fibrillation, are usually not life-threatening situations and may be treated electively. Other arrhythmias which respond to cardioversion include ventricular tachycardia and ventricular fibrillation. These are emergency situations and are considered more fully in Chapter 4.

As elective cardioversion is usually preceded by a trial of drug therapy, these patients are generally already in hospital. Patients with a history of atrial fibrillation are frequently receiving anticoagulant medication both before and after cardioversion to avoid postconversion embolization. Quinidine is often given to patients for at least 24 hours prior to therapy as approximately 10 percent of cases may be converted by this drug alone. Digitalis and beta-adrenergic blocking agents are generally discontinued on the day prior to cardioversion as overdose of these medications may make the procedure ineffective. Hypokalemia must also be corrected.

After the patient is comfortably settled in bed, essential monitoring equipment (ECG, blood pressure) is applied. Supportive and resuscitative equipment as outlined for ECT must be readily available. A peripheral vein is cannulated and adequate pulmonary ventilation maintained with an enriched oxygen supply.

Prior to application, it is important to clean the paddles and check for formation of oxide on the surface which may impede the delivery of adequate energy. Light anesthesia or sedation, which should be managed by an anesthesiologist, is induced with small doses of sodium pentothal (2–3 mg/kg) or diazepam (5–10 mg). Muscular contractions may be caused by cardioversion but are much less severe than during ECT. However, cases have been reported of torn spinous processes, and it is therefore our routine to use small doses (0.3–0.5 mg/kg) of succinylcholine chloride and support ventilation. Deep general anesthesia is not required if energies of 100 watt-sec or less are employed. The duration of shock is 2.5 msec and pain is not generally severe. The unanesthetized patient may complain of a sensation of touching an exposed electrical outlet. However, repeated conversion at higher output levels in apprehensive elderly patients requires more sedation.

The paddles of the cardiovertor are applied over the precordium and on the patient's back (anterolateral positions may be used but these require slightly higher energy outputs). Cardioversion can only be successful when adequate amounts of conductive paste are used, the paddles are far enough apart with no bridge of gel or sweat between them, and firm contact is applied.

Initial treatment for arrhythmias of recent onset should start with low-energy current (about 20–40 watt-sec). If the first discharge is not successful, successive shocks of 50–100 watt-sec, followed by increments of 100 watt-sec are given until the arrhythmia converts. Final discharge is 400 watt-sec.

Although slight, there is a risk of electrocution and therefore, the patient is not touched when the shock is delivered. The complications and treatment of problems which may be related to cardioversion are listed in Table 13-3.

Diagnostic Nerve Blocks

The ability to provide a sterile environment and skilled monitoring make the recovery room a suitable area for performing many types of blocks. Some of the more commonly administered nerve blocks are listed in Table 13-4.

Epidural injection either as a single shot or as a continuous technique through a catheter affords good postoperative pain relief, particularly valuable in addicted patients in whom avoidance of narcotics is preferable. It may also be used as a diagnostic tool to assess the effect of pharmacologic (and therefore temporary) interruption of pain pathways prior to perma-

Table 13-3. Complications and Treatment of Problems Related or Caused by Cardioversion

Complication	Precipitating Factors	Therapy
A-V nodal arrhythmias	cardioversion	none—usually resolve spontaneously
Ventricular arrhythmias	digitalis, quinidine, hypokalemia, hypoventilation, metabolic acidosis	lidocaine 1-2 mg/kg; correct cause
Cardiac arrest	any of above	closed chest massage; cardiac pacing
Hypotension	multiple shocks high energy levels	vasopressors, (norepinephrine, dopamine); cardiac pacing
Pulmonary edema	myocardial damage	sedation; digitalis, diuretics
Burn injuries	inadequate gel application	local treatment

nent surgical or chemical section. A marked sympatholytic effect, as evidenced by increase in temperature of the lower extremities, not only indicates the benefits of surgical sympathectomy in the ischemic limb but ensures maximal blood flow to reattached tissue.

The technique involves insertion of a large bore needle (16-gauge) into the epidural space at the appropriate level. A catheter is threaded into position and the needle withdrawn. Solutions of local anesthetic agents may then be infused as necessary and the block may be maintained for hours or even days. When therapy is discontinued, the catheter should be carefully inspected to ensure its intactness and this finding noted in the patient's record.

Intercostal nerve blocks are given to relieve the pain of rib fractures and to provide analgesia after abdominal surgery and thus facilitate deep breathing and coughing. Because of overlapping of the distribution of nerves, three nerves must be injected to provide complete anesthesia for one dermatome.

Subarachnoid block is usually done for relief of chronic pain associated with cancer. In the terminal stages of this illness, subarachnoid alcohol block is used to cause a chemical posterior rhizotomy. Other techniques include the use of cold, hypertonic saline injections into the subarachnoid space. Pain relief has also been reported following barbotage of cerebrospinal fluid. Injection of local anesthetic agent combined with steroids such as methylprednisolone or dexamethasone may be effective in decreasing pain by an antiinflammatory effect. Injection is made adjacent to the suspected site of the lesion.

A small-gauge needle (22- or 25-gauge) is inserted under sterile conditions into the subarachnoid space at the appropriate level and a local anesthetic solution (usually tetracaine, which may be combined with epinephrine for longer action) is injected.

Operations involving the hands and arms are frequently performed after block of the brachial plexus which may be done by either a supraclavicular or axillary approach. As this anesthetic technique has a relatively slow onset of action (about 20 to 30 minutes until total blockade), the procedure may be performed in a holding area or in the recovery room. The technique involves placement of a small-gauge needle within the sheath of the brachial plexus and injection of about 20-40 ml of local anesthetic solution. Brachial plexus block has also been used successfully in the therapy of angina pectoris involving pain in the left arm.

Stellate ganglion block is used in the treatment of peripheral vascular disease. By abolishing sympathetic supply to the upper extremity, maximal vasodilation is achieved which is advantageous for preserving blood supply in newly anastomosed vessels or in the treatment of Reynaud's disease. It is performed by direct injection of small volumes of anesthetic solution around the stellate ganglion in the neck.

Celiac plexus block is used in the management of chronic pain from upper abdominal viscera (usually cancer pain). If several control blocks indicate good effect, the plexus may be destroyed by injection of 25 ml of alcohol 50 percent.

Prior to performing a nerve block which is usually done by an anesthesiologist or neurosurgeon, an intravenous route must be secured. Baseline vital signs should be recorded and appropriate monitoring (ECG, blood pressure) established. Equipment for emergency resuscitation should be available.

Table 13-4. Blocks Administered in the Recovery Room

Block	Indication
Epidural	pain relief; sympatholytic effect
Intercostal nerves	postoperative pain relief; *Herpes zoster*
Subarachnoid	intractable pain
Brachial plexus	preoperative—anesthetic technique; severe angina
Stellate ganglion	sympatholytic effect; Raynaud's disease
Celiac plexus	chronic pain

Other requirements include:

1. Well-lit area
2. Sterile field
3. Block sets as indicated
4. Local anesthetic solutions—usually lidocaine 0.5-1 percent; tetracaine 1 percent or chloroprocaine 0.5-3 percent
5. Epinephrine 1 ml 1:1,000 (to retard absorption of local anesthetics)

Reactions and complications after blocks are rare and are listed in Table 13-5. Local effects may be due to direct puncture of the nerve, nearby blood vessels, or inadequate sterility. Systemic reactions are directly related to the concentration of the anesthetic in the blood which is determined by the absorption, distribution, and metabolism of the agents. Injection into highly vascular areas or direct intravascular infusion will result in high blood concentrations. Complications usually involve the cardiovascular and central nervous systems. Myocardial depression, bradycardia, and severe hypotension may occur. Although local anesthetic agents have a sedative effect on the central nervous system at low blood levels, at higher levels, excitation and frank seizures may develop with respiratory impairment.

True allergy is extremely rare and limited mainly to ester type drugs like procaine. Again cardiovascular collapse and respiratory dysfunction (especially bronchospasm) may occur. Therapy includes cardiorespiratory support, sedation, and vasopressor infusions (e.g., neosynephrine 0.02 percent infusion, ephedrine 12.5 mg) as indicated.

Table 13-5. Reactions and Complications after Nerve Blocks

Local effect in the immediate area of the block	Pain Hematoma Paresthesias Infection

Systemic reaction affecting the body as a whole	Local anesthetic action
	  Cardiovascular collapse
	  Seizures
	  Allergic phenomenon
	Vasopressor action
	  Tachycardia
	  Hypertension
	  Sweating
	  Apprehension

More commonly, reaction may result from overdose of added vasoconstrictor substances. Treatment includes administration of alpha- and beta-adrenergic blocking drugs such as phentolamine and propranolol, sedation, and constant reassurance.

Blood Patches

A distressing complication of subarachnoid puncture is headache. Although this symptom usually resolves with bed rest, analgesics, and adequate hydration, occasionally, the pain may be incapacitating. An epidural injection of normal saline (30-50 ml) or of the patient's own blood may be beneficial. A catheter is inserted into the same interspace at which the subarachnoid puncture was performed and fluid injected slowly until the headache abates. Adequate hydration must be maintained and the patient should be nursed supine for 24 to 48 hours.

Blood Transfusions

Again for reasons of sterility, appropriate monitoring and availability of skilled personnel, the recovery room may be used as a convenient location to admit patients who require frequent and repeated blood transfusions. These patients are often debilitated with other severe medical problems such as renal failure, metastatic carcinoma, leukemia, and hemophilia.
Requirements for blood transfusion include:

1. Warm, quiet area—preferably with a view through a window
2. ECG and blood pressure monitoring
3. Facilities for hand washing
4. Intravenous trays
5. Equipment for warming blood

Occasionally patients prefer some light sedation prior to receiving blood. If a television set or radio is available, this provides excellent diversion. Warming blood prior to infusion decreases the incidence of cardiac arrhythmias and patient discomfort from cooling. Some filtration system in the administration set is also essential. However, platelets should not be given through a blood filter.

During transfusions, patients should be kept warm, the electrocardiogram monitored for arrhythmias due to cold or hyperkalemia, and the infusion site frequently inspected for infiltration or other reactions.

Hemolytic reaction, an immediate complication of blood transfusion, is caused by incompatibility between antibodies in the recipient's plasma and antigen contained in the donor erythrocytes (see Table 13-6). General hemolysis follows. The commonest causes of this reaction are mistakes in typing, cross matching, initial sampling, or unit administration. The hemolytic process may rapidly progress to disseminated intravascular coagulopathy (DIC). Signs and symptoms include fever, shivering, chills, apprehension, hypotension, tachycardia, and hemoglobinuria.

Treatment, which is aimed at control of bleeding and prevention of renal damage is along these lines:

1. Stop the transfusion. Return the blood to the bank.
2. Describe the patient's symptoms to the bank technician or supervisor.
3. Support the cardiovascular system. Give fluids including protein and hetastarch until compatible blood is available. Administer vasopressors as necessary.
4. Monitor the blood and urine for free hemoglobin.
5. Give mannitol (0.5-1 g/kg intravenously) and follow with furosemide 40-80 mg intravenously to ensure renal output of at least 100 ml per hour.
6. An arterial cannula should be placed and blood gases monitored.
7. Acidosis and hyperkalemia should be corrected.
8. Steroids may be given to modify the antigen antibody reaction. Antihistamines may also be used (diphenhydramine 50 mg).
9. Platelet count, partial thromboplastin time, and complete blood counts should be followed hourly. Hematologic consultation should be sought early.
10. Should DIC develop, supportive therapy must be maintained.
11. All steps must be carefully documented on the hospital record.

If blood is transfused too rapidly, especially if there is preexistent cardiac disease, circulatory overload may develop. Useful drugs which improve cardiac function and allow the vascular system to better tolerate expansion include calcium chloride, dopamine, and digitalis preparations. Diuretics such as furosemide may be necessary. Occasionally ventilatory support is indicated.

By-products of bacteria which persist after sterilization are termed "pyrogens." Use of disposable equipment has essentially eliminated this problem. However, errors in technique of blood collection may result in contamination, especially with gram-negative bacteria and their endotoxins. If septicemia develops, the outcome is usually fatal despite vigorous therapy. Prevention includes adequate refrigeration, dating procedures, careful biologic control, and discarding of open bottles.

Allergic reactions due to the presence in the donor blood of an antigen or antibody whose immunologic counterpart is present in the recipient occurs during about 1 percent of transfusions. The reactions are

Table 13-6. Common Complications Associated with Blood Transfusions

Disease transmission	hepatitis (serum, infectious)
	malaria
	AIDS
	syphilis
	brucellosis
Hemolytic transfusion reaction	shivering
	apprehension
	hypotension
	hemoglobinuria
	DIC
Cardiac failure	hypotension
	tachycardia
	pulmonary edema
Bacteremia	fever
	chills
Allergic reactions	urticaria
	flushing
	tachycardia
	fever
	bronchospasm

usually transient and the transfusion may be continued. Rarely angioneurotic edema or bronchospasm may require emergency therapy with epinephrine, steroids, and respiratory support.

Preoperative Placement of Invasive Monitoring Systems

Monitoring during anesthesia frequently involves measurements from catheters in veins and arteries. In the interest of efficient use of time, these cannulas may be inserted preoperatively under sterile conditions in the recovery room. Although emotional support of the patients is necessary, general anesthesia is usually not required. Central venous, Swan-Ganz, and arterial catheters may all be conveniently placed. Requirements include sterile techniques, cardiovascular monitoring, and suitable transducers and other recording apparatus.

LEGAL ISSUES

All procedures performed in the recovery room must be outlined in the hospital's manual. Although the physician performing the procedure (e.g., the psychiatrist for ECT, the cardiologist for cardioversion) assumes medical responsibility for the patient in the recovery room, the department of anesthesiology is in charge of the recovery room in many hospitals. Therefore, all such therapies should be scheduled with the anesthesiologist who usually will either perform the test (e.g., blocks, cannula insertion) or be in attendance (e.g., ECT, cardioversion).

All procedures (except blood transfusion) require a signed and witnessed surgical consent. It is the recovery room nurse's responsibility to verify the consent form.

SUGGESTIONS FOR FURTHER READING

Covino BG, Vassallo HG. Local anesthetics mechanisms of action and clinical use. New York: Grune and Stratton, 1976.

Lichtiger M, Moya F. Introduction to the practice of anesthesia. 2d ed. New York: Harper and Row, 1978.

Stark DCC. Practical points in anesthesiology. 2d ed. New York: Medical Exam Publishing, 1980.

14
Cardiopulmonary Arrest
Marcelle M. Willock

Cardiac arrest is not a common complication in the recovery room, although life-threatening emergencies frequently occur there. These are mostly respiratory or cardiovascular events, but surgical, neurologic, metabolic, and pharmacologic reasons may abound, and early recognition of these problems may avoid more serious sequelae. Training for nurses and physicians in recovery room management has always addressed these emergencies. "Standards and Guidelines for Cardiopulmonary Resuscitation (CPR) and Emergency Cardiac Care (ECC)" was first published by the American Heart Association (AHA) in 1974 and was updated in 1980.

These guidelines are divided into two components: basic life support (BLS) and advanced cardiac life support (ACLS). BLS covers airway maintenance, breathing, and circulation at a minimum level; ACLS covers the use of adjunctive equipment and drugs to improve ventilation and cardiovascular and metabolic consequences of the initial problem. All physicians and nurses should be certified in basic CPR skills. It is highly recommended that all anesthesiologists also be certified in ACLS, and that the course be given to recovery room nursing staff, with or without a requirement for certification. Since the outcome of patients when ACLS follows BLS promptly is significantly improved, and the necessary equipment and drugs as well as staff knowledgeable in their use are always available in the recovery room, BLS and ACLS are integrated here for recovery room care.

AIRWAY

The tongue is the most common cause of upper airway obstruction in unconscious patients in the supine position. The causes of loss of tone and airway obstruction in the recovery room are myriad and include: (1) unconsciousness secondary to residual anesthetic agents, either inhalational or intravenous; (2) residual muscle relaxant effect; (3) preoperative condition of the patient; (4) intraoperative events; (5) shock; (6) medications given in the recovery room; (7) surgical causes, e.g., type of operation, hemorrhage, and edema.

With loss of tone, the tongue falls back against the posterior pharyngeal wall and obstructs free passage of air into and out of the lungs. Extending the head and lifting the chin (head tilt-chin lift) is the simplest method to open the airway. Alternatively, extending the head and thrusting the mandible forward (head tilt-jaw thrust) by placing the thumb and third fingers behind the angles of the mandible or lifting the chin can accomplish the same goal. For patients who have cervical spine injuries, the jaw thrust without head tilt is preferred. In the recovery room it is common to nurse patients in the lateral position, which allows the tongue to fall forward. If the patient suffers a cardiopulmonary arrest, the patient should be turned supine, for it is easier for the rescuer to perform the above maneuvers with the patient in the supine position. Should there be surgical causes of airway obstruction, e.g., hemorrhage into the neck or airway, then evacuation of blood is mandatory.

If the tilting, lifting, or thrusting maneuvers fail to relieve the obstruction or do so only temporarily, it is necessary to use adjuncts, i.e., nasopharyngeal or oropharyngeal airways, or endotracheal tubes. The nasopharyngeal airway is usually better tolerated by semiconscious patients. If the oropharyngeal or nasopharyngeal airway is insufficient to relieve the obstruction, as may be the case in epiglottic obstruction, then endotracheal intubation is indicated. The esophageal obturator airway (EOA) and the esophageal gastric tube airway (EGTA) are devices designed for out-of-hospital use and have no place in the recovery room.

BREATHING

Once the airway is patent, the adequacy of breathing must be ascertained. Adequacy is defined as normal alveolar ventilation for each patient in terms of rate and tidal volume and, as sometimes measured, blood gases. Many of the causes of airway obstruction will also depress respiration and reduce alveolar ventilation. Closely allied to the mechanical ability to maintain an adequate minute ventilation is the lung's ability to oxygenate the blood. Patients in the recovery room receive supplemental oxygen and occasionally mechanical ventilation. When a patient in the recovery room develops cardiac or pulmonary arrest, immediate ventilation must be instituted, using resuscitation ventilation bags. These are designed to fit onto masks or endotracheal tubes, to self-inflate, and when squeezed to deliver varying amounts of gas into the lungs. There is a one-way valve at the mask or tube end so that the patient's expired gas passes to the atmosphere.

These bags are commonly known by their trade names, e.g., AMBU and Hope. The oxygen concentration can be increased to 50-60 percent by adding oxygen at a flow rate of 10 to 15 liters per minute through tubing attached to the inflow nipple. If a reservoir (either a bag or length of tubing equal in volume to the bag) is also added, the oxygen concentration in the bag may be increased to almost 100 percent. In cases of cardiopulmonary arrest, a bag configured to deliver 100 percent oxygen must be used in order to achieve the highest PaO_2 possible. Thus adjuncts for ventilation include:

1. Oxygen
2. Oral airways
3. Nasal airways
4. Endotracheal tubes
5. Masks
6. AMBU bags

CIRCULATION

Support of depressed circulation is usually achieved by pharmacologic means except in early hypovolemic shock, when fluids, Trendelenburg position, or antishock garments are used, and in cardiogenic shock, when an intraaortic balloon for counterpulsation is used. When the circulation stops, as in cardiac arrest, compression of the chest is mandatory to provide an instant cardiac output. Adjuncts for artificial circulation include

1. Bed board
2. Manual chest compressor
3. Automatic chest compressor
4. Antishock garments
5. Intraaortic balloon

The technique of cardiac compression is described in the AHA guidelines and should be perfected by practice on mannequins. The recommended cardiac compression rate is 60 per minute in the adult, with a breath interspersed on the upstroke of every fifth compression. A compression-relaxation ratio of 50:50 can be accomplished easily by manual compression. A bed board should be placed under the patient's back.

Manual or automatic mechanical compressors are on the market. The cardiac press is manual and consists of a backboard attached to a compressor that is manually adjustable to compress the sternum 1.5-2 inches. This device relieves the staff of the exhausting task of compression, but has a tendency to slip from its initial position and for the tightening screw to loosen, resulting in less excursion and inadequate compression. The automatic chest compressor has a backboard, but its plunger is powered by compressed gas. In addition, it can be set to ventilate the lungs in relation to cardiac compression. Recent data seem to indicate that a slightly longer compression-relaxation ratio and compression with the lungs inflated result in better blood flow and blood pressure.

Closed-chest massage is the preferred method of cardiac resuscitation. However, in the recovery room, surgical procedures in the thoracic cavity may result in conditions (e.g., cardiac tamponade) that are best treated by opening the chest and directly compressing the heart. If the patient has anatomic deformities of the chest which interfere with effective closed-chest compression, open-chest massage should be considered. Open-chest massage has other advantages, especially in hypovolemic shock, for it facilitates the diagnosis of an empty heart. The use of fluids or antishock garments may facilitate resuscitation.

The antishock garment (e.g., MAST, military antishock trousers) is a one-piece outfit with separate compartments for the legs and abdomen and can be inflated to a maximum internal pressure greater than 100 mm Hg. The legs should always be inflated prior to the abdominal section, and the thoracic cage should never be encircled by the garment. Inflated, the garment increases venous return and cardiac output. If this autotransfusion results in hemodynamic and clinical improvement, there is reasonable certainty of hypovolemia, and fluids should be administered. After correction of the hypovolemia, the garment should be deflated slowly in the reverse order, i.e., abdomen first and legs last. The patient's blood pressure should be continually monitored; a fall in pressure means more fluid is needed. It may be necessary to reinflate the garment in the interim.

If inflation of the antishock garment does not result in hemodynamic and clinical improvement, other causes of shock should be sought. The use of this device is contraindicated in cardiogenic shock, for the autotransfusion will only augment pulmonary congestion.

For those patients with cardiogenic shock refractory to fluid and pharmacologic therapy, an intraaortic balloon may be helpful. This device must be inserted surgically after the patient has been heparinized. It consists of a catheter with an elongated balloon that is placed in the descending aorta. Position is checked by X-ray or fluoroscopy. The balloon is mechanically and automatically operated. A sensor reads the ECG and the balloon is inflated, occluding the distal aorta right after closure of the aortic valve and improving coronary perfusion. At the onset of ventricular asystole, the balloon is deflated, lessening impediment to left ventricular ejection and reducing left ventricular stroke work. If the use of the balloon results in hemodynamic and clinical improvement, duration of full counterpulsation is variable before weaning from counterpulsation and eventual withdrawal of this mechanical support to the circulation. Surgical closure of the arteriotomy is necessary, as is checking the distal pulses, either by palpation or Doppler to ascertain good distal perfusion.

INTRAVENOUS FLUIDS

Every patient in the recovery room should have at least one patent free-flowing intravenous cannula in place. Fluid balance is part of the admission history, and thus if a cardiac arrest occurs, the staff will have a fair estimate of the fluid state. If hypovolemia is present, one or more routes are needed for volume expansion with any of the following solutions: normal saline, Ringer's lactate, plasma protein fraction, albumin, or blood. Central lines, e.g., jugular, subclavian, or femoral, may be needed for certain drugs. If the arrest is not associated with hypovolemia, then fluids should be given with caution.

DRUG THERAPY

The aims of drug therapy are as follows:

1. Correct hypoxemia
2. Correct metabolic acidosis
3. Increase perfusion pressure
4. Increase myocardial contractility
5. Control ventricular ectopy
6. Improve cardiac output
7. Control blood pressure
8. Treat pulmonary edema
9. Alleviate pain

Of major importance is the correction of hypoxemia by adjunctive airway equipment, administration of 100 percent oxygen, and measurement of arterial blood gases to determine adequacy of oxygenation and ventilation. With FiO_2 1.0, PaO_2 should be at least 80 mm Hg. If it is less, the endotracheal tube, oxygen flow rate, and resuscitation bag must be checked to determine that the tube is properly located and oxygen is flowing and connected to the resuscitation bag. If hypercapnia is present, the patient's minute ventilation must be increased. Repeated blood gas determinations are necessary.

Inadequate perfusion and oxygenation lead to metabolic acidosis. When resuscitation after cardiac arrest is begun promptly in a previously normal patient, acidosis will not be present initially, and sodium bicarbonate is not required immediately. However, acidosis will ensue with time even when cardiac compression is carried out according to AHA protocol because a low flow state exists. It is estimated that cardiac output is only about 25-30 percent of normal after external chest compressions. Both left and right ventricular outputs are depressed. Problems in oxygenation as well as CO_2 elimination may occur, and there is a buildup of carbonic and lactic acids.

Providing 100 percent oxygen and adequate minute ventilation are essential to correct the respiratory component of problems associated with cardiac arrest. But these are not enough if the arrest is greater than two minutes duration or if the patient previously had metabolic acidosis. It is important to assess the relative contributions of carbonic and lactic acid to the acidotic state. This can be done by using the three golden rules of the AHA (Table 14-1).

First the respiratory factors must be quantified. It is known that for every 10 mm Hg increase or decrease in $PaCO_2$ there is a respective decrease or increase in pH of 0.08 (golden rule 1). This formula is used to correct the actual pH for the respiratory component and then to determine the metabolic component. Golden rule 2 states that for each 0.15 pH increase or decrease there is a concomitant increase or decrease of 10 mEq/liter base. After the base deficit has been determined, total body bicarbonate deficit is calculated by the formula BE(mEq/liter) times weight (kg) divided by 4 (golden rule 3). In cases of cardiac arrest a full calculated amount of sodium bicarbonate should be given to raise the pH to a level conducive to successful defibrillation. However, once the heart has been restarted, the dose of sodium bicarbonate should be cut in half for several reasons. With better circulation and oxygenation, the metabolic acidosis will self-correct to varying degrees. Second there are numerous hazards associated with the rapid administration of sodium bicarbonate. Dysrhythmias or convulsions may occur secondary to rapid ion shifts across

Table 14-1. AHA Golden Rules to Assess Acidosis

Rule 1: Respiratory acidosis
↑ $PaCO_2$ 10 mm Hg → ↓ pH 0.08
↓ $PaCO_2$ 10 mm Hg → ↑ pH 0.08
Rule 2: Metabolic acidosis
↑ pH 0.15 → ↑ base 10 mEq/liter
↓ pH 0.15 → ↓ base 10 mEq/liter
Rule 3: Total body base deficit
$$TBD = \frac{BE(mEq/liter) \times wt\ (kg)}{4}$$

cell membranes. Metabolic alkalosis may occur with a shift in the hemoglobin dissociation curve. Hypokalemia, hypernatremia, and hyperosmolality are also possible consequences. Third, the reaction of sodium bicarbonate as it forms HCO_3^- must be understood.

$$HCO_3^- + H^+ \rightarrow H_2CO_3 \rightleftharpoons H_2O + CO_2$$

Thus after administration of large doses of sodium bicarbonate, the patient must be hyperventilated to expire the excess CO_2 thus produced.

Epinephrine is the drug of choice to improve perfusion pressure and promote spontaneous or better myocardial contractility. It is given in large doses, 1 mg every 5 minutes, at which dosage the alpha effect predominates. If an intravenous route is not available, the same dose should be given via the trachea. The intracardiac route is the least preferred because it takes time to perform and is associated with complications such as failed administration, lung puncture, and myocardial damage.

Epinephrine will also convert fine fibrillation to coarse fibrillation, which is more amenable to defibrillation. In asystole, epinephrine has been found to initiate electrical and mechanical activity; in other pulseless rhythms such as electromechanical dissociation (EMD), it can augment myocardial contractility.

Oxygen, sodium bicarbonate, and epinephrine are the three first-line drugs that can be administered after a cardiac arrest without awaiting a more specific diagnosis. Other first-line drugs—lidocaine, procainamide, bretylium, verapamil, calcium chloride, atropine, and morphine—are targeted to a diagnosis.

DYSRHYTHMIA

Once a diagnosis of cardiac arrest has been made and basic or advanced cardiac life support started, an important step is the identification of the cardiac rhythm. The AHA guidelines require that persons providing advanced cardiac life support be able to recognize the following ECG patterns:

1. Sinus tachycardia
2. Sinus bradycardia
3. Premature atrial complexes
4. Atrial tachycardia
5. Atrial flutter
6. Atrial fibrillation
7. Junctional rhythms
8. Premature ventricular complexes (frequent, multifocal R or T phenomena)
9. Ventricular trachycardia

10. Ventricular fibrillation
11. Ventricular asystole
12. Atrioventricular (AV) block; first degree, second degree (Mobitz I and II), and third degree
13. Ventricular and supraventricular rhythms with aberrant conduction

The common arrhythmias are discussed in Chapter 4. Immediate life-threatening dysrhythmias — ventricular tachycardia, ventricular fibrillation, and ventricular asystole — and electromechanical dissociation are discussed here.

By definition, ventricular tachycardia (VT) is three or more sequential ventricular complexes occurring at a rate greater than 100 per minute. The rhythm may be regular or irregular, and may or may not generate a pulse. Normal sinoatrial (SA) node activity may continue and can result in a variety of pictures on the ECG screen. P waves may occur but show no relationship to the QRS complex. SA node discharge may be received by the AV node and HIS-Purkinje system when these are nonrefractory, and therefore, a "normal" QRS complex (a capture beat) may occur. It is also possible that the ventricle will be depolarized from an aberrant focus at the same time, resulting in a fusion beat. Last, the ventricles may depolarize the atria by retrograde conduction, and in this case there may be a constant relationship between the QRS and P waves.

When a patient with VT by monitor has a pulse and is hemodynamically stable, intravenous lidocaine is the drug of choice. Initial dose is 1 mg/kg, followed immediately with an infusion of 1 mg per minute. If the arrhythmia is not terminated by the first bolus, repeated 50-mg boluses can be given every 5 minutes, up to 225 mg total. If the patient does not respond to lidocaine, procainamide is the next drug of choice. The dosage is 100 mg every 5 minutes given at a rate of 20 mg per minute. The endpoint of this medication is any of the following: (1) the dysrhythmia ceases, (2) hypotension, (3) QRS increase by 50 percent of original width, or (4) total of 1 gm given. If the VT is refractory to both lidocaine and procainamide, bretylium is indicated. The dosage is 5-10 mg/kg over 8-10 minutes. If the abnormality persists, the dose can be repeated an hour later.

When the patient with VT is pulseless or otherwise hemodynamically unstable (hypotension or pulmonary edema), immediate DC-synchronized cardioversion is indicated. Initial dosage is 20 joules. If the first shock is unsuccessful, repeated shocks should be given, the energy being increased incrementally to a maximum of 200 joules. In cases of recurring VT or VT refractory to drug therapy, a transvenous pacemaker, set for overdrive pacing, may relieve the dysrhythmia.

Ventricular fibrillation (VF) is a dire, life-threatening complication. Depolarization of the ventricles is random, resulting in chaotic contraction of the myocardial fibers and no stroke volume ejected. The ECG may show small wave amplitude (fine VF) or large wave amplitude (coarse VF). When VF appears in a patient being monitored, one precordial thump should be given immediately. If this is not successful in stopping the dysrhythmia, defibrillation should be instituted immediately, prior to starting basic life support, with an initial energy setting of 200-300 joules. If the first shock is unsuccessful, another should be given immediately. If this is unsuccessful, basic life support should be started, epinephrine and sodium bicarbonate given, and countershocks at a maximum of 360 joules applied. If the chest is open and the paddles applied directly on the heart, then the initial dose is 5 joules and is incrementally increased to a maximum of 40 joules if repeated shocks are needed.

Ventricular asystole means cardiac standstill. There is neither electrical nor mechanical activity in the heart, although P waves may rarely be seen. Asystole may occur spontaneously or may follow VF. Basic CPR should be started, the patient intubated quickly, ventilated with 100 percent oxygen, and epinephrine 0.5-1.0 mg given intravenously. This may initiate cardiac action. If acidosis is suspected, sodium bicarbonate 1 mEq/kg should be given followed by atropine 1-2 mg intravenously. If there is no improvement, calcium chloride 500-1,000 mg intravenously is administered. Cardiac compression must be continued throughout the resuscitation to provide an effective circulation. Defibrillation may be tried, for it is sometimes difficult to distinguish fine fibrillation from asystole on the ECG.

Electromechanical dissociation (EMD) is a condition whereby the electrical depolarization of the heart is not followed by mechanical contraction. Once diagnosed, basic CPR with intubation and administration of 100 percent oxygen are followed by epinephrine 0.5-1.0 mg and sodium bicarbonate 1 mEq/kg. If no pulse results, calcium chloride 500-1,000 mg is given. Should no change result, acidosis should be corrected and further doses of epinephrine and calcium chloride given. Isoproterenol may be helpful. In the recovery room especially, other causes of pulselessness should be considered: cardiac tamponade, myocardial rupture, ruptured aneurysm, and so on.

What happens after successful defibrillation? The patient should continue to be ventilated with 100 percent oxygen, and carotid pulse should immediately be palpated as a guide to the adequacy of the circulation. An artery should be cannulated as soon as possible to allow continuous monitoring of systemic arterial pressure and frequent blood gas and electrolyte determinations. A number of arrhythmias may occur. There may be a supraventricular rhythm, sinus or otherwise, with a normal or fast rate. A lidocaine bolus 1 mg/kg followed by a continuous infusion of lidocaine 1-4 mg per minute should be administered. There may be bradycardia with junctional escape or atrioventricular arrhythmia.

Adequacy of oxygenation should be checked and acidosis corrected if present. Should these measures fail to result in a rate greater than 50 beats per minute, atropine 0.5 mg intravenously should be given to a maximum of four doses, or 2.0 mg. Isoproterenol may be effective, and epinephrine or norepinephrine may be needed to raise arterial blood pressure. A pacemaker may also be considered. Cardiac standstill may follow ventricular defibrillation. First, adequacy of ventilation should be ascertained and acidosis corrected, then the usual procedures for asystole followed. Ventricular fibrillation may recur after a successful defibrillation. Oxygenation and acid-base balance must be checked and corrections made as needed, and cardiac compressions should be reinstituted. Epinephrine 0.5–1.0 mg is given and defibrillation is again attempted at 200 joules. If fibrillation persists, then bretylium 5–10 mg/kg is given. Table 14-2 lists the first-line drug dosages and actions.

DEFIBRILLATORS

The many different defibrillators on the market all operate on the same principles. They may be electrically or battery operated, but are all DC defibrillators. The energy is stored in capacitors and passes through current-limited inductors to the paddles. The optimal paddle shape and size for adults seem to be a round shape of 13 cm diameter.

For external defibrillation there is a choice of paddle placement: standard and anterior-posterior. In standard placement, one paddle is to the right of the sternum and below the clavicles, and the other is at the apex of the heart. In the anterior-posterior placement, one paddle is over the precordium while the other is under the back directly behind the heart. This requires a flat paddle for the posteriorly positioned one. For open-chest defibrillation, one paddle is placed over the right atrium and the other at the apex of the heart.

The skin poses resistance to the current reaching the heart, and therefore, some means of reducing this resistance is necessary. This may be accomplished by using commercial defibrillator pads, saline-moistened sponges, or electrode paste between the paddles and the patient's skin. The sponges should be moistened but not so wet that the saline flows all over the chest. Similarly, the electrode paste should be only under the paddles, for when the current is applied it may bridge over rather than transverse the chest. In open-heart defibrillation, saline-moistened sponges are placed on the right atrium and apex of the heart under the paddles.

Operating the defibrillator is relatively easy after it is switched on. Some have "quick-look" paddles, i.e., the ECG can be picked up via the paddles and displayed on the defibrillator screen. The energy is selected and the capacitor switch is activated to charge it to the preselected level.

Table 14-2. First-line Drugs: Their Dosages and Actions

Drug	Dose	Action
Oxygen	15 liters/min	correct hypoxia
Sodium bicarbonate	1 mEq/kg	correct acidosis
Epinephrine	0.5–1.0 mg	increase perfusion pressure; enhance myocardial contractility; promote coarse fibrillation; increase myocardial automotivity
Lidocaine	1 mg/kg (maximum 225 mg)	suppress ventricular automaticity
Procainamide	100 mg q 5 min (maximum 1 gm)	suppress ventricular dysrhythmias
Bretylium	5–10 mg/kg (maximum 20 mg/kg in 2 hours)	elevate fibrillation threshold
Atropine	0.5–2.0 mg (maximum 2.0 mg)	reduce vagal tone
Verapamil	0.075–0.15 mg/kg (maximum 15/mg 30 min)	block slow (calcium) channels
Calcium chloride	5–7 mg/kg	increase myocardial contractility
Morphine	2–5 mg q 5–30 min	relieve pain; increase venous pooling; decrease systemic vascular resistance

Once the desired energy level is achieved, the paddles are placed with firm pressure on the patient's chest. The operator should ensure that everyone is clear of the patient and then depress the buttons discharging the energy into the patient. After defibrillation, the ECG and pulse are checked. If fibrillation is still present, the defibrillator must be recharged in order to discharge another shock. If the fibrillation is successfully termianted, then the defibrillator should be turned off. Steps in defibrillation are:

1. Identify VF on ECG monitor.
2. Turn defibrillator on.
3. Select energy level.
4. Charge capacitor.
5. Apply defibrillator pads, saline-soaked sponges, or electrode jelly to patient's chest.
6. Place paddles on patient's chest in proper position with firm pressure.
7. Recheck rhythm on ECG monitor.

8. Check that everyone is clear of patient.
9. Call out "All clear."
10. Defibrillate by depressing both buttons on paddles simultaneously.
11. Recheck rhythm on ECG.
12. Feel for carotid pulse.

In cases of ventricular and superventricular tachydysrhythmias, a synchronized cardioversion is indicated, in which case the operation of the defibrillator is slightly different. The synchronizing switch is activated, which prohibits the operator from discharging the energy. Instead, the defibrillator is programmed to be activated by the R wave of the ECG. The energy level is selected at 200 joules, the capacitor charged to that level, and the paddles applied firmly on the patient over an appropriate skin-resistant reducing substance. The ECG on the defibrillator is checked to ensure that a prominent R wave is visible, and both buttons are depressed on the defibrillator. The defibrillator will discharge after being activated by the R wave. After the shock is given, the ECG should be checked for rhythm and the pulse palpated. It may be necessary to repeat the synchronized cardioversion, in which case, all the steps must be followed again. Should ventricular fibrillation occur after a synchronized cardioversion, the synchronizer switch must be turned off, and the process for defibrillation followed. Steps in synchronized cardioversion are

1. Identify VT or SVT on ECG monitor.
2. Turn defibrillator on.
3. Activate synchronizer switch.
4. Select energy level.
5. Charge capacitor.
6. Apply defibrillator pads, saline-soaked sponges, or electrode jelly to patient's chest.
7. Place paddles on patient's chest in proper position with firm pressure.
8. Recheck rhythm on ECG monitor, look for R wave.
9. Check that everyone is clear of patient.
10. Cardiovert by depressing and holding down both buttons on paddles until discharge occurs.
11. Recheck rhythm on ECG.
12. Feel for carotid pulse.

Patients who manifest AV nodal reentrant tachydysrhythmias may benefit from verapamil. The initial bolus is 0.075–0.15 mg/kg over 1 minute. If this is not successful in terminating the arrhythmia, a repeat dose of 0.15 mg/kg may be given within 30 minutes after the first dose, with a caveat that the total dose within 30 minutes not exceed 15 mg.

POSTRESUSCITATION MANAGEMENT

What happens after resuscitation depends on the patient's immediate response, the duration of the resuscitative effort, and the patient's prearrest status.

Assuming a previously healthy individual with a short period of resuscitation who awakens rapidly, is appropriately responsive, has stable hemodynamic values, and breathes spontaneously, normal recovery room care (i.e., monitoring of vital signs and the ECG and administration of oxygen) should be continued while a diligent search for the cause of the arrest is made. A complete neurologic examination should be performed to assess the patient's status and to compare it to the prearrest or preoperative state. A chest X ray should be done and the film reviewed to rule out any pulmonary problems and to confirm placement of any central cannulas. A 12-lead ECG should be recorded, dated, and timed for a comparison with previous and subsequent strips. Blood for serum electrolytes, arterial blood gases, and cardiac enzymes should be drawn. The patient should be closely watched in the recovery room for some time, and the decision to transfer him from the recovery room to another unit should be made after reassessing his status through multidisciplinary consultation.

Patients may manifest single or multisystem failure after resuscitation. The base-line recovery room care remains the same, but these patients may require endotracheal intubation with any of the various modalities of mechanical ventilation and varying concentrations of oxygen. Close monitoring of arterial blood gases is needed. Support of the circulation may call for vasoactive, cardiotonic, or diuretic drugs (Table 14-3). Measures to forestall occurrence of dysrhythmias should be started. In these cases, arterial and pulmonary artery pressures should be monitored and cardiac output determined. A transvenous pacemaker may also be needed. A Foley catheter in the bladder provides a means of assessing renal function and fluid balance.

The central nervous system will have suffered a great insult by the cardiopulmonary arrest. After 2-4 minutes of arrest, brain glucose and glycogen stores fall, and after 5 minutes, adenosine triphosphate (ATP) is gone, resulting in inactivation of the intracellular sodium pump mechanism and increase in intracellular water. Not only does intracellular edema occur, but there are also changes in cellular and vascular permeability, and autoregulation of the cerebral circulation is lost. Blood flow to the brain will depend on an effective perfusion pressure, i.e., mean arterial pressure minus intracranial pressure (ICP). It may be necessary to monitor ICP directly. Therapy is aimed at maintaining adequate cerebral perfusion pressure (CPP) at 80-100 mm Hg with well-oxygenated blood (PaO_2 greater than 80 mm Hg) and a $PaCO_2$ between 28 and 32 mm Hg. Elevating the

Table 14-3. Second-line Drugs: Their Dosages and Actions

Drug	Dose	Action
Norepinephrine	16 μg/ml titrated	increase myocardial contractility
Dopamine	2-20 μg/kg/min titrated	increase cardiac output; increase blood pressure
Dobutamine	2.5-10 μg/kg/min titrated	increase myocardial contractility
Isoproterenol	2-20 μg/min titrated	increase heart rate; increase myocardial contractility; decrease systemic vascular resistance
Metaraminol	0.4 mg/ml titrated	increase blood pressure
Propranolol	1-5 mg titrated	decrease heart rate; suppress dysrhythmias
Nitroglycerin	10-50 μg/min titrated	dilate coronary arteries; decrease blood pressure
Nitroprusside	0.5-8 μg/kg/min titrated	decrease blood pressure

head 30 degrees promotes venous drainage and decreases cerebral edema. Osmotic and loop diuretics are given to reduce cerebral edema. There is controversy regarding the use of corticosteroids in this phase of management.

If coma persists, other causes should be sought, e.g., hyperosmolar state, diabetes, severe electrolyte imbalance, and catastrophic intracranial events, and appropriate therapy instituted. Fever must be controlled, but although hypothermia is theoretically beneficial, it is not routinely used. Should convulsions occur, these must be controlled with barbiturates, diphenylhydantoin, or diazepam.

General supportive care is important. The eyes should be coated with methylcellulose and protective measures taken to avoid corneal abrasions or ulceration. Tracheal suctioning should be done quickly, for ICP rises with each suction. The hands and feet should be supported in functional positions. A nasogastric tube should be inserted and its output checked for volume and signs of bleeding. Cimetidine may be indicated because of the high incidence of gastric stress ulceration.

EQUIPMENT

Every recovery room should have a defibrillator and a crash cart. The cart should be stocked with airway equipment as well as minor surgical and thorocotomy trays. The number of each item must be adjusted to meet the size and needs of the unit.

First-line drugs should be stocked on the crash cart in easily opened and administered packages and in standard doses. Second-line drugs are commonly found in the medicine cabinet, and it may not be necessary to have these on the cart.

The crash cart and defibrillator should be checked at least once daily and on every shift in those units open 24 hours. Once a month the Bioengineering Department should check the accuracy of the output and note this on the defibrillator.

SUMMARY

The guidelines of the American Heart Association for BLS and ACLS are presented, tailored to the specific needs of the recovery room. It is highly recommended that all anesthesiologists and recovery room nursing personnel take a full course in ACLS.

SUGGESTIONS FOR FURTHER READING

American Heart Association. Standards and guidelines for cardiopulmonary resuscitation (CPR) and emergency cardiac care (ECC). JAMA 1980; 244: 453–509.

American Heart Association. Textbook of advanced cardiac life support. Dallas: AHA, 1981.

15
Criteria for Establishment of Brain Death
Ashok Kumar

The recovery room nurse may be involved in the care of the brain-dead patient under several circumstances. Patients who have suffered irreversible brain damage and who are potential organ donors may be transferred to the recovery room because of its proximity to the operating room. Occasionally, all criteria for brain death may not have been met and the patient may be nursed at this location for hours or even days. Patients may have been moribund preoperatively or suffered an intraoperative catastrophe. Examples of this would include the patient with massive pulmonary embolism scheduled for umbrella insertion or the patient who develops disseminated intravascular coagulopathy in response to multiple blood transfusions. Another example is the patient who has undergone posterior fossa exploration which carries potential risk of brain stem injury. Occasionally fatally injured multiple trauma victims may be transferred directly from the emergency room to the recovery room for attempted preoperative stabilization or monitoring or simply because of lack of other suitable bed space. Rarely a patient may sustain an overwhelming postoperative complication such as myocardial infarction or massive aspiration.

The need to accurately identify death of the brain became apparent some 30 years ago with the advent of transplant surgery. For obvious reasons, not least among them the legal considerations, it is essential that extensive measurement, observation, and documentation demonstrate that there can be no return of cerebral function before life support systems are withdrawn.

Brain death refers to death of a single organ. These patients have sustained an acute irreversible structural brain damage and are profoundly comatose and apneic. Without intervention, anoxia causes dysfunction of the heart and other organs and death of the individual. With modern technology, ventilation, renal status, and nutritional requirements can be adequately met, but brain function cannot be revitalized.

Death has been traditionally viewed as cessation of heart action. However, cardiac function can be taken over by machines or even by a transplant. The state of the scientific art is far from envisioning brain transplantation, and thus death of that organ is considered the terminal event.

In any definition of death, there is no assumption that death of an organ involves death of all cells in that organ or in other organs. The hair and nails continue to grow after cardiac arrest. Skin and cornea can be removed after 24 hours of circulatory arrest for viable transplant. Bone or arterial grafts are still functional if they are harvested within 48 hours.

The main criterion for establishing brain death is *cessation of brain stem function*. It is well known that an anencephalic child with no cerebral hemispheres can breathe spontaneously and swallow and patients in "coma vigil" in whom there are no functioning connections between the cortex and the midbrain may survive for years without mechanical ventilation. In contrast, a brain dead individual in deep irreversible coma cannot breathe and has no sign of neural activity above the foramen magnum. Thus criteria to determine death revolve around tests of brain stem function.

BRAIN STEM DEATH

The functions of the brain stem are:

1. Initiation of spontaneous respiratory activity.
2. As a two-way relay station to allow cortical function and maintain consciousness.
3. Maintenance of global cerebral metabolism and blood flow.
4. Maintenance of systemic blood pressure.
5. A site for the nuclei of the cranial nerves. Neurologic testing of the cranial nerve reflexes identify areas of viability in the brain stem. (Table 15-1).

The diagnosis must be approached systematically. There are several conditions under which brain stem death needs to be considered; e.g., comatose, apneic patients who require ventilatory support and in whom there is no response to painful stimuli. The cause of the brain damage should be identified as irreversible. Thus a history, physical examination and special investigations should be available. Occasionally, this information is not available and reliance must be placed on chemical analysis and

Table 15-1. Brain Stem Nuclei

Cranial Nerve	Function
I. Olfactory	smell
II. Optic	vision
III. Oculomotor	eyeball movements
IV. Trochlear	
V. Trigeminal	sensation face; muscles of chewing
VI. Abducens	eyeball movements
VII. Facial	taste; front of tongue, muscle of face
VIII. Acoustic	hearing, balance
IX. Glossopharyngeal	taste; back of tongue, muscles of pharynx
X. Vagus	viscera; muscles of larynx
XI. Spinal accessory	muscles of neck
XII. Hypoglossal	muscles of tongue

The nuclei contained within the brain stem must be tested individually to determine if any areas of viability remain.

failure to improve with supportive treatment and the passage of time. Potentially reversible conditions include drug intoxication, hypothermia, and metabolic or endocrine disorders. Controversy exists over the time delay which must be realized before brain stem testing in drug overdose situations becomes valid. Plasma half-lives are guidelines (e.g., alcohol metabolism 10 ml per hour; morphine 10-50 ml per hour; phenobarbital 100-150 ml per hour; aspirin 30 ml per hour). Moreover, brain concentration tends to lag behind plasma levels.

Effects of muscle relaxants after anesthesia, especially in patients with renal failure, may present a picture which mimics brain death.

Clinical Tests to Establish Brain Stem Death

Before brain death is established, all tests must demonstrate that brain stem reflexes are lost.

1. Ventilatory function. After disconnection from respiratory support and in the presence of a normal $PaCO_2$ and PaO_2 the patient must not breathe spontaneously.
2. Motor function. If focal or general seizures are observed this implies that nerve impulses are passing through the brain stem, proving viability. Decorticate (arms flexed, legs extended) or decerebrate (arms and legs extended and rotated) movements also indicate a living brain stem. Flaccidity in all four limbs must be demonstrated.

3. Eye movement. With the eyelids held open, the head is turned quickly from one side to the other. If the brain stem is intact, the eyes will focus straight ahead briefly before moving in the direction of rotation. Without brain stem function, the eyes move with the head (Doll's eyes maneuver.) This test should not be performed if a cervical fracture is suspected.
4. Brain stem reflexes. There should be no pupillary response to shining a bright light into the eyes or to corneal stimulation. Putting cold fluid in one ear normally causes the eyes to rotate to that side. If the brain stem is dead, there is no response to this cold caloric testing. There should be no bucking response to insertion of a catheter to the endotracheal tube. Pressure on the supraorbital margins should not cause grimacing.

Special Tests of Brain Stem Death

The electroencephalogram (EEG) might seem appropriate and even essential as the nerve cell activity of the brain stem is being evaluated. However, its value is limited by electronic interference from other equipment in the area, static generated by apparel worn by personnel, and the availability of technical staff. One rather facetious study even suggested that similar EEG patterns are obtained both from a bowl of jello and a dead brain when scalp electrodes are used.

Nevertheless, because this test provides documentation, it is still the one most frequently employed in the United States to establish brain death.

If no blood flow can be shown on a four-vessel cerebral angiogram, proof-positive of a nonviable brain stem is established. Technical problems such as vascular spasms and the need to distinguish external from internal carotid blood flow dictate that this test, which is time-consuming, only be performed by highly specialized individuals.

PROTOCOLS

One of the first guidelines for the establishment of brain death was published by an Ad Hoc Committee of the Harvard Medical School. The Harvard criteria dictated that the following conditions should be documented:

1. Unreceptiveness and unresponsiveness
2. No movements or respiration
3. No reflexes

4. Flat EEG
5. Tests repeated and found unchanged in 24 hours
6. No evidence of hypothermia or central nervous system depressant drugs

It was subsequently suggested that the diagnosis of brain death could be made on the basis of clinical judgment. These so-called Minnesota criteria required:

1. Known but irreversible intracranial lesion
2. No spontaneous movement
3. Apnea
4. Absent brain stem reflexes
5. All findings unchanged after 24 hours

The American Medical Association, in attempting to ensure that responsibility stayed with the physician rather than with the state, noted:

1. A statutory definition of death is neither desirable or necessary.
2. Death shall be determined by the clinical judgment of the physician using the necessary available and currently accepted criteria.
3. Permanent and irreversible cessation of function of the brain constitutes one of the various criteria which can be used in the medical diagnosis of death.

With such divergent views on what constitutes brain death, the problem is best resolved locally in the institution by a committee of the Medical Board who should establish guidelines which can be periodically renewed or updated as circumstances dictate.

An example of such guidelines which have been approved at the Albert Einstein College of Medicine are:

I. In cases of coma of known etiology
   A. The possibility of recovery of any brain function must be excluded. The cessation of all brain function must have persisted for an appropriate period of observation or trial of therapy, i.e., at least 6 hours of absence of brain function documented by clinical observation and an EEG. In cases of anoxia, the period of observation should be 24 hours.
   B. Barbiturate blood levels must be below 1 mg%.
   C. The patient must have a rectal temperature greater than 36°C.
   D. The patient should not be in shock or hypoxic.
   E. The patient must be older than 5 years of age.

F. Clinical criteria: The following criteria must be verified by a neurologist or a neurosurgeon who is not part of a transplant team.
  1. No spontaneous activity of the patient at any time during or after the neurological examination.
  2. No response to loud noise.
  3. No pupillary light reflexes.
  4. Absent oculocephalic and oculovestibular reflexes.
  5. Absent corneal and oropharyngeal reflexes.
  6. No cardiac response to eyeball compression.
  7. No decorticate or decerebrate posturing.
  8. No spontaneous respiration determined by turning off the respirator while the patient is maintained with diffusion oxygenation for 10 minutes (an oxygen cannula inserted loosely into the trachea). (Spinal reflexes such as extensor plantar reflexes, deep tendon and flexor withdrawal reflexes may be preserved in the presence of cerebral death and are compatible with the diagnosis of cerebral death.)
G. EEG criteria: The EEG must be recorded at the time of or after the neurological examination which meets those clinical criteria. This EEG must be recorded by and interpreted by individuals qualified to perform these functions. Electrocerebral silence must be demonstrated according to the standards outlined by the American EEG Society.
  1. A minimum of eight scalp electrodes and earlobe references covering the major brain areas.
  2. Electrode resistance under 10,000 ohms and over 100 ohms.
  3. Interelectrode distances of at least 10 cm.
  4. Sensitivity increased from 7.5 $\mu v/ml$ to 2.0 $\mu v/ml$ or better during part of the recording, with inclusion of appropriate calibration.
  5. The use of time constraints of 0.3 to 0.4 seconds during most of the recording.
  6. Test for reactivity to intense stimuli such as pain, loud sound, and strong light.
  7. Recording time of at least 30 minutes. The integrity of the entire recording system must be checked at the beginning and at the end of the recording, and a noncephalic lead must be employed to monitor electrical activity not of cerebral origin.
H. Other procedures: Four-vessel intracranial angiography is definitive for diagnosing cessation of circulation to the entire brain.
I. Age consideration
  1. For all children down to the age of 5 years, the criteria for adults are acceptable.

2. Below the age of 5 years, a repeat electroencephalogram after 24 hours is mandatory or cerebral angiogram showing no flow.
II. In case of coma of unknown etiology: When the possibility exists that the patient has or might have taken drugs that suppress central nervous system function, four-vessel intracranial angiography is recommended.

LEGAL AND INTERNATIONAL STATUS OF BRAIN DEATH

The international situation can be summarized as follows: (1) There is legal recognition that brain death constitutes death in 33 states of the United States, and in France, Canada, and Australia. (2) Brain death is accepted medically as death but without legal statute in the remaining states of the United States and in the United Kingdom. (3) Brain death is not recognized as synonymous with death in Denmark, Israel, and Japan.

Presently, 12 countries (including Canada, Britain, and Australia) rely on clinical tests only. The most recent report in the United States from the President's Commission for the Study of Ethical Problems in Medical, Biomedical, and Behavioral Research concluded that "if the brain stem completely lacks function, the brain as a whole cannot function."

Whatever the final legal or medical outcome of the criteria for the definition of death, the concept of organ death rather than cell death must be understood. Irreversible cessation of brain stem function does not imply death of every nerve cell in the brain stem or whole brain.

SUGGESTIONS FOR FURTHER READING

Anonymous. What and when is death? JAMA 1968; 204:219-20.
Korein J. The problem of brain death development and history. Ann NY Acad Sci 1978; 315:19-38.
Molinari GF. Brain death, irreversible coma and words doctors use. Neurology 1982; 32:400-402.
Veatch RM. The definition of death: ethical, philosophical and policy confusion. Ann NY Acad Sci 1978; 315:307-321.
Veith FJ, Fein JM, Tendler R, et al. Brain death—a status report of medical and ethical considerations. JAMA 1977; 238 (15):1651-1655.

III
ADMINISTRATION

16
Planning the Physical Structure of the Recovery Room
Margaret DeFranco

The fundamental purpose of the recovery room (RR), or postanesthesia care unit, is to provide direct and continuous patient observation during emergence from general or regional anesthesia. During this period the RR nurse is responsible for the constant monitoring of the patient's vital functions including cardiovascular, respiratory, and neurological status. Administration of oxygen therapy, intravenous fluids, and blood, and inspection of tubes, drains, and dressings is also performed simultaneously. Prevention or prompt recognition and treatment of postoperative complications are also objectives during this phase of the surgical experience. In addition to the specific nursing actions unique to the RR, nurses in this critical care unit must provide for the care of the patient requiring advanced life support measures following surgery. In this situation mechanical ventilation, invasive pressure monitoring (systemic arterial, pulmonary artery, intracranial), cardiac arrhythmia detection and treatment, administration of intravenous vasoactive medications, peritoneal dialysis, intra-aortic balloon counterpulsation, or cardiopulmonary resuscitation may be indicated.

The dynamic and critical environment of the RR necessitates that the structural format facilitate the demanding nature of patient care. To meet the primary objective, that of continuous observation of the postanesthesia patient, guidelines for the design and furnishing of a RR are provided.

GENERAL PHYSICAL CONSIDERATIONS

The available floor space, location of support services and facilities, financial status of the institution, building and fire codes, and anticipated surgical patient volume and population determine the structure and function of the individual RR. It is essential that medical and nursing personnel who are experts in the care of the postanesthetic patient collaborate with the architect when planning the design of this area. This ensures a unit which is architecturally acceptable and optimally functional.

Structural Configuration of the Unit

The four geometrical considerations involved in the layout, or floor plan, of the RR, are the circle, semicircle, square, and rectangle. Each has its advantages and disadvantages. All are capable of providing space for efficient and functional patient care environment.

Circle

The circular configuration (Figure 16-1) is a completely round unit, usually with the nurses' station in the center. The nurses' station in the core provides complete visual surveillance of all patients. The distance from this

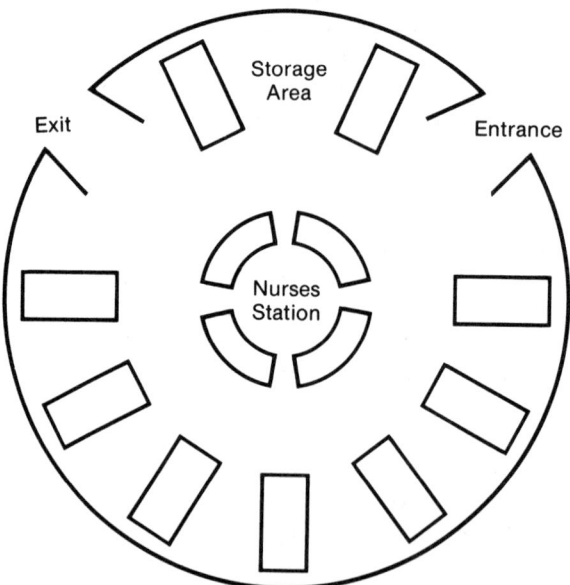

Figure 16-1.   Circle.

PLANNING THE PHYSICAL STRUCTURE OF THE RECOVERY ROOM   253

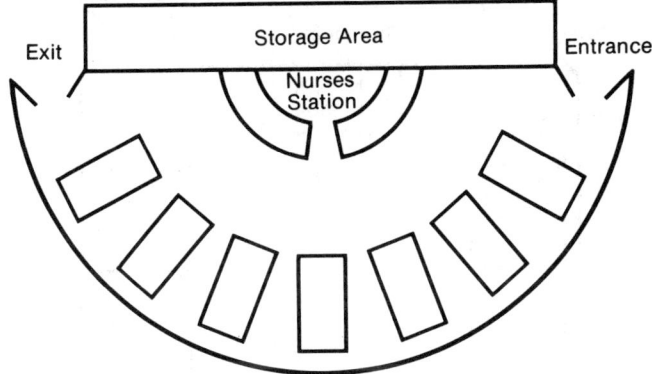

Figure 16-2.   Semicircle.

central station to any one patient is equal and usually minimal, allowing immediate access to the patient's bedside when necessary.

Often with the circular design, storage space is limited or is physically removed from the main area. Thus, the nurse cannot watch the patient when retrieving supplies. The circular setup is not recommended for a unit that requires more than a six- to eight-bed capacity, as this would decrease efficient space use. The central nurses' station is a potential source of noise and excess activity. This problem may be avoided by enclosing the station within a glass partition.

Semicircle

The semicircle (Figure 16-2) is similar in form to the circle except that the nurses' station is located along the straight wall of the half-circle. The supply area can be located along this wall on either side of the nurses' station, providing the nurse with access to supplies and equipment while simultaneously observing the patient.

If the nurses' station also conforms to the semicircle, it has the same patient observation advantages as the circular plan. If it is located along the wall, the distance between the station and each patient varies. The semicircle also is not intended for a unit requiring a large bed capacity.

Square

A square unit (Figure 16-3) is capable of providing efficient patient visualization and adequate storage space. If the nurses' station is located in the center of the square, the advantages are comparable to the circular plan. If the station is along one wall of the square, the disadvantages are similar to that of the semicircle. Often the supply area in this format is located

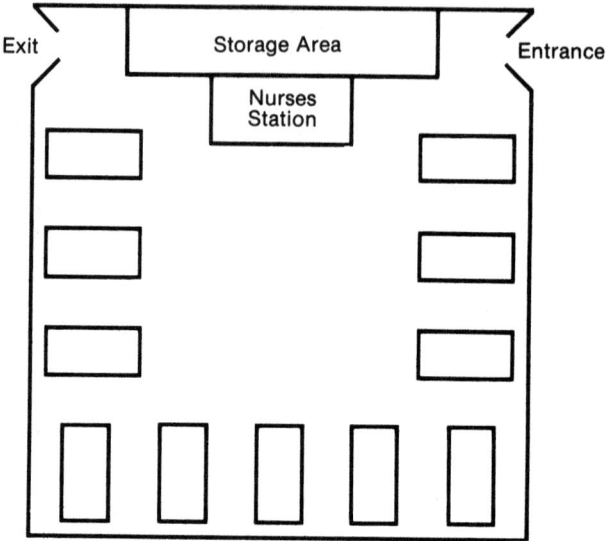

Figure 16-3. Square.

behind the nurses' station, requiring the nurse to lose sight of the patients to obtain equipment and supplies. Bed capacity with the square configuration depends on location of the nurses' station.

Rectangle

The rectangular floor plan (Figure 16-4) provides adequate storage space and is capable of accommodating a large bed capacity, often 20 beds or more. Depending on the size of the room, two nurses' stations located on either end may be advisable to provide the necessary patient observation requirements. If one central nurses' station is used, patient visualization as well as the distance between nurses' station and the patient will vary.

Patient Observation

The issue of bed placement in the patient care station has historically involved controversy. The head of the bed may be located proximal to the nurses' station, allowing the nurse immediate access to the patient as well as visualization of all patients while at the bedside. This placement, however, may be cumbersome when working with suction, oxygen, and X ray apparatus. These obstacles may be avoided if preplanning of the unit involves placement of oxygen, suction, and electrical outlets on ceiling-suspended columns which are raised and lowered as needed.

The alternative bed position is with the head located distally to the nurses' station. If equipment and supplies are located along the wall, this placement is more practical for the administration of nursing care. Complete visualization of the patient's head and chest from the nurses' station is not always possible, particularly if the patient is lying down.

Support Structures

Pillars and support columns should not interfere with the visualization of or access to patients. As mentioned previously, ceiling-suspended equipment columns are often desirable, especially where space is limited, as they can be raised out of the way when not in use.

Central Nurses' Station

The main nurses' station should be located in an area of the unit which is equidistant from all patients to assure adequate visualization. This will vary according to the geometrical shape of the unit. The high activity level which occurs at the nurses' station is a constant source of noise pollution in the RR. This area may be enclosed in a glass barrier to reduce the noise level; however, this may also result in the loss of vital auditory cues from the patient in actual or potential distress. The top of the nurses' station desk should allow an unobstructed view of the entire patient unit. Chairs should be mobile and adjusted to a height which allows the nurse to see over the desk.

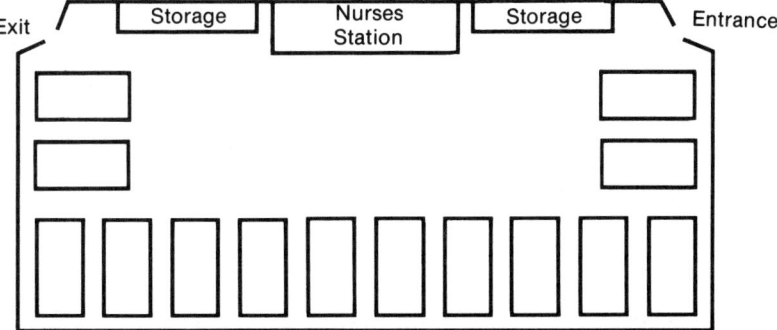

Figure 16-4. Rectangle.

The majority of the RR nurse's time is spent at the patient bedside rendering direct patient care; complete patient observation cannot be accomplished from any other location. Each staff nurse should be provided with a chair at the bedside for physical relief from routine walking and standing, as well as to avoid congregating of the staff at the main nurses' station. The chairs should be at the patient's bed level and freely mobile. This type of chair, with the addition of a small connected desk, provides the additional advantage of a flat surface for documentation of patient observations.

Dividing Walls

Dividing walls between patient units provide privacy, prevent cross contamination, and control noise. It is recommended that the upper portions of these partitions be glass to allow observation of other patients. Dividing walls, especially if solid, often require an increase in the number of staff necessary for optimum patient care. Often glass walls are used to divide the unit into halves or thirds. Any type of dividing wall, however, will reduce critical auditory patient observations.

LOCATION OF EQUIPMENT AND SUPPLIES (FIGURE 16-5)

Nurses' Station

Ideally the nurses' station should contain a central electrocardiogram (ECG) monitoring console with readout capabilities. Clinical supplies, phones (at least two per desk), and an addressograph machine are required items. Adequate desk space for physicians' and nurses' documentation is also necessary.

Medications

A medication storage and preparation area should be located in close proximity to the nurses' station. Provision must be made for a single- or double-locked cabinet for storage of controlled substances. Some hospital pharmacies are capable of providing unit-dose medications on an immediate demand basis. If this is not possible a stock medication inventory should include commonly used analgesics, corticosteroids, diuretics, antibiotics, anesthesia reversal agents, antiarrhythmics, antiemetics, cardiotonics, antihypertensives, and a surplus of emergency drugs. In addition to the above categories of drugs, the following medications are highly recommended stock items for the RR:

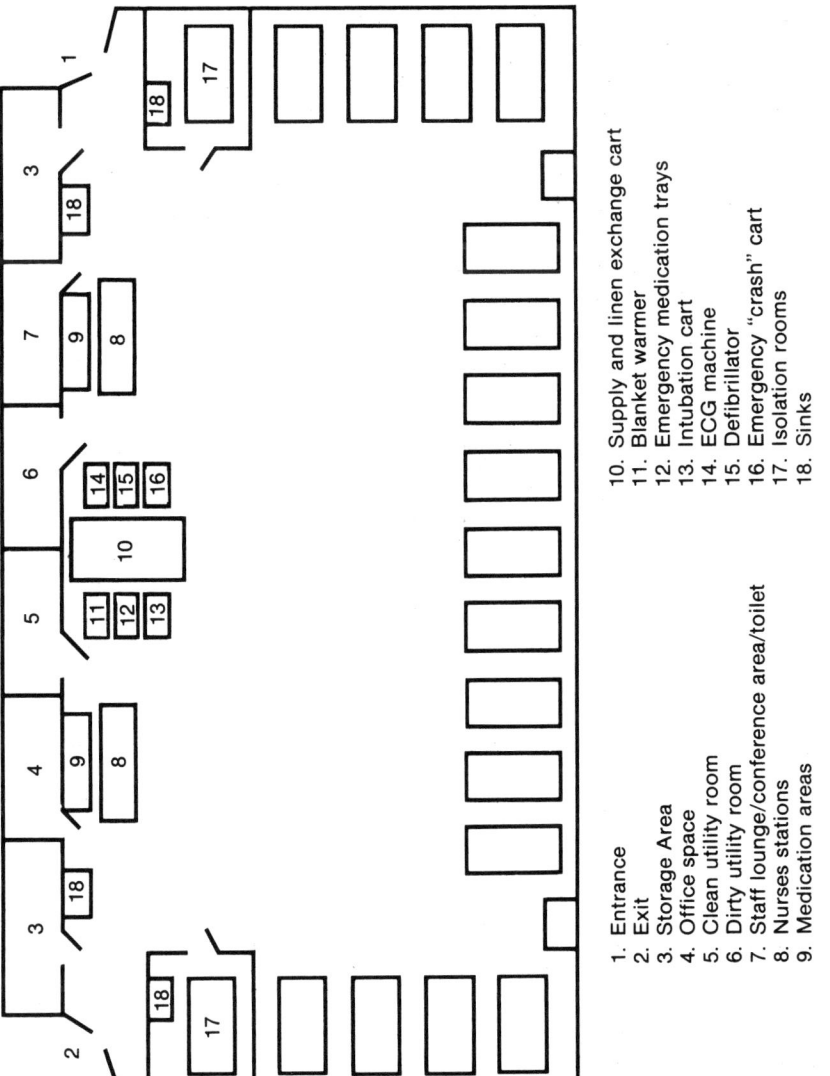

Figure 16–5. Schematic Representative of Recovery Room.

Acetaminophen suppositories
Apresoline hydrochloride (Hydralazine)
Aminophylline
Aspirin suppositories
Atropine sulfate
Aquamephyton (vitamin K)
Calcium chloride
Calcium gluconate
d-Tubocurarine chloride (Curare)
Dexamethasone (Decadron)
Dextrose 50 percent
Digoxin
Diazoxide (Hyperstat)
Diphenylhydramine hydrochloride (Benadryl)
Dopamine
Doxapram hydrochloride (Dopram)
Droperidol (Inapsine)
Edrophonium chloride (Tensilon)
Ephedrine sulfate
Furosemide (Lasix)
Hydrocortisone
Insulin (regular)
Mephentermine sulfate (Wyamine)
Naloxone hydrochloride (Narcan)
Neostigmine (Prostigmine)
Nitroglycerine — sublingual, paste, Transderm
Oxytocin (Pitocin)
Pancuronium bromide (Pavulon)
Phenylephrine hydrochloride (Neo-Synephrine)
Phenytoin sodium (Dilantin)
Procainamide hydrochloride (Pronestyl)
Prochlorperazine (Compazine)
Promethazine hydrochloride (Phenergan)
Protamine sulfate
Propranolol (Inderal)
Physostigmine (Antilirium)
Sodium heparin
Succinylcholine chloride (Anectine)
Trimethobenzamide hydrochloride (Tigan)
Parenteral narcotics and controlled substances:
Codeine
Diazepam (Valium)
Hydromorphine hydrochloride (Dilaudid)
Meperidine hydrochloride (Demerol)
Morphine sulfate
Phenobarbital

Emergency Equipment

An adult emergency "crash" cart should always be available for immediate use. The following medications should be located on the cart or be immediately available on the unit. It is also suggested that an extra supply of these medications be stored in the RR.

Atropine sulfate
Bretylium tosylate (Bretylol)
Calcium chloride
Dobutamine hydrochloride (Dobutrex)
Dopamine hydrochloride
Epinephrine, intravenous and intracardiac
Isoproterenol hydrochloride (Isuprel)
Lidocaine, single intravenous dose and intravenous infusion
Nitroglycerine, intravenous drip infusion

Procainamide hydrochloride (Pronestyl)
Sodium nitroprusside (Nipride)

The emergency cart should also contain equipment necessary for endotracheal intubation, and central venous, systemic arterial, and pulmonary artery catheter insertion. The adult emergency cart is acceptable for use in pediatric emergencies; however, a list of pediatric drug dosages and specific pediatric intubation equipment should be readily available.

A portable defibrillator with adult and pediatric paddles and a 12-lead ECG machine should be located in the RR.

Due to the comparatively high incidence of respiratory emergencies in the RR, it is advisable to have a separate intubation cart or tray for adults and children. This eliminates use of the entire emergency "crash" cart for respiratory emergencies. The adult intubation tray should contain:

Laryngoscope handle
Extra laryngoscope batteries
Laryngoscope blades: sizes medium and large; example: Miller #2 and 3 straight, Macintosh #3 and 4 curved
Extra blade lamps
Stylette or guidewire (malleable metal or plastic)
Water-soluble lubricant
Lidocaine ointment
Oropharyngeal airways: sizes small, medium, large; example: Guedel #3, 4, 5, 6
Nasopharyngeal airways: sizes small, medium, large; example: Guedel #28, 30, 32 French
Manual resuscitator bag (preferably capable of administering 100 percent oxygen); example: PMR 2 manual resuscitator
Manual resuscitator bag masks: sizes small, medium, large; example: B.O.C., Foregger #3, 4, 5
Cuffed endotracheal tubes: sizes 6.5 to 10.0 mm I.D.
Syringe
Tongue blade
Succinylcholine: 10-ml vial
2-x-20-ml syringes of sodium pentothal (replaced daily)

The pediatric intubation cart or tray should contain the same equipment as the adult tray but should be slightly modified for pediatric use. The following guidelines are suggested:

Laryngoscope blades; examples: premature newborn; #0 Miller (straight); full-term newborn; #1 straight; 3 to 5 years; #2 curved; over 5 years; #3 curved
Uncuffed endotracheal tubes: sizes 2.5 to 6 mm I.D.

Oral airways: sizes premature to small adult; examples: Guedel #000 to 3
Manual resuscitator bag: sizes baby, adult
Manual resuscitator bag masks: sizes premature, infant, child; examples: Rendell-Baker Soucek, B.O.C., AMBU type — sizes #0 (premature newborn), 1, 2
Suction catheters: sizes 6 to 12 French
Nasopharyngeal airways: sizes 26 to 30 French

A malignant hyperthermia crisis tray should be available for immediate use and must contain the following:

Sodium bicarbonate
Furosemide
Mannitol
Dantrolene sodium
Procainamide hydrochloride
Regular insulin
Dextrose 50 percent

The following equipment should be available immediately to treat malignant hyperthermia:

Foley catheter insertion equipment
Nasogastric tube
Electronic temperature recorder and probe
Cooling blanket
Iced normal saline solution for infusion and irrigation
Iced Ringer's lactate solution for infusion
Rectal tube
IV insertion equipment; central venous catheter
Blood study equipment (blood chemistries, gases, enzymes)
100 percent oxygen source

A chemonucleolysis anaphylaxis tray should be available in those institutions where this procedure is performed. Contents of this tray include:

Sodium bicarbonate
Epinephrine 1:10,000 (intravenous and intracardiac)
Hydrocortisone
Diphenylhydramine
Cimetidine
Blood gas determination supplies

In addition to this emergency equipment, at least one ventilator (preferably volume cycled) should be in the RR at all times. If this is not possible, mechanical ventilators should be immediately available from the Respiratory Therapy Department. A portable ECG monitor/defibrillator unit must be available for the transport of critically ill patients who require continuous monitoring.

Supply Cabinets

Storage areas for supplies should be situated to allow the nurse to obtain needed supplies or equipment without losing sight of the patient. Equipment which may be housed in these areas includes: intravenous solutions and tubings, oxygen therapy supplies, dressings, tapes, monitoring equipment, drainage tubes and bags, irrigation kits, monitoring transducers. Exchange carts which are centrally supplied and restocked daily are ideal for the RR. They are mobile, may be approached from either side, and may be placed anywhere in the unit where space permits. Linens may also be stored and stocked in the same fashion.

Plumbing

All plumbing systems are subject to the National Standard Plumbing Code, chapter 14, "Medical Care Facility Plumbing Equipment."
 A staff toilet located within the RR unit is necessary and contributes to the continuous immediate availability of RR personnel.
 There should be a clinical sink with elbow or foot controls for every three to four patient units. An automatic wall-mounted soap dispenser of approved germicidal soap and disposable towels and waste receptacles for each sink are also necessary.
 A "dirty" utility room for disposal of wastes and testing of specimens must be provided. This room contains the flushable bed pan hopper, receptacles for measurement of drainages, and materials for specimen testing.

Electrical Safety

In the event of interruption of normal electric power supply the emergency generator must be brought to full voltage and frequency within 10 seconds.

Miscellaneous

Due to the particular susceptibility of the postanesthesia patient to hypothermia, a blanket-warming machine is a necessity. An automatic ice machine is also desirable for local cold applications.

An X-ray film illuminator unit facilitates viewing of postoperative X-ray films.

The ambient temperature in the RR should be maintained at 23°C (75°F), with a relative humidity of 50 to 60 percent. A minimum of two air changes of outdoor air per hour are required to be supplied to the room.

SENSORY DEPRIVATION

If at all possible, the construction of the RR unit should involve the inclusion of windows which allow daylight to be visible. This provides a natural source of visual relief for the RR personnel. It also provides a day/night orientation for the awakening patient or the patient who must remain in the RR for an extended period of time either for physical or logistic reasons.

Because of the relative geographic isolation of the unit, RR personnel are continuously subject to a lack of environmental diversion. The confining nature of the self-contained unit, the close working relationships of the relatively small staff, the critical level of nursing care delivered, and the limited opportunities to leave the unit, all contribute to a heightened anxiety atmosphere. It is thus essential that, whenever feasible, the physical environment be manipulated to reduce physical and psychological stressors.

A separate lounge or conference area which is physically removed from the RR but is in close proximity to the unit is highly recommended for relaxation, stress reduction, and teaching sessions.

SENSORY BOMBARDMENT

Noise pollution is inherent to the nature of the RR environment. Mechanical devices, excessive personnel and patient traffic, and the acute nature of the medical and nursing care delivered, all contribute to the increased noise level. To reduce sensory stimulation for both staff and patients, lighting, whenever possible, should be soft and diffuse. If fluorescent overhead lighting is used it should be a shade which closely simulates daylight to assure accurate clinical observations. Colors of walls, wallpaper, and draperies should be pastels or beige. Ceiling patterns should be simple and involve shapes that do not resemble twisting or complex configurations which could contribute to visual distortions by the patient emerging from anesthesia.

PLANNING THE PHYSICAL STRUCTURE OF THE RECOVERY ROOM

INDIVIDUAL PATIENT CARE UNITS

Stretchers (Beds)

Each patient care unit should have one stretcher. These should be stored in an area out of the direct line of traffic flow but accessible to the operating room. Pneumatically controlled stretchers provide ease of use and relatively low maintenance requirements. The stretcher must be capable of being maneuvered into several positions, including elevation of head, knees, and feet, total elevation, Trendelenburg, and reverse Trendelenburg. A chart rack or foot board provides convenience for the nurse as well as patient safety. If a head board is a component of the stretcher, it should be capable of being easily and rapidly removed in emergency situations. The mattress should be of firm, durable, and washable material. Stretchers with many crevices and intricate lines are not easily cleaned or disinfected and pose a threat to infection control.

Size and Number

Each patient care unit should be at least 10 feet long to allow maneuverability of the bed in and out of the unit. There should be 4 feet of space between each unit to accommodate personnel and equipment necessary to render total patient care.

The RR should contain at least one and one-half to two patient care units for every surgical suite.

Equipment and Supplies

Mandatory

The following articles and equipment are basic requirements for any size RR. The items below are ideally wall mounted to prevent excess congestion of supplies and equipment at the bedside.

Sphygomanometer: one per unit
Vacuum/suction outlets: at least three per unit (nasogastric, endotracheal, chest)
Oxygen source: at least two per unit (oxygen administration for the non-intubated patient, mechanical ventilation)
Compressed air outlet: one per unit
X-ray receptacle: one per two units

Emergency call button: one per unit
Monitors (hemodynamic): one per unit

Monitors should be capable of continuous ECG monitoring, with readout capabilities. At least half the monitors should contain one or two additional monitoring modes and transducer equipment for pulmonary artery, systemic arterial, right atrial, apnea, or intracranial pressure monitoring.

The following items may be located in individual unit cabinets or on counter tops and shelves:

Suction catheters: #14 French whistle tip and straight designs
Yankhauer suction tip (tonsil suction)
Oxygen delivery system: nasal catheter, cannula, or prongs; nebulizer (cool and heated) with face tent or mask; masks (nonrebreathing), adult and pediatrics; and tracheostomy collars
Tongue blades
Water-soluble lubricant
Emesis basins
Sterile water: individual 50–100-ml containers for rinsing suction catheters
Syringe: 20 ml
Sterile disposable gloves
Unsterile disposable gloves

The following are ideally ceiling mounted or suspended:

Overhead surgical lamp: one per unit
Dividing drapes or curtains
IV pole: one per unit

Highly recommended are:

Sterile dressing supplies
Washcloths, facial tissues, plastic disposable bed pads ("CHUX")
Noninvasive blood pressure monitoring machine ("Dynamap"): one per RR
Volumetric infusion pump: one per RR

PROXIMITY OF SUPPORT SERVICES AND FACILITIES

Operating Room

Ideally the operating room (OR) corridors should communicate directly with the entrance to the RR. The critical period involving transfer of the patient from the OR to the RR should be accomplished within minutes. This decreases the incidence of postanesthesia complications which must be managed during transit when vital supplies, equipment, and personnel are not readily available. The close proximity of the OR to the RR allows the RR nurse to physically enter the OR for consultation with the OR nurse, anesthesiologist, or surgeon when indicated.

A communication system (telephone, intercom) which allows the RR nurse to contact OR personnel is essential. This system should allow communication with each individual OR suite, as well as with a central OR control office. An overhead page system which is audible in the OR corridors is also necessary.

Anesthesia Services

Access to the anesthesia office and lounge should also be available through a verbal communication system. These areas should also be within a reasonable distance (seconds) to the RR to enable prompt response from the anesthesiologist in an emergency and for direct communication between the RR nurse and anesthesiologist concerning specific patient management.

Blood Bank and Clinical Laboratories

The blood bank should be located adjacent to the OR for immediate retrieval of blood products. If this is not possible, an acceptable blood storage refrigerator containing blood products for the day's surgical case load should be located within the OR. Dispensing of the blood in this case should be monitored by a designated staff member.

Facilities for blood gas determinations and hematocrit estimation should be located in the immediate vicinity of the OR or RR. Laboratories for blood chemistry, hematology, microbiology, and urinalysis are ideally located on the same floor as the RR. If this is not possible, ancillary personnel should be available to expedite delivery of laboratory specimens to the appropriate areas.

Surgical Intensive Care Unit

To minimize transfer-induced patient trauma and postoperative complications, the surgical intensive care unit (SICU) should be located on the same floor as the OR and RR department. Equipment and personnel necessary for the continuous monitoring of cardiac status, blood pressure, and ventilatory support during transport of the patient to the SICU must be readily available.

Elevators

Designated patient elevators should be available for transporting patients from the RR to the patient care areas. They should be equipped with a device which permits the cars to bypass all landing button calls and be dispatched directly to any floor. The RR nurse should be provided with a key to operate these elevators.

Entrances and Exits

All RR doors should be wide enough to accommodate the widest bed used in the hospital (with the siderails in the raised position) and the tallest traction or orthopedic bed. The size of other mechanical-assist devices (mechanical ventilators, intraaortic balloon pumps) should also be considered when determining door width and height. Ideally doors leading to and from the RR should be double width with an electronic switch for automatic operation.

To decrease traffic congestion, it is recommended that traffic flow in one direction. This would require that the entrance and exit doors be located at opposite ends of the RR.

INFECTION CONTROL

Isolation Rooms

At least one isolation room for every 10 to 12 beds is recommended.

> Patients requiring isolation (as detailed by the Infection Control Committee or Department) will be cared for in a designated area in the PAR, (preferably a separate room), apart from other patients. If such an area is not available, continuous nursing care will be provided elsewhere in the hospital. The quality of care in this situation will be equal to that available in the PAR.
> Those patients requiring strict or respiratory isolation must be housed in a private room. [ASPAN Guidelines for Standards of Care, Section IV, G,H.]

Alternative isolation locations in the absence of a RR isolation room include an operating room suite, a surgical intensive care unit room, or the

PLANNING THE PHYSICAL STRUCTURE OF THE RECOVERY ROOM

patient's own private room. It is essential that if an area other than the RR is used for isolation of a patient postanesthetic care be rendered by a qualified RR nurse. Another alternative is to use the RR and confine the patient to an area which is not in the direct line of traffic. Portable screens or barriers may be used to confine the patient. The next closest patient should be at least two patient units away.

General Guidelines

Additional infection control guidelines are given below. For information regarding specific infection control parameters (hemodynamic monitoring, intravascular, oxygen and suction equipment) it is recommended that the individual hospital Infection Control Department and the Center for Disease Control be consulted.

1. Personnel with active infections (eye, skin, respiratory, gastrointestinal) should not work in the area.
2. Eating, drinking, and smoking must be restricted to a designated area.
3. Hospital furnished uniforms must be worn by personnel rendering direct patient care. These are worn once only and then laundered or discarded.
4. Shoes which are worn exclusively in the hospital are allowed in the RR without shoe covers.
5. When leaving the RR area, personnel should wear a buttoned lab coat or cover gown. These should promptly be removed upon return to the RR.
6. Whenever possible, disposable equipment should be used.
7. RR beds or stretchers must be stripped of linen between each patient use. Mattress and bed frame must be wiped down with an approved detergent germicide immediately after use.
8. All horizontal surfaces and equipment are cleaned daily.
9. Floors should be of a smooth surface and cleaned with an approved detergent germicide by the wet vacuum system. Carpeting is not recommended for the RR.

FIRE REGULATIONS AND CODES

Recommended basic fire prevention methods and codes are presented below. For specific minimum standards, the National Fire Protection Association should be consulted.

Walls

All walls which enclose the RR unit should be the smoke stop partition type. These walls provide a 90-minute smoke delay.

Doors

Doors leading to and from the RR, utility rooms, locker rooms, offices, or lounges within the RR should be B rated. These provide a 60-minute smoke delay. In the event of a fire emergency, the RR entrance and exit doors should close automatically. Doors leading to other rooms within the unit should remain closed at all times.

Fire Extinguishers

There are four types of fire extinguishers that may be used in the RR. These extinguishers are Type A (water), Types B,C (carbon dioxide), and Halon. If the Type A and Types B,C extinguishers are chosen to supply the area, the following guidelines must be followed:

Type A: One extinguisher is required every 200 square meters (2200 square feet); a staff member should always be within 25 meters (75 feet) of the device.

Types B,C: One is required every 200 square meters (2200 square feet); a staff member must be within 15 meters (50 feet) of the device.

Recently the trend has been toward the use of the Halon fire extinguisher. This device is highly recommended when considering the furnishing of a contemporary RR. A 14-pound Halon fire extinguisher replaces one Type A and four Types B,C extinguishers. An added advantage is the provision of one extinguisher which is appropriate for use on any type of fire. The Halon extinguisher also has the advantage of a 30-foot stand-off distance, the distance between user and fire source required to effectively extinguish the fire. In comparison, the stand-off distance for a carbon dioxide extinguisher is 3 meters (8 feet).

Fire Blankets

Fire blankets for fires involving an individual patient are not required to date. However, it is suggested that for future planning each RR have one fire blanket per two to four patients.

Sprinkler Systems

Automatic sprinkler systems are presently not required in the RR. It is anticipated that revision of fire codes in the near future will result in sprinkler system requirements. This should be taken into consideration when planning a new unit. However, it is recommended that sprinkler devices be located in storage areas, janitor closets, and utility rooms.

CONCLUSION

When planning the physical environment of the RR, it is essential that the personnel who will be caring for the postanesthesia patient have input into the decision-making process. Experts in each related field should be consulted for the most current information. The nature and volume of surgery will determine the specific needs of the RR. In order to achieve the primary goals of the RR, i.e., scrupulous patient observation and prevention, early recognition, and treatment of complications in the postanesthetic period, basic minimum standards must be met.

SUGGESTIONS FOR FURTHER READING

Britt BA, ed. Malignant hyperthermia. Internat Anesth Clin 1979; 17(4).
Cook KG. Assessment and management of anxiety in recovery room patients. Curr Rev Rec Room Nurs 1983; 5(7).
Drain CB, Shipley SB. The recovery room. Philadelphia: WB Saunders, 1979.
Dripps RD, Eckenhoff JE, Vandam LD. Introduction of anesthesia. The principles of safe practice. 6th ed. Philadelphia: WB Saunders, 1982.
Levin RN. Pediatric anesthesia handbook. 2d ed. New York: Medical Examination Publishing Co, 1980.
National Fire Protection Association. Code 101: Life Safety, 1982.
Roizen MF, ed. Chemonucleolysis anaphylaxis: recognition and treatment. Chicago: Smith Laboratories, 1983.
Snow JC. Manual of anesthesia. 2d ed. Boston: Little, Brown, 1982.

17
Nursing Requirements in the Recovery Room
Karen D. Spadaccia

This chapter delineates those responsibilities of patient care falling under the realm of nursing and the measures for achieving them. The purpose of recovery room nursing is to provide skilled individualized care to the patient in the immediate postoperative period. The recovery room nurse is an integral member of the health team who communicates and collaborates with other team members to deliver safe, effective care.

POSITION REQUIREMENTS

Head Nurse

The position of head nurse has a dual role — that of clinician and manager. The head nurse must be knowledgeable in medical and surgical nursing, as well as proficient in the practice of recovery room nursing. This proficiency must include an appropriate knowledge of human physiology and the effects upon it of surgical interventions, anesthetic agents, and related drugs.

In addition to this clinical base, the head nurse must also have managerial skills that allow for appropriate staff assignments, counseling of subordinates, an appropriate rapport with other departments, and the ability to function within the chain of command (Figure 17-1).

The suggested requisites for the role of head nurse are:

1. Minimum of 5 years of medical-surgical recovery room nursing
2. Minimum of 2 years of management experience

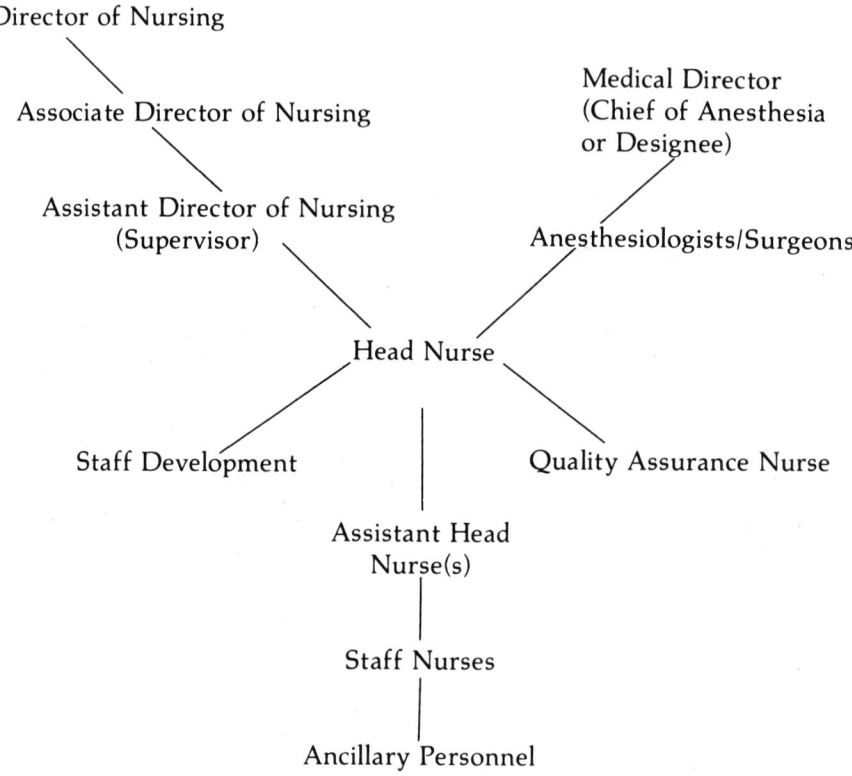

Figure 17-1. Chain of command.

3. Bachelor of science in nursing
4. Basic life support
5. Coronary care certification
6. Displayed experience with budgeting

The Joint Commission on Accreditation of Hospitals (JCAH) requires written evaluations of all nursing personnel at the end of their probationary period and at least annually. These evaluations must be criteria based and individualized. They must directly reflect particular performance and be stated in measurable goals and objectives. The responsibility of these evaluations falls to the head nurse.

Nursing Staff

The recovery room is a critical care area and as such should be staffed by professional nurses that have been selected by keeping in mind the acuity level of the patients in this area. The ability to use the nursing process is essential in this setting (Figure 17-2).

Due to the short-term relationships between nurses and patients and the continually changing needs of these patients, the nurse must be flexible and able to adapt easily to changes. Therefore, the suggested requisites for staff nurse are:

1. Registered professional nurse
2. Minimum of 3 years of medical-surgical nursing
3. Basic life support
4. Coronary care certification
5. Ability to function as a team member

The role of licensed practical nurses (LPNs) in the recovery room is limited by their training. They can play an important part in data collection and in direct patient care. However, it falls to the professional nurse to make assessments and plan intervention. Therefore, constant supervision is mandatory should LPNs be employed in a recovery room area.

Nursing assistants, orderlies, and clerks can play a vital role in this area as they can perform nonnursing functions and thereby allow the nurse to function in her expected role. Responsibilities falling to these personnel include:

1. Assisting with transport
2. Maintaining equipment
3. Stocking
4. Keeping of logs
5. Telephoning
6. Cleaning
7. Communicating with family members
8. Writing requisitions

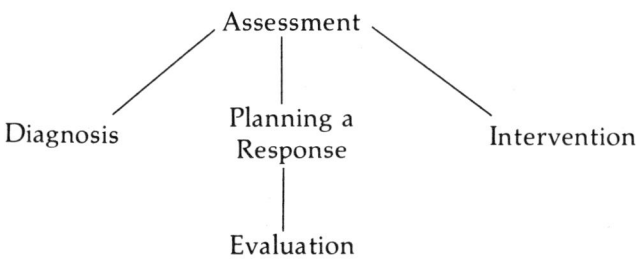

Figure 17-2. Steps of nursing process.

All staff assigned to this area must have a comprehensive orientation program and ongoing education to update their skills and knowledge on all levels. An in-depth approach to this is discussed in Chapter 18.

STAFFING PATTERNS

Staffing needs will vary from institution to institution, as they are based on size, census, and hours of operation. Perhaps of most importance is the type of patients receiving care. It would be ideal to staff based on acuity level; however, most institutions would not lend themselves to this type of staffing. It would require advanced knowledge of the operative schedule as well as a medical history of each patient. This is not always feasible and would not lend itself to projected long-term staff scheduling.

Prior to determining staffing needs for your unit, certain criteria and parameters must be established. First of all, a classification system for all patients must be designed to determine the acuity level of the patient (Table 17-1). This system can also be used to make assignments. A log should be maintained documenting acuity levels of patients on admission and discharge and length of stay. This keeps an ongoing record, and staffing patterns can be adjusted accordingly. Involvement in a smaller unit requires that a policy be established whereby patients requiring long-term intensive care nursing may be transferred directly to that unit from the operating room, thus eliminating the possibility of one staff member being involved in the care of one patient for an entire shift.

Staffing according to census appears to be the most plausible in this setting. It allows for coverage during peak hours and can lend itself to the use of alternative methods of staffing, i.e., per diem pool, staggered shifts, and "on call." A good rule of thumb to follow is one nurse for each two beds in use (Figure 17-3).

Unless direct access to emergency assistance is available, there should be two personnel in the recovery room when there is a patient. One of these staff members must be an RN. This may mean that smaller institutions must develop an on-call system. The personnel involved may not work regularly in the recovery room. Therefore, teaching sessions must be provided for these other nurses.

DOCUMENTATION

The Record

The recovery room record is sole documentation of the care a patient has received during this phase of the perioperative period. Therefore, it should reflect accurately and completely what has occurred. It is a nursing record

Table 17-1. Classification System

Classification I (1:1 nurse–patient ratio)	Classification II (1:2 nurse–patient ratio)	Classification III (1:3 nurse–patient ratio)
1. All pediatric patients	1. Frequent vital signs	1. Vital signs q 15 minutes
2. All patients on admission	2. ECG monitoring	2. Evaluation periodically
3. Mechanical ventilation	3. Confusion and/or restlessness	3. Admission score of 9–10
4. Presence of ET tube	4. Obtundation of gag reflex	
5. Continual ECG or hemodynamic monitoring	5. Periodic medications	
6. Frequent medications	6. Frequent nursing intervention	
7. Frequent assessment	7. Admission score of 5–8	
8. Constant nursing intervention		
9. Admission score of 1–4		

	Monday to Friday		Weekends and Holidays	
7 am to 3 pm	3 RNs	1 aide	2 RNs	1 aide
10 am to 6 pm	3 RNs	1 aide	—	—
3 pm to 11 pm	2 RNs	1 aide	1 RN	1 aide
11 pm to 7 am	1 RN	1 aide	1 RN	1 aide

Type of unit: 16-bed unit; average weekday census 48; average of 9.4 classification 1 patients; OR schedule 7-4 pm, but often runs until 7 or 8 pm. Used as overflow for ICU; average overnight stays 2.3. Emergency cases only after 5 pm and weekends.

	Monday to Friday		Weekends and Holidays	
7 am to 3 pm	1 RN		1 RN	1 aide
8 am to 4 pm	2 RNs		—	
9 am to 5 pm	1 RN	1 aide	—	
or				
10 am to 2 pm	1 RN			
10 am to 6 pm	1 RN		—	

Type of unit: 8-bed unit; average week day census 22; average of 2.3 classification 1 patients; OR schedule 7-3 pm, but often runs until 5 pm. ICU used on evenings, nights, and weekends other than Saturdays 7-3.

Figure 17-3. Examples of staffing pattern using census.

and so should indicate all phases of the nursing process. The record should lend itself to ease of documentation as well as ease in discerning data collected.

A flowsheet type of record is mandatory, as time for documentation is limited. The use of admission and discharge checklists is advisable (Figures 17-4 and 17-5). This gives a concise picture of the patient's status. The record itself can be designed in any fashion to meet the needs of the institution (Figure 17-6). Preestablished criteria for categories on these checklists and the use of scoring systems eliminates a good portion of the subjectivity of these records, thus making them a more universal reflection of patient status (see Appendix 2).

A carbonized record is advisable, and this copy should be kept with a copy of the anesthesia record. JCAH requires a minimum of six staff meetings per year to evaluate care given in the recovery room. Retaining a copy of both records allows for accurate auditing and the isolation of problems or potential problems.

Sole responsibility of documentation on this record falls to nursing personnel. However, the anesthesiologist must make use of this record, along with his own observations and with verbal input from the staff when evaluating patient progress, and in making notation in the progress notes.

```
Preop diagnosis _____
Procedure _____
Anesthetic:  General _____ Spinal _____ Local _____ Sedation _____
Preop vital signs:    T _____ BP _____ P _____ R _____
Initial assessment:                    Activity           Score
                                       LOC                _____
                                       Respirations       _____
                                       Color              _____
                                       Movement           _____
                                       Circulation        _____
                                              Total       _____
EBL _____
Intraoperative Fluids:                 Type              Amount
                         Solutes       _____          _____
                                       _____          _____
                         Colloids      _____          _____
                                       _____          _____
                                       _____          _____

Dressing:            Type _____     Status _____
Drains:              Type _____     Status _____
                     _____          _____
                     _____          _____

O₂ therapy:          Type _____     FIO₂ _____
Monitoring equipment: ECG _____
                      Arterial line _____
                      SG _____
                      ICP _____
```

Figure 17-4. Admission checklist. LOC = Level of Consciousness; EBL = Estimated Blood Loss; ECG = Electrogardiogram; SG = SWANN GANZ; ICP = Intracranial Pressure.

It is not possible in every institution to have a physician or a nurse anesthetist assigned to the recovery room. Therefore, it is essential to establish standing orders and protocols by which the nursing staff can function. These should include the following areas:

1. Oxygen therapy
2. Medications
    Intravenous or intramuscular
    Reversal agents
    Split doses
3. Weaning criteria
4. Extubation

```
Discharge vital signs:  T _____ BP _____ P _____ R _____
Final assessment:                        Activity          Score
                                         LOC               _____
                                         Respirations      _____
                                         Color             _____
                                         Movement          _____
                                         Circulation       _____
                                              Total        _____
Fluid therapy in RR:                     Type            Amount
                            Solutes     _____           _____
                                        _____           _____
                            Colloids    _____           _____
                                        _____           _____

Dressing:  Status _____
Drains:    Type _____      Status _____
                _____              _____
Medicated: Drug _____ Dose _____ Time _____
           and
           Route _____      _____      _____
O₂ therapy: Type _____ FIO₂ _____
```

Figure 17-5. Discharge checklist.

5. Fluid management
6. Emergency measures
   Cardiac arrest protocols: adult and pediatric
   Malignant hyperthermia
7. Discharge criteria
8. Verbal orders

Documentation of these protocols should be maintained in the policy manual and reviewed periodically by the head nurse and the medical director of the unit. In this fashion, care given and recorded on the record is legally covered by these existing policies.

NURSING STANDARDS OF CARE

Guidelines for standards of care are currently in existence. It is advisable to be conversant with these and have copies in the policy manual. These guidelines have all been published with a statement saying that these are

NURSING REQUIREMENTS IN THE RECOVERY ROOM

RECOVERY ROOM RECORD

DATE _____

WRITE OR IMPRINT PATIENT INFORMATION ABOVE

REMARKS

Pre-Op B/P

Name of Operation			
Surgeon		Anesthesiologist	
Anesthetic			

Fluids Given	In Operating Room	In Recovery Room
Lactated Ringer's		
Lactated Ringer's with Dextrose 5%		
Dextrose 5%		
Blood		
Albumin		
Intake Total		
EBL Total		
Urine Output Total		

Medications	Dose	Time	Sig.	Medications	Dose	Time	Sig.
1.				4.			
2.				5.			
3.				6.			

ARRIVAL	DISCHARGE
Dressings	
Urinary	
Lt./Sump	
Other	
Ventilation	
O_2	
Monitor	

TIME:

POST ANESTHETIC RECOVERY SCORE

	Norm. Score	Pat. Score Arr.	Disch
Activity	2		
Respiration	2		
Circulation	2		
Consciousness	2		
Color	2		
TOTAL	10		

DISCHARGE NOTE: Time _____ A.M./P.M.

Signature _____ M.D.

Signature _____ R.N.

SYMBOLS

DeSalvo-Wayne Form No. 31329-B

Figure 17-6. Example of recovery room record.

only guidelines and must be adjusted to meet the needs of each institution. However, in spite of this disclaimer, it is very possible, given the professional nature of the organizations that have published them, that they will be interpreted as standards. Therefore, deviations may be considered unacceptable by a jury of lay persons. A list of some of the current guidelines is given under further readings at the end of the chapter. It is advisable to check with your state recovery room associations for the existence of such guidelines.

Following the trend that nursing is taking in establishing itself as an accountable profession, rather than the historical role of one of delegation, it has become apparent that there is a need to define quality nursing care. To this end, each recovery room should develop nursing standards of care. The standards should follow the nursing process (see Figure 17-2) and establish the minimum level of care that will be allowed for each patient.

Prior to the writing of nursing standards, certain criteria must already have been established.

1. Policies and procedures
2. Areas of responsibility: nurse, anesthetist, and surgeon
3. Monitoring criteria: frequency, method, and established parameters

In addition, a working knowledge of the nursing process and a development of assessment skills — observation, palpation, percussion, auscultation, and interviewing — is essential (Table 17-2).

The format used for these standards may vary from institution to institution but should remain constant within one institution. They must also be attainable and reflective of actual care given. When writing these standards, begin with those areas most commonly seen or dealt with in the recovery room, i.e., admission, discharge, patients who require ventilatory support. Standards can and must reflect universally accepted recovery room practice and those established by each institution (Appendix 3). Based on these established standards, review of care is conducted.

Table 17-2. Nursing Assessment

1. Collecting data or information
2. Using all available sources of information
   a. Primary: patient
   b. Secondary: physician, chart, staff members, values from equipment used
3. Identifying problems
4. Establishing priorities
5. Setting goals

QUALITY ASSURANCE PROGRAMS

It is essential to the proper functioning of a recovery room that a quality assurance program be designed. As the care given in the recovery room is jointly one of medical and nursing, the program designed must be multidisciplinary. To further promote the concept of a team approach, the auditing, monitoring, assessment, and actions taken must be a collaborative effort.

The process involved for review can be retrospective or concurrent, but must include each of the following:

1. Established criteria, based on standards of care with no room for individual interpretation. This provides the staff with an expected performance level and the reviewer with tools to evaluate the level of compliance.
2. Method for monitoring. Monitoring can be retrospective or concurrent and should be designed to check on step-by-step compliance with established criteria. An audit is perhaps the easiest method (Figure 17-7).
3. Establishing problems. Following collection of data, review and evaluation must take place. Determination of deficiency is made and area of responsibilty — nursing or medical — is determined.
4. Action. Problem-solving techniques are designed and action to be taken established. Deadlines for compliance are made as well as a method for reevaluation.

Upon completion of an audit, statistics, and documentation of follow-up, it is essential to integrate this with the institution's quality assurance program.

On January 1, 1981, the JCAH implemented the quality assurance standards and assesses quality assurance programs in the hospitals it surveys based on these standards. They may be found in the *Accreditation Manual for Hospitals* and should be reviewed prior to setting up programs.

SUMMARY

Written standards of care, job descriptions and delineations, policies and procedures, and documentation of care given are essential to an effective recovery room. Without clear definitions of professional practices and compliance, patient care can and will suffer.

Objectives:
1. To evaluate adequacy of present documentation of care given in the recovery room.
2. To determine level of compliance with current format.

Criteria: YES   NO   NA
1. Did the patient's name and financial number appear?
2. Type of surgery indicated?
3. Type of anesthesia used indicated?
4. Admission assessment done?
    LOC
    Respirations
    Color
    Circulatory status
    Activity
5. Oxygen therapy indicated?
6. Vital signs monitored at least q 15 minutes?
7. Ventilatory status reevaluated?
8. LOC reevaluated?
9. Status of wound indicated?
10. Fluid status indicated?
    Intraoperative
    Postoperative
11. Status of drains indicated?
12. Medication administered?
    Type
    Dose
    Route
    Effect
13. Documentation of anesthesiologist assessment?
14. Nursing discharge assessment done?
15. Record signed — RN?
    MD?

Figure 17-7.   Sample audit.

SUGGESTIONS FOR FURTHER READING

American Association of Critical Care Nurses. Standards for nursing care of the critically ill. Reston, VA: Reston Publishing Co., 1980.

Accreditation Manual for Hospitals 1983. Joint Commission of Accrediting Hospitals. Chicago, IL.

Block D. Criteria, standards, norms—crucial terms in quality assurance. J Nurs Admin 1977; 7(Sept):20-30.

Campbell C. Nursing diagnosis and intervention. New York: John Wiley and Sons, 1978.

DeKornfeld T, Israel J, eds. Recovery room care. Springfield, IL: Charles C Thomas, 1982.

Drain CB, Shipley S. The recovery room. Philadelphia: WB Saunders, 1979.

Guidelines for standards of care. American Society of Post Anesthesia Nurses, 1983.

Guidelines for recovery room care. New York State Society of Anesthesiologists, New York State Association of Nurse Anesthetists, and New York State Recovery Room Nurses Association, 1982.

Halloran EJ. Staffing assignment: by task or by patient? Nurs Manag 1983; 14(August):16-18.

Mason E. How to write meaningful nursing standards. New York: John Wiley and Sons, 1978.

Practice advisory for recovery room. American Society of Anesthesiologists. Anesthesia Practice Advisory No 2 May 1978.

Seaman DJ. Post anesthesia room transfer. Nursing 83, 1983; 13(9):47-49.

18
Educational Program for Recovery Room Personnel
Dorothy M. Williams

The professional nurse should gain clinical experience under the direction of the head nurse, clinical instructor, preceptors, and senior staff nurses through participation in selected progressive clinical experience. The recovery room preceptorship program is designed to provide a nursing orientation at the unit level that will facilitate the integration of the beginning recovery room practitioner into the recovery room routines and the assimilation of the recovery room's philosophy, policies, and procedures into the new nurse's performance. The most important purpose is the development of competence and expertise in recovery room nursing.

ROLE AND RESPONSIBILITIES OF THE CLINICAL INSTRUCTOR

The clinical instructor is responsible for facilitating the orientation process of new recovery room staff nurses. This includes planning, coordinating, and evaluating the recovery room orientation. The clinical instructor is also responsible for assessing and evaluating the orientee's clinical performance for the first month of employment in collaboration with the head nurse and preceptor as well as participating in the three-month performance appraisal process of the new staff nurse.

1. The clinical instructor participates with the head nurse in selecting a preceptor for each orientee.

2. After specific assignment of the preceptor, the clinical instructor meets with the head nurse and preceptor to discuss scheduling of time and areas in which the preceptor will need assistance from the clinical instructor and head nurse to implement the role.
3. The clinical instructor facilitates the orientee's assessment of specific learning needs by requesting the orientee to complete the registered nurses's orientation skills checklist (Appendix 4).

The clinical instructor is a behavioral role model for both the orientee and the preceptor. Guidance is provided for the preceptor by the clinical instructor through ongoing feedback, support, and evaluation of the preceptor's role and preceptor's performance. At the end of the orientation, the clinical instructor meets with the head nurse and preceptor to discuss positive and negative aspects of the role and to revise implementation of the role as necessary.

PRECEPTOR SELECTION AND TRAINING

All preceptors involved in the recovery room orientation should be selected based on demonstrated proficiency in technical, intellectual, and interpersonal skills. They must also express an interest in teaching and being involved in the appraisal process.

All preceptors should be given training and guidance by the head nurse and clinical instructor in the following:

1. Using the orientation checklist
2. Assessing the learning needs of new employees
3. Giving and receiving feedback
4. Developing effective written objectives
5. Writing meaningful and objective evaluations

The preceptor in the recovery room should continually collaborate with the clinical instructor and head nurse during the entire three-month orientation for the purpose of:

1. Assessing the learning needs of the orientee
2. Planning an orientation specific to the identified learning needs of the orientee
3. Implementing the teaching plan by providing the orientee with the necessary supervised clinical experiences using the checklist as a guide.
4. Evaluating the nursing care of the orientee, giving constructive feedback and writing a formal appraisal at the conclusion of the orientation

The preceptor will:

1. Serve as a role model by delivering quality nursing care in accordance with the policies and procedures of the Department of Nursing.
2. Assist the orientee to integrate socially and professionally into the unit by providing information regarding the roles and responsibilities of all members of the multidisciplinary team while introducing the orientee to the team members.
3. Assess the beginning learning needs of the orientee through questioning and observing the orientee during the first few days in the unit.
4. Schedule weekly meetings with the orientee to review the checklist, develop weekly expectations for the orientee, and discuss problems and concerns. Keep written records of all conferences.
5. Assist the orientee to identify the orientee's own learning needs and direct the orientee to the appropriate resource.
6. Continue to serve as a resource person and evaluator by using the orientation checklist as a guide to experiences pertinent to the orientee's development.
7. Prepare a written evaluation at the end of the first month. Review with the head nurse and participate in oral presentation to the orientee. Participate in subsequent advisory and counseling sessions as indicated.
8. Review with the orientee near the conclusion of the day orientation expectations and available resource personnel on all shifts. The majority of the clinical experiences on the recovery room checklist should be supervised and signed off by the clinical instructor, and preceptor while the orientee is on the day shift.
9. Meet with the assigned preceptor on evenings or nights before the orientee is transferred to discuss progress and identify future learning needs of the orientee.
10. The new shift preceptor will fulfill all of the responsibilities of the day preceptor as indicated. The orientee and new preceptor will be assigned to work in the same zone and on the same evenings or nights during the one-month orientation to the shift.

WEEKLY ORIENTATION OUTLINE FOR PRECEPTOR PROGRAM

Week 1

Monday, Tuesday, Wednesday

Orientee in classes with the clinical instructor.

Thursday, Friday

Preceptor orientation to the unit layout and routines. At the end of these two days, the orientee will be responsible for:

1. Locating equipment and specific access within the unit.
2. Identifying members of the multidisciplinary team.
3. Locating and reading reference manuals.
4. Reviewing the organization of the patient's chart.
5. Understanding the format and use of the recovery room record.

Weeks 2 to 6

The orientee will shadow the preceptor and be responsible for becoming familiar with the recovery room structure and function and will become knowledgeable about:

1. Special records and charting. Orientee will review and be supervised using the recovery room record, the continuous ventilation record, and the standards of charting in the recovery room.
2. Monitoring equipment. Orientee will review and be supervised using the monitoring system, defibrillator, electrocardiogram (ECG), and recovery room alarm system.
3. Checking equipment. Orientee will review and be supervised using emergency carts, pediatric cart, ordering narcotics, plasma supply, reordering stock drugs, ventilators, hypothermia machine, portable suction and blood warmers.
4. Arterial lines. Orientee will review and be supervised assisting with insertion, the nursing care, and drawing of arterial blood samples from the cannula.
5. Central venous pressure (CVP) monitoring. Orientee will review and be supervised with assisting at insertion of CVP lines, doing CVP dressing changes, drawing blood samples, and removing CVP lines.
6. Swan-Ganz catheters. Orientee will review and be supervised assisting at insertion, nursing care, measurement of pulmonary artery pressure, wedge pressure, and CVP.
7. Respiratory care. Orientee will review and be supervised assisting with intubation, caring for the intubated patient, caring for the patient on the ventilator, intermittent mandatory ventilation (IMV), and positive end-expiratory pressure (PEEP), weaning patients from respirators, use of the Wright respirometer, Radford nomograms, sterile suctioning procedure, extubating patients, insertion of airways.
8. Blood samples. Orientee will review and be supervised doing arterial punctures for arterial blood gases, lactate and pyruvate, ionized

calcium, prothrombin time (PT), partial thromboplastin time (PTT), coagulation profile, hematocrit readings, pseudocholinesterase levels, and serum electrolytes.
9. Miscellaneous equipment. Orientee will review and be supervised in the use of the IVAC pump, venodyne boots, use of the doppler, and pediatric specific-gravity urometer.
10. Patient apparatus and equipment. Orientee will review and be supervised in the care of patients with chest tubes, care of patients on total parenteral nutrition (TPN) and TPN catheters, care of patients with continuous bladder irrigation, administration of blood and blood products, whole blood, packed cells, fresh frozen plasma, platelets, reconstituting packed cells.
11. Electrical safety. Orientee will review with clinical instructor, plugs, grounding, beds, and all pertinent electrical equipment.
12. Physiologic considerations in the recovery room. Orientee will review with the clinical instructor and be responsible for: respiratory anatomy and physiology, cardiovascular anatomy and physiology, renal anatomy and physiology, gastrointestinal anatomy and physiology, integumentary anatomy and physiology.
13. Concepts in anesthetic agents. The orientee will review with the clinical instructor and be responsible for: postoperative care of patients who have received inhalation anesthetics, intravenous anesthetics, muscle relaxants, regional anesthetics. Drug interactions in the recovery room are also reviewed.
14. Postoperative nursing care. The orientee will review with the clinical instructor and be responsible for:
    a. Physical assessment of the recovery room patient, airway management, management of unconscious patient.
    b. Recovery room standards of care.
    c. Postoperative care following ear, nose, neck, and throat surgery.
    d. Postoperative care following thoracic surgery.
    e. Postoperative care following vascular surgery.
    f. Postoperative care following orthopedic surgery.
    g. Postoperative care following neurosurgery.
    h. Postoperative care following thyroid and parathyroid surgery.
    i. Postoperative care following gastrointestinal, abdominal, and anorectal surgery.
    j. Postoperative care following genitourinary surgery.
    k. Postoperative care following gynecologic surgery.
    l. Postoperative care following breast surgery.
    m. Postoperative care following plastic surgery.
15. Special considerations. The orientee will review with the clinical instructor and be responsible for:
    a. The geriatric patient.
    b. The pediatric patient.

c. Postoperative nausea and vomiting.
d. Shock and disseminated intravascular coagulation.
e. Cardiopulmonary resuscitation.
f. Chemotherapy.
g. Radiation therapy.
h. Immunosuppressed patient.
i. Pain medication and anesthetic drugs.
j. Care of the patient with invasive monitoring.
k. ECG interpretation.
l. Acid-base and hypoxia.
m. Pulmonary edema.
n. Congestive heart failure.

Weeks 6 to 8

Under the guidance of the preceptor, orientees will spend time gaining experience in the organizational skills needed to coordinate their patient care assignments which will gradually be increased to working a zone as staff members of the recovery room on the day shift. Orientees will continue to expand their knowledge base and expertise in clinical practice. The following experiences will be provided if they have not already been reviewed in previous weeks:

1. One day rotation to the special care unit
    a. Use of the following equipment:
        1. Bear and Jet ventilators
        2. Laminar flow
        3. Swan-Ganz catheters
        4. Mass spectrometer
2. One day rotation following a patient through surgery
    a. Holding area
    b. Operating room
    c. Recovery room
3. One day shadowing the rehabilitation therapist to learn chest physiotherapy.

Weeks 8 to 10

Upon transfer to an assigned shift, a new preceptor will be assigned to the orientee. To assure continuity in the orientation process, the original preceptor will meet with the newly assigned preceptor, the orientee, clinical instructor, and the head nurse. The progress of the orientee and the checklist will be reviewed. The orientee will be assigned to work the same nights or evenings with the preceptor for one month. The orientee's patient assignment will be determined by the preceptor in collaboration with the charge nurse. During this time, the orientee will:

1. Meet the nursing and medical personnel on an assigned shift.
2. Become familiar with the shift routines.
3. Become familiar with the expectation of the registered nurse in recovery room care on an assigned shift.
4. Observe the preceptor's clinical and organizational skills in delivering patient care to one to five patients.
5. Deliver safe, quality patient care to assigned patients.

Weeks 10 to 12 and Thereafter

The orientee will be responsible for using the preceptor and all other nursing resources as needed in the ongoing process of planning for and delivering quality patient care.

SUGGESTIONS FOR FURTHER READING

American Society of Anesthesiologists. Practice advisory for recovery room. ASA Newsletter. 1978; 2 (May).

Drain CB, Shipley S. The recovery room. Philadelphia: WB Saunders, 1979.

Israel JS, DeKornfeld TJ. Recovery room care. Springfield, IL: Charles C Thomas, 1982.

Plasse NJ, Lederer JR. Preceptors: a resource for new nurses. J Nurs Leadership Manag 1981; (June)

Recovery room clinical preceptor program. Memorial Sloan Kettering Cancer Center, Department of Nursing, New York, 1980.

Smith CE. Planning, implementing and evaluating learning experiences for adults. Nurse Educator. 1978; (Nov-Dec).

19
A Role for the Recovery Room Nurse in the Wards
Ann Marie Terra

HOLISTIC NURSING

The involvement and interaction of the recovery room nurse on the unit is a primary facet in a multidisciplinary approach complementing holistic care. Modern technology has influenced and necessitated the expansion of recovery room nursing practice to incorporate critical care expertise. This evolutionary factor is essential to ensure the patient's safe and smooth passage through the crisis of surgical intervention. Juxtaposed is the increased scope of knowledge and skills required in the formulation of nursing diagnoses and utilization of the nursing process assuring effective, efficient, quality care.

Terminology

Health, defined epidemiologically, is the state of complete well-being of the physical, mental, and social processes, not merely the absence of disease. *Disease* results from an imbalance in equilibrium as governed by the environment and is a state of unwellness, a manifestation of pathology. *Holistic* is termed more than the sum total of parts. *Holistic medicine* includes the metaphysical or spiritual approach and deals with the well individual who becomes unwell (Figure 19-1).

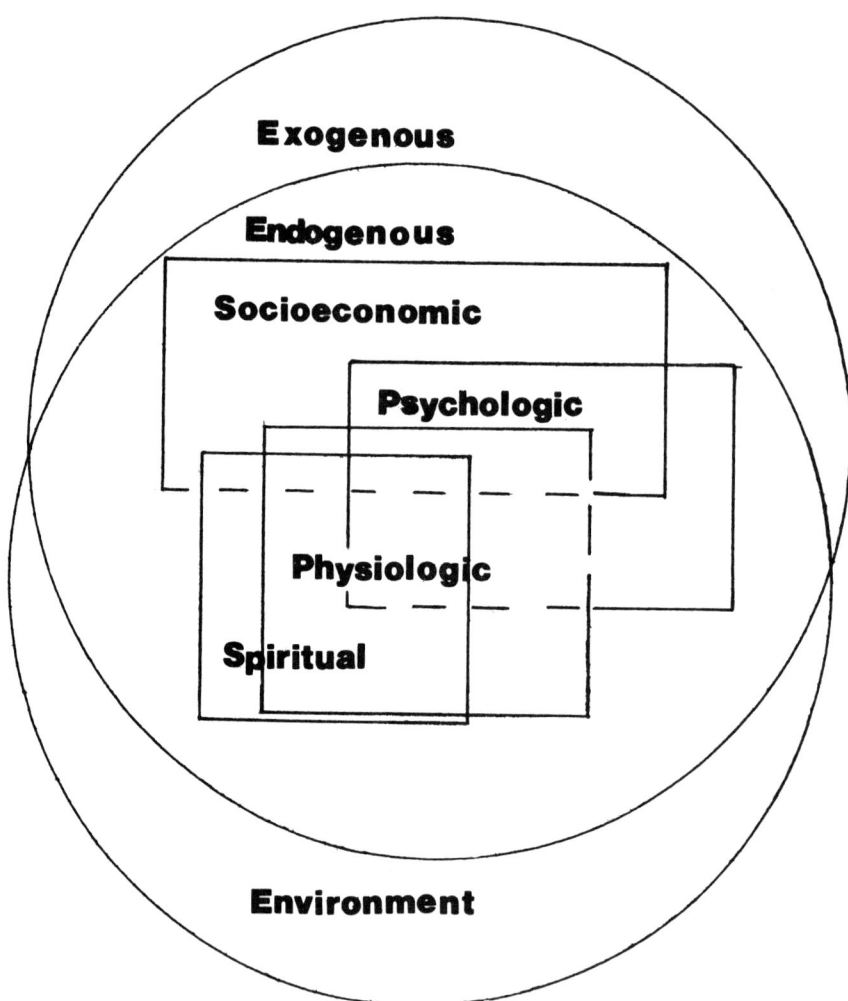

Figure 19-1. Holistic concept of man and environment.

Positive → Negative
Well → Unwell

In our efforts to maintain equilibrium, various coping mechanisms attempt to compensate for stress, strain, and the unwellness of the disease state (Figure 19-2). Holistic nursing may be defined as the concept involving total care of the patient in an integrated manner encompassing all patient systems in the well/ill continuum. The goals are based on the standards of care.

A ROLE FOR THE RECOVERY ROOM NURSE IN THE WARDS 295

Holistic Approach

1. Emphasis is on the interrelatedness of all systems subject to vascillation, effected by the exogenous and endogenous environment.
2. Structure and application of the nursing process as a tool with the patient as the framework.
3. Identification of patient needs and coping mechanisms such as fear, anxiety, loss of control over self; these will effect learning and recovery (return to wellness). Physiologic and emotional support is then required.
4. Utilization of a perioperative role (Figure 19-3).

Methodology

1. Collect data from the chart and unit nurses.
2. Preoperative visit: establish rapport with patient and family; observe all systems; listen and obtain history; initiate or reenforce patient teaching; discuss expectations.
3. Postoperative visit and phone calls: evaluate care delivered; reenforce teaching.

Communication

An exchange of information enhances communication and understanding with the unit nurses regarding the client. This is useful in fostering the

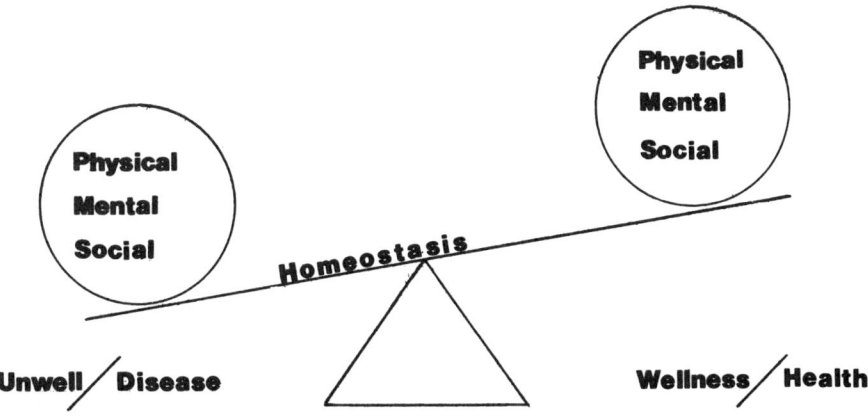

Figure 19-2. Maintenance of homeostasis.

Surgical experience

Phase	Process	Description
Preop	Assessment	Preop visits Patient teaching
Intraop	Planning	Identification of patient problems (anesthesia, positioning, surgical complications)
Postop	Implementation Intervention	of goals formulated (nursing care plan, patient teaching)
	Evaluation	and surveillance of post-anesthetic care, requires continuous reassessment

Figure 19-3. The nursing process: Perioperative role of the recovery room nurse.

teamwork concept, vital for quality care and an holistic approach. In addition, it promotes: a safe environment and effective and efficient nursing care.

The nursing diagnosis originating on the unit can be transferred to the operating room and recovery room with appropriate reassessment. Previously identified problems in other settings can become the basis of a nursing care plan and assist in determining a baseline (Figure 19-4).

Age, sex, value systems, and beliefs as well as life experience are influential factors in determining the patient's accommodation to the proposed surgical experience.

Preparation for preoperative teaching should include review of chart, identification of previous surgery and type, and a brief discussion with the unit RN.

Preoperative Teaching

The recovery room nurse can help the patient in the following ways:

1. Understand proposed surgery and outcome (this validates informed consent). Appropriate explanation and discussion in laymen terminology can be positive reenforcement.

2. Discuss routine preoperative preparation (i.e., shave, antiseptic shower, premedication, transfer to the operating room, family waiting area, etc.).
3. Explain the environment: holding area; operating room (narrow OR bed, surgical lights, personnel dress); and recovery room (recovery from anesthesia until stable for transfer to unit or intensive care).
4. Explain nature and type of equipment attached to the patient (i.e., Foley catheter, nasogastric tube, airway, intravenous).
5. Explain general nature of discomfort upon reacting from anesthesia, reassurance of availability of pain relief medication.
6. Reenforce patient teaching on deep breathing, coughing, leg exercises, changing position.
7. Review incision and type of dressing.
8. Assist in coping with feelings of anxiety, fear, and depression by encouraging verbalization on sexuality, body image, loneliness, powerlessness, etc. This is of prime importance, since learning and retention are related to the level of stress and coping adaptability.
9. Set achievable goals in dealing with illness and surgery.

Types of Learning

Knowledge and assessment of the type of learning the patient requires is necessary to determine the manner of presentation:

1. Cognitive learning: need for information
2. Affective learning: need to learn (or change) attitudes, behavior.
3. Psychomotor learning: need to acquire new skills.

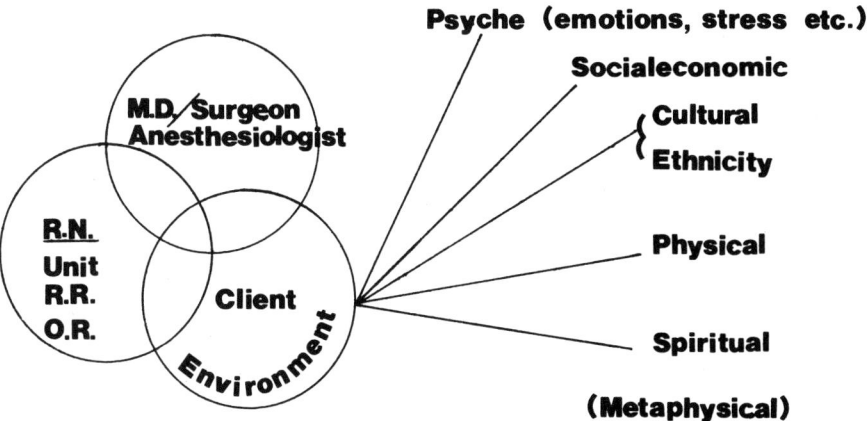

Figure 19-4. Interrelatedness of team (holistic) approach.

Teaching Aids

Recommended teaching aids that can be adapted according to availability of financial resources and staffing patterns are as follows:

I. Preoperative interview
   A. Objectives
      1. Instruct patient and family.
      2. Identify patient needs and assist with problem solving.
      3. Document patient needs (ensures continuity of care).
      4. Establish rapport and trust.
      5. Collect data: (a) obtain history and perform physiologic assessment (physical impairment, handicaps, limitations) and psychologic assessment (mental status, orientation, fears, apprehension).
      6. Develop and implement individualized nursing care plan.
      7. Coordinate care plan with other members of health team.
      8. Increase job satisfaction.
      9. Reduce postoperative level of stress and complications.
      10. Minimize hospital stay.
   B. Methodology
      1. Observe patient's color, respiration, muscle activity, circulation.
      2. Listen and encourage client verbalization.
      3. Question and obtain a history, elicit patient participation.
   C. Types of interviewing techniques
      1. Direct: assertive, direct questioning, uses confrontation and interpretive methods.
      2. Nondirect: Rogerian, less assertive approach, encourages patient to initiate communication regarding perceptions and concerns without blocking him or assuming what his fears are.
      3. Transactional analysis employing the three defined levels (child, parent, mature adult) requires cognizance regarding role interchanges.
   D. Recommendation: Conduction of the preoperative interview should occur sitting at the patient's level and initiated by self-introduction. Specific questions concerning surgery or anesthesia can be referred to the appropriate physician. Application of effective communication skills, both verbal and nonverbal (body language), contribute to the accomplishment of established goals.
II. Group classes: Planned, regularly scheduled classes for prospective surgical patients and families can be arranged preoperatively or before admission. Coordination of classes with presurgical testing may be convenient. Patient education and staff development departments

can assist in conjunction with OR and RR inservice personnel in the development and implementation of informative classes. Staff participation should be encouraged and utilized to promote efficacy of the program and self-actualization. Suggested modalities for adaptation and presentation of classes are:
1. Self-teaching instructional modules
2. Lectures
3. Role playing
4. Pictures, posters
5. Booklets and/or pamphlets

III. Audiovisual aids: Presentations recorded or filmed on site or obtained commercially can range from simple to elaborate, depending on institutional resources available. Ingenuity and adaptability are primary ingredients in initiating an effective, and rewarding program. Considerations include:
1. Slide presentation (with or without documentary, taped or lecture)
2. Video tapes
3. Movies, films
4. Closed-circuit television

IV. Tours: Recommended times are geared toward personnel availability and traffic hours. Obvious areas to include are:
1. Presurgical testing (labs, radiology)
2. Ambulatory surgery unit
3. Surgical units
4. Holding area
5. Operating room
6. Recovery room
7. Family waiting area
8. Intensive care areas (optional)

Classes or tours can be held at predetermined intervals compatible with patient and staff scheduling and arranged via the Admitting Office.

V. Recommended sources of assistance for initiation and implementation of proposed programs are:
1. Patient Education Department
2. Audiovisual Department
3. Volunteer Department
4. Surgical Specialty Department
5. Social Service Department
6. Public Relations Department
7. Multidisciplinary committees
8. Nursing committees
9. Community relations committees
10. Specialty committees (i.e., OR and RR committee)

PEDIATRIC PATIENTS

Elective surgery for the pediatric patient involves consideration and focus on stages of growth and development in addition to the family unit. Education of child and parents will allay fear and anxiety and accelerate the child's return to homeostasis with minimal negative incidence. Public awareness through creative avenues of education satisfies attainment of goals.

Class participation can be elicited via contact with the local school's health education departments. Initially a brief presentation to the class can include:

1. Dress in "scrubs"
2. Discussion and visual aids integrated with the human body system currently being studied.
3. Discussion regarding surgery and role of the OR and RR nurse.
4. Introduction of proposed poster contest illustrating these discussions
    Prize awards for most outstanding, etc. (i.e., T-shirts, ribbons)
    Prearranged poster display at school or at local mall in conjunction with Health Education Week or Health Fair
    Publicity through school and newspaper coverage.

Preoperative preparation ideally begins in the surgeon's office, where the child and parents should have specific needs identified and addressed. A preparatory hospital tour is highly indicated, and a "show and tell" is also beneficial.

Recommendations

During the preoperative visit, the child should be addressed directly. At this time, determination of language and comprehensive skills can be assessed. Nickname, age, height, and weight are ascertained to formulate an individualized teaching care plan (Table 19-1).

Availability of medical equipment for handling is suggested, i.e., anesthesia masks, blood pressure apparatus, stethoscope. Based on indications as well as the preference of the anesthesiologist, premedication for pediatric patients may not be ordered. If ordered however, preferable administration is one hour prior to transport to the holding room to allow for full effect. The holding area should be quiet and screened; parents should be encouraged to remain with the child. Research regarding parental presence in the recovery room has demonstrated stress reduction in the postanesthetic phase. Alleviation of the child's fear of separation appears to be of consequence.

Table 19-1. Assessment and Implementation for the Teaching Plan

Development Level	Consideration
1. *Preschool children* (4–6 years)	
Have limited time concept	demonstrate with dolls or drawings
Short attention span	note any comfort object, i.e., blanket, animal, doll, etc.
Ritualistic	
2. *School age* (6–12 years)	
Higher cognitive level	demonstrate equipment
Ability to focus on several sequential concepts	encourage play sessions (to act out fears and fantasies)
Greater attention span	provide simple explanation
3. *Adolescent* (12–18 years)	
Increased complexity of understanding	increase complexity of explanation
Fear of body exposure	use visual aids
	assure protection of privacy

AMBULATORY PATIENTS

Preoperative teaching and preparation can be initiated and coordinated with preadmission (presurgical) testing. Focus on the short-term aspect of hospital stay requires definitive instructions regarding the admission procedure and preoperative instructions. General, stand-by, or local anesthesia is of considerable importance to the disposition of the patient and length of stay. Discharge instructions are essential. Standard admission and specific preoperative protocol regarding preparation and instructions should be documented. Avoid miscommunication and unnecessary delays and inconvenience to all concerned.

Communication by telephone both preoperatively and postoperatively provides:

1. Reenforcement of instructions
2. Clarification of information
3. Reassurance

SUMMARY

A holistic approach using the nursing process can enhance the postanesthetic recovery of adult and pediatric patients. Adaptation is dictated by need, institutional size, and budgetary allowance. The key is innovativeness and creativity of those involved to devise, coordinate, and implement from a variety of effective programs and techniques.

SUGGESTIONS FOR FURTHER READING

Ayers C, Walton L. A guide for the preoperative visit. AORN J 1974; 19:413-418.
Bille DA. Preoperative teaching: rights and responsibilities. Today's OR Nurse 1979; (Oct):9-13.
Blom GE. The reactions of hospitalized children to illness. Pediatrics 1958; 41:59-60.
Boegli EH, Boegli RG. Can preop learning be improved? AORN J 1972; 16:43-45.
Crain WC. Theories of development: concepts and applications. Englewood Cliffs, NJ: Prentice-Hall, 1980.
Diniaio MJ, Ingoldsbry B. Parental presence in the recovery room. AORN J 1983; 38:685.
Dunn R, Dunn K. Practical approaches to individualized instruction. West Nyack, NY: Parker Publishing Co., 1972.
Edwards B. Preop home visits: patient perception and nurse self-image. AORN J 1974; 19:419-422.
Hercules PR. Nursing in the postoperative care unit. AORN J 1978; 28:1047.
Hercules P. O.R. experience teaches continuity of care. AORN J 1983; 32:299.
Hudak CM, Gallo BH, Lohr T. Critical care nursing. Philadelphia: JB Lippincott, 1973.
Kanda NL. Staff development for R.R. nurses. AORN J 1977; 26:664-667.
Korsch B. The child and the O.R. Anesthesiology 1975; 43:251-257.
Lockhart CH. Practical consideration in the preoperative psychological preparation of the pediatric patient. In: Emotional and Psychological Responses to Anesthesia and Surgery. F Guerra, JA Aldrete, eds. New York: Grune & Stratton, 1980.
Lorig K. An overview of needs assessment tools for continuing education. Nurse Educ 1977; (March/April):12-26.
McClintoc J. Preoperative care of the pediatric patient. Today's OR Nurse 1980; 2(5):7.
Ridgway M. Preop interviews assure quality care. AORN J 1976; 2:1083.
Rozman F. Nursing process in the recovery room. AORN J 1976; 2:1069-1075.
Schmidt FE, Woolridge PJ. Psychological preparation of surgical patients. Nurs Res 1973; (March/April):108-115.
Steward DJ. Premedication for the pediatric patient. Annual refresher course lectures. American Society of Anesthesiologists, 1979, pp. 1-3.

20
Liabilities of the Recovery Room Team
Stefanie Putkowski

From both a medical and legal standpoint the recovery room is considered to be one of the areas of highest risk in a hospital setting. This is due to the extremely precarious physical condition of a patient who has just undergone surgery, often of a major type, who is still under the lingering effects of anesthesia. This delicate situation places both the patient and the nurse in a very vulnerable position: the former in a life-threatening one, and the latter in a legal situation. It is because of this unique relationship that a chapter dedicated to the legal aspects of recovery room nursing is essential.

MALPRACTICE

The earliest documented medical malpractice case occurred in 1377, when a doctor was sued for improper treatment of a leg. Since that time both the best and the worst of nurses and physicians have endured the distress of being sued. Since the mid 1970s the number of lawsuits instituted against individual nurses and doctors has skyrocketed, heralding what has been referred to by insurance companies as the "medical malpractice crisis."

When one makes the statement that a physician or nurse has been found "guilty of malpractice," a picture of a criminal is often conjured up in the minds of those unfamiliar with the law. This notion is quite far from the truth and shows the need for a basic understanding of the issues.

Definition of Malpractice

Medical malpractice is a form of negligence that occurs when a professional, in treating or caring for a patient, does not conduct himself with reasonable prudence and skill. There are three essential elements to a medical malpractice case: (1) that a relationship existed between physician or nurse and patient; (2) that there was a departure from the accepted standard of care; and (3) that this departure was the proximate (direct) cause of the injury being alleged.

Persons Involved in a Lawsuit

The *plaintiff* is the person who brings on the complaint, and initiates the lawsuit. Generally, it is the patient who is the plaintiff. However, in the case of a deceased patient, the plaintiff is often a spouse or other family member, and is referred to as the *executor* of the decedent plaintiff's estate. In the case of an infant (any person who has not reached majority is considered an infant under the law) it is usually the parent who, as the *guardian*, brings about the lawsuit on behalf of the infant plaintiff.

The *defendant* is the person or hospital against whom the lawsuit is brought. This is the *party* to the suit who must be defended in the courtroom. Usually, the decision as to which hospital personnel are to be named as defendants is made by the plaintiff's attorney, not by the plaintiff. It is common for a plaintiff to sue physicians and nurses with whom he has a good relationship because his attorney convinces him that it is necessary for the prosecution of a case. Some attorneys will name only those people who had a direct role in an alleged injury, whereas others will name everyone who cared for the patient and whose name appears in the medical record. Either way, a defense must be prepared for each of the defendants.

Standard of Care

The term "standard of care" is a most important concept in a malpractice suit. It is determined by what a reasonably prudent person acting under similar circumstances might do.

To determine the standard of care the attorneys will use the knowledge of an *expert witness*. Because the jury will not be familiar with the standard of care, the expert witness will explain if and where there was a deviation. It is customary for several expert witnesses to be brought into the courtroom by both sides. For example, in a lawsuit alleging that a child was brain damaged as a result of labor and delivery at a defendant hospital, it would be typical to bring in expert witnesses in the fields of obstetrics, obstetrical nursing, pediatrics, genetics, pharmacology, and psychiatry. Each side will bring in as many experts as necessary in an attempt to prove or disprove to the judge and jury that the standard of care practiced by the defendants was in keeping with the medical community.

Statute of Limitations

The statute of limitations is the period of time during which a plaintiff can institute a lawsuit. The statutory period begins when an injury occurs, although in some cases (usually involving foreign objects left in the body) the statutory period begins when the injured person discovers the injury.

The statute of limitations is a great concern to both defendants and plaintiffs because, depending on the nature of the particular malpractice case, several years may elapse before institution of the suit. This can be beneficial for the plaintiff but extremely problematic for the defendant. The difficulty is that with the passage of time memories fade and hospital witnesses move away. It is crucial for the hospital staff to report any unusual incidents or probable future lawsuits to the hospital's risk management department. Careful, factual documentation is essential.

The statute of limitations varies from state to state. In New York, for example, an adult patient may sue up to 2.5 years from the time that the alleged malpractice took place. If a patient dies as a result of medical or nursing treatment, the executor of the estate can bring about a suit up until 2 years from the date of death. If a patient undergoes a surgical procedure, continues to complain of discomfort for several years, and then learns through surgery or an X ray that a sponge was left behind, another full year may elapse before the statute of limitations has run out. In the case of an infant, the statute is either 10 years or until the infant has reached majority plus 2.5 years.

Obviously, the statute of limitations need not be memorized at this juncture, but suffice it to say, the plaintiff can sometimes wait several years. The importance of early reporting by the hospital staff cannot be overemphasized, so that witnesses can recount the occurrence while memories are fresh.

NURSING LIABILITY

The professional nurse is legally responsible for any harm brought about by negligence or imprudence. The following are some of the most common major allegations brought against nurses:

1. Failure to adequately monitor the patient
2. Failure to administer medications promptly and properly
3. Failure to follow physician's orders promptly and properly
4. Failure to report significant changes in a patient's condition
5. Failure to take correct telephone orders
6. Failure to protect the patient from falls
7. Failure to follow established nursing protocol

Failure to Adequately Monitor the Patient

Mrs. G. was a 31-year-old woman who entered the hospital to undergo elective plastic surgery on her breasts. The surgery was performed under general anesthesia with endotracheal intubation, and no unusual intraoperative events were reported. She was brought to the recovery room already extubated, with orders for vital signs to be taken every 15 minutes.

The nurse took the patient's vital signs on admission and noted them as: blood pressure 120/80, pulse 70, respiration 20. However, she also noted that the patient was "unreactive." She then left the patient and returned 15 minutes later to take the vital signs. She found the patient to be grossly cyanotic with no obtainable vital signs. Despite extensive resuscitative attempts the patient expired.

This case is an example of a departure from the accepted standard of care: i.e., an unreactive patient must be constantly observed and monitored. The nurse, in *abandoning* the unreactive patient, failed to act in a prudent manner.

Another problem often found lies not in the monitoring but in the lack of documentation of it. If the medical record is devoid of notes relative to the nurse's observations, it will be quite impossible to try to prove to the judge and jury that it was done. Take every step to write observations clearly and concisely. Note the site and condition of all drains, tubes, and surgical incisions. If an oral airway is in place, it must be noted. Mention if the patient is intubated or already extubated. Document the site of all intravenous lines (i.e., infusing in dorsum of left hand).

Failure to Administer Medications Promptly and Properly

The professional nurse is responsible for handling and dispensing medications. Not only must the nurse understand the indications for the medications, she must also know the side effects and the proper route of administration. She will be held accountable in a court of law for knowing this information with regards to any medications she has administered.

Mrs. M., a 78-year-old woman, was admitted to the hospital for treatment of her hypothyroidism. Her medication regimen included, among other things, "Lugol's solution, 1 gtt., po, b.i.d." The evening nurse misunderstood the order and administered 1 gtt. of Lugol's solution to the patient's right eye. The patient sued for corneal damage.

This is a clear-cut case of nursing negligence in that the nurse obviously did not understand the indications of the medication which she administered, nor did she properly follow the doctor's orders.

Failure to Follow Physician's Orders Promptly and Properly

The nurse is responsible for reviewing the medical record to ascertain whether the doctor's orders have been modified. In the case of *Toth* v. *Community Hospital at Glen Cove*, twin girls born prematurely were placed under oxygen. One baby suffered total blindness while the other suffered severe damage to one eye. The physician ordered 6 liters of oxygen per minute for the first 12 hours, then 4 liters per minute thereafter. Unfortunately, the nurses continued to give 6 liters of oxygen for several weeks. The jury found the nurses guilty of malpractice for not following the doctor's orders correctly.

Nurses can also be found negligent if they carry out an order which is unsafe or erroneous. If the order appears questionable, it is incumbent upon the nurse to have the order clarified *by the physician who wrote it*. In the Louisiana case of *Norton* v. *Argonaut Insurance Co.* the courts focused attention on the nurse's responsibility to seek clarification. In this case a 3-month-old infant girl was admitted to the hospital because of a congenital heart problem. At the time of her admission, it was agreed that the mother could continue to administer the baby's daily dose of oral Lanoxin. One evening the assistant director of nursing was making rounds and found the nurse in pediatrics to be busy with an emergency. In an attempt to assist the floor nurse, the assistant director decided to review the stack of charts at the nursing station to see if any medications needed to be administered. With regards to Baby Girl Norton, she found that the physician's order for "3 cc of Lanoxin today" had not yet been carried out. The nurse was not familiar with the pediatric elixir, intended for oral use, and it occurred to her that 3 cc of injectable Lanoxin might be excessive for a 3-month-old baby. She discussed the matter briefly with two other physicians on the unit, who said that if that was ordered by the attending physician, then that was what was meant to be given. The problem was that the physicians interpreted the order to be for oral elixir, so they did not share the nurse's concern. She administered the 3 cc of injectable Lanoxin, and the baby died an hour later. It was held by the court that there was a departure from the accepted standard of competent nursing care in that the nurse did not seek clarification from the physician who wrote the order.

Failure to Take Correct Telephone Orders

Since the physician, unlike the nurse, usually does not maintain a vigil by the patient's bedside, telephone orders often become a necessity. Because it is incumbent upon the nurse to transcribe the orders, every effort must be made to be careful and accurate. "Orders should be repeated, once transcribed, for verification purposes. Verification of an order by another nurse on a second phone is helpful."

Failure to Report Significant Changes

In the case of *Goff v. Doctor's Hospital*, a patient in the recovery room was seriously bleeding because the doctor failed to suture properly. Although the attending physician was no longer present in the hospital once the bleeding was recognized by the nurses, he was the only physician who was contacted. The patient died. The court held that the nurses were negligent in their failure to report the condition in a way that could be handled promptly.

It is not enough merely to report a changing condition to the appropriate personnel. The nurse must also document all observations and nursing actions taken while awaiting the physician's arrival. Many a lawsuit has been lost simply because of a lack of documentation in this area. In the case of a patient who, for example, is suddenly showing signs of respiratory distress, writing "Patient dyspneic. Dr. Smith paged stat," is not adequate. A note regarding a patient whose condition is significantly changing should be as specific and detailed as possible. A good nursing note would read something like this:

9:00 p.m. Patient complaining of difficulty in "catching his breath." B/P 120/80, P-90, R-30. Dr. Smith, Anesthesia, paged stat. Head of bed raised. O_2 at 5 L via face mask. Color good.
9:03 p.m. B/P 100/70, P-90, R-30.
9:05 p.m. Complaining of chest pain. Pale. Diaphoretic. B/P 90/60, P-irregular 90, R-30. Dr. Smith not arrived. Paged again stat. Emergency cart at bedside. ECG being done now. Mrs. Chu, Nursing Supervisor, paged stat.
9:07 p.m. B/P 90/60, P-?60, R-shallow.
9:10 p.m. Dr. Smith here. B/P palpable at 80. Pulse-? Cardiology called stat.
9:12 p.m. Intubated by Dr. Smith. Dr. Jones, Cardiology, arrived.

The above sample note not only illustrates the detail involved, but also gives an idea as to how to document when a physician does not respond to an emergency page. The nurse must note what she is doing for the patient while awaiting the doctor, and who else she has paged. In this case a full 10 minutes elapsed before the doctor arrived, and this must be factually documented. However, as the anesthesiologist on call may be involved in other emergencies elsewhere in the hospital, the nursing supervisor should be called simply to offer assistance in locating other physicians.

It is important to understand that the medical record is admitted into evidence in the courtroom. Often, the jury will be shown portions of the original record, and any discrepancies will be brought out and exposed. To minimize exposure, the professional nurse can take certain general measures when documenting. They are as follows:

Be objective. Do not label your patient (or the physician) as being "obnoxious" or "demanding." Even though this might be the case, remarks like this will infuriate a jury, and cause them to look upon the author of the note in a disfavorable light. Brief, factual notes are essential.

Do not obliterate. If an error in charting has been made, simply draw a line through the sentence. It should be initialed by the person who both wrote the note and made the correction. Any attempts to obliterate or white out a note will be viewed in the courtroom as an attempt to falsify the record.

Avoid discrepancies. Read the note before yours. If the information is contrary to your findings, document that you are aware of the discrepancy and that the doctor will be made aware.

Use addendums when necessary. If the nurse wishes to add something to a previously written note, it must be done in a separate note, dated and timed when the additional note is written. The addendum should never be written in the margin or in between lines, as this will be viewed by a jury as an attempt to "doctor" the record.

Medical malpractice litigation is a sad but true reality, reflecting modern society and the changing trends in the public mind. It can never be completely avoided, because as long as there are human beings involved, human error will exist. Meticulous record keeping, prudent judgment, and early reporting of cases will help to minimize exposure.

SUGGESTIONS FOR FURTHER READING

Bertolet M, Goldsmith L, eds. Hospital liability: law and tactics. 4th ed. New York: Practicing Law Institute, 1980.

Help with legal aspects of nursing practice. 1st ed. Chapel Hill, NC: WL Ganong Company, Health Care Management Consultants, 1979.

Pozgar GD. Legal Aspects of Health Care Administration. 2d ed. Aspen Systems, 1983.

Willig SH. The nurse's guide to law. New York: McGraw Hill, 1970.

IV
APPENDICES

APPENDIX 1

Guidelines for Blood Component Therapy

Product	Content	Indications	Volume	Shelf Life	Comments
Whole blood	red cells, leukocytes, platelets, plasma	acute massive blood loss; neonatal exchange transfusion	500 ml	35 days in CPDA-1 at 106° C	~ $50 per unit. Not available in all hospital blood banks.
Red blood cells	red blood cells, leukocytes, some plasma	anemia	200–350 ml	35 days in CPDA-1 at 106° C	~ $50 per unit.
Red blood cells frozen-thawed	red blood cells, very few leukocytes, platelets, plasma	anemia; prevent reactions to white blood cells, platelets, plasma proteins; storage of rare bloods	170–190 ml	frozen, 3 yr thawed, 24 hr	Rare bloods are frozen in large reference centers. expensive (~ $90 per unit)

(Continued)

Product	Content	Indications	Volume	Shelf Life	Comments
Red blood cells (leukocyte-poor)	red blood cells, few leukocytes, some plasma	prevent febrile reactions due to white blood cell antibodies; anemia	200–250 ml	35 days CPDA-1 at 106° C	Try before using frozen-thawed red blood cells in patients with febrile transfusion reaction.
Platelet concentrate	platelets, few leukocytes, some plasma	bleeding due to low platelet count or poor platelet function	20–50 ml	72 hr	Red blood cells contaminate most units of platelets. (Use Rh-negative units for Rh-negative recipients).
Leukocyte concentrate	leukocytes, platelets, few red blood cells	serious infections in leukopenic patients	500–300 ml	24 hr	Patients may experience febrile reaction to transfused leukocytes.
Fresh frozen plasma	clotting factors, no platelets	clotting disorders	220–250 ml	frozen, 1 yr thawed, 6 hr	Discouraged for simple volume expansion.
Cryoprecipitated AHF (antihemophiliac factor)	factor VIII, factor XIII, fibrinogen, von Willebrand's factor, fibronectin	deficiencies in: factor VIII, factor XIII, von Willebrand's factor	10–25 ml	frozen, 1 yr thawed, 6 hr	
Purified AHF concentrate	factor VIII	factor VIII deficiency	lyophilized powder	determined by manufacturer	300–1,600 units/vial $30–$150/vial

Product	Composition	Indication	Volume/Form	Shelf life	Comments
Autoplex	activated procoagulants	inhibitor to factor VIII	30 ml sterile water; lyophilized powder	2 yr	Prohibitively expensive. Hepatitis and DIC risk. Use only with consultation of hematologist.
Factor IX	factors II, VII, IX, X; 500 or 1000 units factor IX	factor IX deficiency (Christmas disease) factors II, VII, IX X deficiency	20–40 ml sterile water; lyophilized powder	determined by manufacturer; store at 2.8° C	Hepatitis risk great. Cost, $60 or $140/vial
Albumin	5% albumin or 25% albumin	plasma volume expansion required	250 or 500 ml 50 or 100 ml	3 yr	Product of choice for volume expansion. Risk of hepatitis minimal.
Plasma protein fraction	albumin alpha and beta globulins	plasma volume expansion required	5% 250 or 500 ml	3 yr	Minimal risk of hepatitis.
Rh(D) immune globulin	gamma globulin rich in anti-D immunized donors	prevention Rh(D) sensitization in Rh-negative patients	1–2 ml	3 yr	To be used in Rh-negative patients without anti-Rh(D) antibody.
Immune serum	gamma globulin	hypogammaglobulinemia or disease prophylaxis	2 ml 10 ml	3 yr	IV preparation recently available.

APPENDIX 2

Postanesthetic Recovery Score
J. A. Aldrete

A. Purpose
  1. To be used as a guideline for the evaluation of the postanesthetic patient.
  2. A set criteria that the postanesthetic patient should meet before discharge from the recovery room.
  3. To provide objective information of the physical condition of patients arriving in the recovery room after anesthesia.
B. Scoring system
  1. *Activity.* The muscular activity is assessed by observing the ability of the patient to move his limbs either spontaneously or on command.
     a. Ability to move all four extremities scores 2.
     b. Ability to move two extremities scores 1.
     c. Unable to move any extremity scores 0.
  2. *Respiration.* No complicated apparatus or sophisticated physical tests are used.
     a. Ability to deep breathe and cough scores 2.
     b. Limited respiratory effort (i.e., splinting) or dyspnea scores 1.
     c. No evident spontaneous respiratory effort scores 0.
  3. *Circulation.* This is the most difficult sign to evaluate by a simple method. Changes in the arterial blood pressure from the preanesthetic level were chosen because it is reliable, it is monitored throughout the anesthetic period, and it is one of the first signs taken on arrival in the recovery room.
     a. Systolic arterial blood pressure 20 percent ± preanesthetic level scores 2.

b. Systolic arterial blood pressure 20 to 50 percent ± preanesthetic level scores 1.
c. Systolic arterial blood pressure 50 percent ± preanesthetic level scores 0.
(Note: Great differences in diastolic blood pressure should be noted.)
4. *Consciousness.* Ability of patients to answer simple questions and follow verbal commands. Only verbal stimuli are to be used.
   a. Full alertness with ability to answer question scores 2.
   b. Patient arousable by calling his name scores 1.
   c. Auditory stimuli fail to elicit any response scores 0.
5. *Color.* Patients are to be scored on their color in the recovery room whether this skin color was present prior to surgery or not (example: jaundiced preoperatively and postoperatively).
   a. Obviously normal or pink skin color scores 2.
   b. Any alteration from the normal pink, but not cyanotic; for example: pale, dusky, blotchy, jaundiced scores 1.
   c. Cyanotic nailbed, lips, and skin scores 0.
(Note: Check patient oral mucosa if any questions.)

C. Results of Postanesthetic Recovery Score
   1. Optimum score is 10. Patient may be discharged from the recovery room with scores of 8, 9, or 10. Nursing judgment must be used since this scoring system is not infallible.
   2. Patients who had scores of 10 preoperatively, but received scores less than 8 during the postoperative state require more constant observation and may need a specialized nursing care area such as the intensive care unit.
   3. Chronically debilitated, senile, or paralyzed patients may never receive an optimum score. Each patient must be treated individually and discharged from the recovery room at the discretion of the attending anesthesiologist.
   4. There are variables which may influence patient's emergence from anesthesia and thus his score. These include:
      a. Type of anesthetic agent used.
      b. Use of paralyzing drugs and narcotics during surgery.
      c. Type of surgery performed.
      d. Duration of surgery and anesthesia.

APPENDIX 3

Nursing Care Standard:
Care of the Patient in the Recovery Room

Patient's recovering from anesthesia will receive short-term intensive nursing care. Through continuous observation, monitoring, assessment, and nursing care, postanesthetic complications will be prevented or be recognized and treated promptly.

Assessment	Plan	Intervention
1. Adequacy of airway	1. On admission to RR and q 15 minutes.	1. If airway not patent suction (oral, nasal, pharyngeal) or insert nasal/oral airway.

2. Adequacy of ventilation
   a. Strength of voluntary muscles
   b. Use of accessory muscles
   c. Respirations, rate, and rhythm
	2. Administer oxygen as ordered by physician. Encourage coughing and deep breathing. On admission and q 15 minutes.	2. Notify anesthesiologist if patient in respiratory distress and requires mechanical assistance or medications.

3. Presence of protective reflexes
   a. Gag
   b. Cough
	3. On admission	3. Stay at patient's bedside until present.

(Continued)

Assessment	Plan	Intervention

4. Cardiovascular status
   a. Pulse, rate, and rhythm
   b. Blood pressure
	4. On admission and q 15 minutes. Apply warm blankets.	4. With any pulse arrhythmias, place on ECG monitor. Notify anesthesiologist and surgeon of significant deviations in vital signs or ECG.

5. Fluid status	5. Monitor intake and output. Administer fluids and blood products as ordered.	5. Notify surgeon of signs and symptoms of dehydration or fluid overload.
6. Allergic reactions	6. On admission and continuously.	6. Notify surgeon or anesthesiologist with any signs or symptoms.

7. Pain
   a. Type
   b. Location
   c. Severity
   d. Effects of nursing care
	7. Proper positioning and support for operative reassurance, psychological support. Medicate as ordered. On admission and continuously.	7. Notify surgeon if plan ineffective, or if pain unexplained.

8. Neuromuscular status A. Nerve blocks: Assess sensation, spontaneous or reflex movement, color, warmth, edema of area around and distal to operative site.	A. Elevate limb/area as indicated. On admission and q 15 minutes.	

B. Spinals, epidurals: Assess upper level of anesthesia, respiratory function, sensations, spontaneous or reflex movements, color, warmth of lower extremities.

9. Level of consciousness
   a. Response to noxious stimuli.
   b. Response to verbal stimuli.
   c. Orientation to person, place, and time.

10. Condition of operative site
    a. Type of dressing or suture line
    b. Drainage tubes
    c. Drainage
    d. Edema

B. Reassure patient of temporary nature of anesthetic effects. Have patient move lower extremities on admission and q 15 minutes until movement is restored.

9. On admission and q 15 minutes.

10. On admission and q 15 minutes.

9. Notify anesthesiologist with decreasing level of consciousness.

10. Notify surgeon of any abnormal finding.

APPENDIX 4

Orientation Checklist

PART I

Week 1

Monday, Tuesday, Wednesday.

Orientee in classes with clinical instructor.

Thursday and Friday.

Preceptor will introduce orientee to the unit layout and routines. At the end of these two days the orientee will be responsible for:

I. Locating the following areas and equipment:
   - _____ 1. Adult emergency carts, pediatric emergency cart, defibrillator, cardioverter, ECG machine
   - _____ 2. Portable suctions, portable oxygen
   - _____ 3. MAI ventilators, respiratory equipment
   - _____ 4. Recovery room supplies
   - _____ 5. Medication and IV area
   - _____ 6. Supply carts, clean utility room
   - _____ 7. Dirty utility room
   - _____ 8. Anesthesia laboratory
   - _____ 9. Recovery room emergency alarm system
   - _____ 10. Special trays, cutdowns, thoracentesis, universal, etc.
   - _____ 11. Ice machine
   - _____ 12. Time schedules, request book
   - _____ 13. Blood tube cart

II. Identifying members of interdisciplinary team:
   _____ 1. Head nurse
   _____ 2. Director of nursing
   _____ 3. Assistant director
   _____ 4. Unit service coordinator
   _____ 5. Unit secretaries
   _____ 6. Surgical chiefs
   _____ 7. Nursing assistants
   _____ 8. Anesthesia Department staff

III. Locating and reading the following reference manuals:
   _____ 1. Nursing Service Manual
   _____ 2. Nurse Reference Manual
   _____ 3. Recovery Room Policy and Procedure Manual
   _____ 4. Isolation Procedure in Recovery Room
   _____ 5. Surgical Procedures Manual
   _____ 6. Intravenous Therapy Admixture Manual
   _____ 7. "Current Reviews of Recovery Room Nursing"
   _____ 8. Posting of educational programs offered at hospital

IV. Reviewing the organization of the patient's chart

V. Understanding the format and utilization of the recovery room record

Part II

Time Frame	Activity	Date Instructed	Supervised Clinical Experience	Comments

1st week	1. Education:
	   a. Classes with clinical instructor
	2. Orientation:
	   a. Location of key areas and equipment
	   b. Introduction to team members
	   c. Reading reference manuals
	   d. Review of patient chart
	   e. Review of recovery room record			

Time Frame	Activity	Date Instructed	Supervised Clinical Experience	Comments
2nd week	1. Emergency and monitoring equipment: a. Monitoring system b. Defibrillation/cardioversion c. ECG Machine (take a 12-lead ECG) d. Pacemaker equipment e. Emergency cart—adult and pediatric f. Recovery room alarm system 2. Recovery room record keeping: a. Vital signs section b. Intake and output section c. Medication section d. Laboratory section e. Continuous ventilation record f. Charting on nurses notes 3. Checking recovery room supplies a. Ordering narcotics b. Reordering stock drugs c. Plasma supply d. Medication slips 4. CVP monitoring a. Assist at insertion b. CVP reading c. CVP dressing change d. Drawing blood samples			

Time Frame	Activity	Date Instructed	Supervised Clinical Experience	Comments

	5. Blood samples:
	   a. Venipuncture
	   b. Arterial puncture for ABGs
	   c. Routine electrolytes and ABG
	   d. Ionized Ca^+
	   e. coagulation profile
	   f. Lactate and pyruvate
	   g. Hematrocrit readings
	   h. Pseudocholinesterase levels
	   i. Interpretation of data
	 6. Arterial lines:
	   a. Assist at insertion
	   b. Nursing care
	   c. Drawing ABG and blood samples
	 7. Infection control:
	   a. Sterile technique
	   b. Aseptic technique
	   c. Care of patient on isolation
	 8. Patient safety:
	   a. Physical safety
	   b. Electrical safety
	 9. Anesthetic agents
	   a. Inhalation anesthetics
	   b. Intravenous anesthetics
	   c. Muscle relaxants
	   d. Regional anesthetics
	   e. Drug-drug interactions in RR			

Time Frame	Activity	Date Instructed	Supervised Clinical Experience	Comments

3rd week	1. Respiratory care:
	 a. Care of patient with tracheostomy or endotracheal tube
	 b. Assisting with intubation
	 c. Care of patient on MA-1 respirator
	 d. Care of patient on Bear respirator
	 e. Care of patient on PEEP
	 f. Care of patient on CPAP
	 g. Care of patient on IMV
	 h. Weaning from respirator
	 i. Insertion and removal of oral and nasal airways
	 j. Use of Wright respirometer
	 k. Suctioning procedure
	   1) Sterile endotracheal or tracheostomy suctioning
	   2) Sterile nasotracheal suctioning
	   3) Nasopharyngeal and oropharyngeal suctioning
	 l. Extubation
	 m. Chest physiotherapy			

Time Frame	Activity	Date Instructed	Supervised Clinical Experience	Comments

	2. Swan-Ganz catheters
	   a. Assisting with insertion
	   b. Nursing care
	   c. Measurement of pulmonary artery pressure, wedge pressure, and CVP
	   d. Interpretation of data
	3. Mixing and administration of IVs
	   a. Mixing IV fluids
	   b. Incompatibilities
	   c. Administering IVs
	4. Administration of blood products
	   a. Whole blood
	   b. Packed cells
	   c. Plasma
	   d. Fresh frozen plasma
	   e. Platelets
	5. Administration of medication:
	   a. Use of IV medication manual
	   b. Administration of IV push medications
	   c. Administration of medications via Soluset/IV Piggyback			

4th week	1. Stoma therapy a. Orientation with stoma therapist and application of information to RR patient			

Time Frame	Activity	Date Instructed	Supervised Clinical Experience	Comments
	2. Admission procedure to RR			
	3. Discharge procedure from RR			
5th–8th week	1. SCU rotation			
	2. Use of following equipment:			
	a. Blood warmer			
	b. IVAC pump			
	c. Hypothermia machine			
	d. Venodyne boots			
	e. Doppler			
	f. Pediatric S.G. urometer			
	g. Hematocrit machine			
	h. Portable suction			
	3. Patient care:			
	a. Physical assessment of the recovery room patient			
	b. General RR care			
	c. Breast surgery			
	d. Neurologic patient			
	e. Pediatrics			
	f. Thoracic			
	g. Head and neck			
	h. Gastrointestinal, abdominal, anorectal surgery			
	i. Genitourinary surgery			
	j. Hepatic artery ligation and intraarterial catheters			
	k. LeVeen shunt			
	l. Celestin tube			

Time Frame	Activity	Date Instructed	Supervised Clinical Experience	Comments
	m. Staging skin flaps and skin grafts			
	n. Vascular surgery			
	o. Orthopedic surgery			
	p. Gynecologic surgery			
	q. Plastic surgery			
	4. Special considerations: Patient care			
	5. Chest physiotherapy by rehabilitation therapist			

APPENDIX 5

Abbreviations, Normal Values, Conversion Factors, and Blood Gas and Acid-Base Analyses

Abbreviations

a	Artery	lb	Pound
ac	Before meals	med	Medial
ad lib	As needed	min	Minute
amt	Amount	mg	Milligram
ant	Anterior	no.	Number
approx	Approximately (about)	noc	Night
		NPO	Nothing by mouth (nihil per os)
bid or bd	Twice a day		
BP	Blood pressure	O_2	Oxygen
C	Centigrade	OB	Obstetrics
c̄	With	OR	Operating room
cc	Cubic centimeters	p	Pulse
DC	Discontinue	Ped, or Peds, Pedi	Pediatrics
ECG (EKG)	Electrocardiogram (tracing of heart function)	po	Per os or by mouth
		postop	Postoperative

EEG	Electroencephalogram (brain wave tracing)	prn	When necessary
		preop	Preoperative
		pt	Patient
		PT	Physical therapy
ER	Emergency room	qd	Every day
F	Fahrenheit	qh	Every hour
f	Frequency	qid	Four times a day
fld	Fluid	qod	Every other day
GI	Gastrointestinal (stomach and intestine)	qs	Quantity sufficient
		r or resp	Respirations
		sol	Solution
gm	Gram	stat	At once
gr	Grain	sup	Superior
gtt	Drop	tab	Tablet
h	Hour	TPR	Temperature, pulse, respiration
Hgb	Hemoglobin		
H_2O	Water	via	By way of
hs	Bedtime	wt	Weight
I and O	Intake and output		
IV	Intravenous		
kg	Kilogram		
lab	Laboratory		
lat	Lateral		

Abbreviations for Respiratory Patterns

SR	Spontaneous respiration
AR	Assisted respiration
CV	Controlled respiration
IPPB(V)	Intermittent positive pressure breathing (Ventilation)
IMV	Intermittent mandatory ventilation
CPAP	Continuous positive airway pressure
PEEP	Positive end expiratory pressure
HFJV	High-frequency jet ventilation

Respiration Abbreviations

	Abbreviation	Example	
A	alveolar gas	PAO_2	Partial pressure of oxygen in the alveolus
B	barometric	P_B	Barometric pressure
D	dead space gas	V_D	Volume of the dead space
E	expired gas	P_{ECO_2}	Partial pressure of expired carbon dioxide
i	inspired gas	F_iO_2	Fraction of oxygen inspired
a	arterial blood	PaO_2	Partial pressure of arterial oxygen
b	blood	Q_b	Rate of blood flow
c	capillary blood	PcO_2	Pressure of oxygen in the capillaries
v	venous blood	$PvCO_2$	Venous pressure of carbon dioxide
$\bar{v}$	mixed venous blood	$P\bar{v}CO_2$	Central venous pressure of carbon dioxide
C	concentration of gas	CaO_2	Arterial concentration of oxygen
F	fractional concentration of gas	F_{ECO_2}	Fraction of expired carbon dioxide
P	pressure of gas		
Q	blood volume	Q_b	Rate of blood flow
V	gas volume		
S	saturation	SaO_2	Arterial saturation of oxygen
TV		tidal volume	
f		frequency	
MV		minute ventilation	

Normal Values

Blood Values

Hematocrit	45% ± 7% males
	40% ± 6% females
Hemoglobin	14–18 g % males
	12–16 g % females
	12–15 g % children
	14.5–24.5 g % newborns
Platelet count	150,000–40,000/ml
Erythrocytes	5×10^6/mm^3 males
	4.5×10^6/mm^3 females
Leukocytes	5,000–10,000/mm^3
Blood volume	69 ml/kg males
	65 ml/kg females
Bleeding time	1–6 minutes
Prothrombin time	12–14 seconds
Alcohol levels	
Intoxication	0.3–0.4%
Stupor	0.4–0.5%
Coma	Above 0.5%
Serum barbiturates	
Coma	1.5 mg/100 ml
Serum electrolytes	
Potassium	3.5–5 mEq/liter
Sodium	136–145 mEq/liter
Chlorides	100–106 mEq/liter
Bicarbonate	21–28 mEq/liter
Phosphate	2 mEq/liter
Sulfate	1 mEq/liter
Organic acids	6 mEq/liter
Calcium	5 mEq/liter
Magnesium	2 mEq/liter

CSF

Albumin	10–30 mg/dl
Cell count	0.8 cells/ml
Glucose	45–75 mg/dl
Protein total	15–45 mg/dl

Urine

pH	4.6–8.0
SG	1.012–1.024

Glucose	negative
Acetone	negative

Vital Signs

Pulse	
Infants	112–130 beats/min
Adult	70–80 beats/min
Elderly	56–62 beats/min
Respiration rate	
Infants	30–50 breaths/min
Adults	12–20 breaths/min
Blood pressure	
Infants	80/58–50/40
Adults	110/60–148/90

Respiration

Rate	12–35/min
Rhythm regular	
Tidal volume	4–8 cc/kg (250 → 500 cc)
Vital capacity	20–50 cc/kg (1.5 → 4 l)
Negative inspiratory pressure	$-40 \rightarrow -80$ cmH$_2$O
Dead space/tidal volume (VD/VT)	< 0.3

Conversion Factors

Measurement Conversion

centimeter = inches × 2.54

inches = $\dfrac{\text{centimeter}}{2.54}$

kilogram = pound × 2.2

pound = $\dfrac{\text{kilogram}}{2.2}$

1 meter = 39.37 inches

Temperature Conversion

Centigrade = Fahrenheit (0.555) − 32
Fahrenheit = Centigrade (1.8) + 32

Pressure Unit Conversions

To Convert From	To	Multiply By
cm H_2O	mm Hg	0.735
	inches Hg	0.0290
	psi	0.0142
mm Hg	cm H_2O	1.36
	inches Hg	0.0394
	psi	0.0193
inches Hg	mm Hg	25.4
	cm H_2O	34.5
	psi	0.491
psi	mm Hg	51.7
	cm H_2O	70.4
	inches Hg	2.04

Arterial Blood Gases

pH	7.35–7.45
$PaCO_2$	35–45 mm Hg
PaO_2	95–100 mm Hg
CO_2 content	26–28 mEq/liter
Bicarbonate (HCO_3)	22–28 mEq/liter
O_2 saturation	
Arterial	94–100%
Venous	60–85%
O_2 content	
Arterial	15–23 vol %
Venous	10–16 vol %

Arterial Blood Gas Analyses

I. Reason
   To determine if the patient is well oxygenated.
   To determine the acid base status of the patient.

II. Obtained from an artery because
Arterial blood is a good way to sample a mixture of blood. (There is incomplete mixing of blood in a venous sample.)
Arterial blood determines how well the lungs are oxygenating the blood.

III. Performing arterial puncture
   A. Equipment
      1. 20- or 22-g needle.
         a. There is less potential for a hematoma with a smaller needle.
         b. Causes less pain for the patient.
      2. Syringe
         a. A glass syringe with a luer block is preferred to prevent disconnection of the needle from the syringe. A glass syringe is preferred because the gases may diffuse out from some types of plastic.
         b. The syringe should be a larger capacity than the volume required for analysis (usually 2-3 ml suffices).
         c. The plunger should slide freely the entire length of the barrel.
      3. Heparin
         The syringe should be coated with heparin (1000 μ/ml). Excess heparin should be discarded. (Too much in the syringe will alter the pH of the blood), but heparin should be left in the needle and hub of syringe.
      4. Rubber tip cap
         Both can be used to seal off the sample from air but the rubber stopper is preferred.
      5. Rubber stopper
      6. Prep pads
         Although alcohol pads are supplied, a betadine prep is preferred.

Disorders of Acid Base Balance

Respiratory acidosis: pH ↓ pCO$_2$ ↑ HCO$_3$ normal or ↑

1. Obstructive lung disease
2. Oversedation and other causes of compromised function of the respiratory center (even with healthy lungs)
3. Other causes of hypoventilation

Respiratory alkalosis: pH ↑ PCO_2 ↓ HCO_3 normal or ↓

1. Hypoxia
2. Anxiety
3. Pulmonary embolus
4. Pregnancy

Metabolic acidosis: pH ↓ pCO_2 normal or ↓ HCO_3 ↓

1. Diabetic acidosis
2. Poisonings: salicylate, methyl alcohol, paraldehyde
3. Renal failure
4. Lactic acidosis
5. Diarrhea
6. Treatment with Diamox

Metabolis alkalosis: pH ↑ pCO_2 normal or ↑ HCO_3 ↑

1. Diuretic therapy, edecrin, furosemide, and the thiazides
2. Steroid therapy
3. Cushing's disease
4. Fluid losses from the upper gastrointestinal tract, vomiting, nasogastric suction resulting in loss of acid

APPENDIX 6

American Heart Association Advanced Cardiac Life Support

ALGORITHMS FOR CARDIAC DYSRHYTHMIAS—ADULT

Unmonitored Ventricular Fibrillation

Recognition: unresponsive, apneic, pulseless
↓
Call for help; initiate CPR
↓
ECG monitor available
↓
Ventricular fibrillation ——No→ to Asystole or Electromechanical Dissociation Algorithm
| Yes
↓
Defibrillate 200 to 300 joules delivered energy
↓
Check pulse
↓
Change in rhythm? ——Yes→ to appropriate algorithm
|
No
↓
Recharge defibrillator immediately 200 to 300 joules and defibrillate
↓
Check pulse
↓
Change in rhythm? ——Yes→ to appropriate algorithm
|
No
↓
Continue CPR; place IV line; intubate trachea if necessary
↓

Epinephrine 0.5 to 1.0 mg IV or intratracheal
+
Sodium bicarbonate 1 mEq/kg (75 mEq initial dose—average-size adult)
or, preferably, according to ABGs
↓
† Defibrillate 360 joules delivered energy (maximal output)
↓
Check pulse
↓
Change in rhythm? —— Yes→to appropriate algorithm
|
No
↓
CPR
↓
Defibrillate 360 joules delivered energy
↓
Check pulse
↓
Change in rhythm? —— Yes→to appropriate algorithm
|
No
↓
CPR
↓
Bretylium 350 to 500 mg or 5 mg/kg IV bolus
↓
after CPR for two minutes
↓
Defibrillate 360 joules of delivered energy
↓
Check pulse
↓
Change in rhythm? —— Yes→to appropriate algorithm
|
No
↓
CPR
↓
Bretylium 700 to 1,000 mg or 10 mg/kg IV bolus
↓
CPR; sodium bicarbonate IV according to ABGs or one-half original
dose if no ABGs available (if 10 minutes have elapsed)
↓
Defibrillate 360 joules delivered energy
↓
Check pulse
↓
Change in rhythm? —— Yes→to appropriate algorithm
|
No
↓
CPR
↓

†Reference point for *Monitored* Ventricular Fibrillation Algorithm

Repeat epinephrine 0.5 to 1.0 mg IV every *five minutes* and bicarbonate at
one-half dose or according to ABGs
and/or
Repeat bretylium 10 mg/kg IV bolus every 15 minutes

Monitored Ventricular Fibrillation

Monitored Arrest
Ventricular fibrillation? ——No→to appropriate
| algorithm
Yes
↓
Establish unresponsiveness and pulselessness
↓
Call for help; precordial thump
↓
Check pulse
↓
Change in rhythm? ——Yes→to appropriate
| algorithm
No
↓
Defibrillate 200 to 300 joules delivered energy
↓
Check pulse
↓
Change in rhythm? ——Yes→to appropriate
| algorithm
No
↓
Recharge defibrillator immediately 200 to 300 joules
delivered energy and defibrillate
↓
Check pulse
↓
Change in rhythm? ——Yes→to appropriate
| algorithm
No
↓
CPR, place IV line, and intubate trachea if necessary
+
Epinephrine 0.5 to 1.0 mg IV or intratracheal + ? bicarbonate IV
↓
To † in Unmonitored Ventricular Fibrillation Algorithm

*Asystole**

CPR
↓

*If patient is hypothermic, core temperature should be normalized.
Be aware that what appears to be asystole may be fine ventricular fibrillation and could respond to countershock.

Intubate, ventilate, establish IV if necessary
↓
Epinephrine 0.5 to 1.0 mg IV or intratracheal
Repeat at five-minute intervals as needed
↓
Sodium bicarbonate 1 mEq/kg (or 75 mEq IV as initial dose average-size adult); repeat at ten-minute intervals at one-half original dose or, preferably, according to ABGs
|
CPR
↓
Atropine 1.0 mg IV
|
CPR
↓
Check pulse
↓
Change in rhythm? ——Yes→to appropriate
| algorithm
No
↓
CPR
↓
Calcium chloride 10% solution 5 mL IV; repeat every ten minutes as needed
|
CPR
↓
Check pulse
↓
Change in rhythm? ——Yes→to appropriate
| algorithm
No
↓
CPR
↓
Repeat epinephrine IV, bicarbonate IV, calcium chloride IV as above
↓
Consider isoproterenol infusion 2 to 20 µg/min
|
CPR
↓
Check pulse
↓
Change in rhythm? ——Yes→to appropriate
| algorithm
No
↓
Repeat epinephrine IV, bicarbonate IV, calcium chloride IV as above
↓
Consider pacemaker

Electromechanical Dissociation

Consider hypovolemia, cardiac tamponade, rupture, or tension pneumothorax as cause. Reassess ventilation, oxygenation.

CPR
↓
Epinephrine 0.5 to 1.0 mg IV or intratracheal
Repeat at five-minute intervals as necessary
↓
Sodium bicarbonate 1 mEq/kg (or 75 mL IV initial dose average-size adult)
Repeat at ten-minute intervals at one-half original dose or,
preferably, according to ABGs
↓
Change in rhythm
and/or return of pulse? ——Yes→to appropriate
    | algorithm
No
↓
CPR
↓
Calcium chloride 10% solution 5 mL
Repeat at ten-minute intervals as needed
↓
Change in rhythm
and/or return of pulse? ——Yes→to appropriate
    | algorithm
No
↓
CPR
↓
Repeat epinephrine IV, bicarbonate IV, calcium chloride IV as above
↓
Isoproterenol infusion 2 to 20 μg/min
(Despite presence of rhythm, continue CPR if no palpable pulse present)
Consider trial of volume infusion

Ventricular Tachycardia

```
Patient with pulse
  │
  ├── Yes ──► Conscious ── Yes ──► Precordial thump
  │             │                    │
  │             │                    ▼
  │             │                  Check pulse
  │             │                    │
  │             │                    ▼
  │             │                  Change in rhythm? ── Yes ──► to appropriate algorithm
  │             │                    │
  │             │                    No
  │             │                    ▼
  │             │                  Lidocaine 100 mg IV bolus (or 1 mg/kg)*
  │             │                    +
  │             │                  Cardioversion 200 joules delivered energy
  │             │                    │
  │             │                    ▼
  │             │                  Check pulse
  │             │                    │
  │             │                    ▼
  │             │                  Reversion to normal rhythm? ── Yes ──► lidocaine infusion 2 to 4 mg/min
  │             │                    │
  │             │                    No
  │             │                    ▼
  │             │                  Bretylium 350 to 500 mg IV or 5 mg/kg over eight- to ten-minute period
  │             │                    │
  │             │                    ▼
  │             │                  Check pulse
  │             │                    │
  │             │                    ▼
  │             │                  Reversion to normal rhythm? ── Yes ──► lidocaine infusion 2 to 4 mg/min
  │             │                    │
  │             │                    No
  │             │                    ▼
  │             │                  Cardioversion 200 joules delivered energy
  │             │
  │             └── No ──► Precordial thump
  │                          │
  │                          ▼
  │                        Check pulse
  │                          │
  │                          ▼
  │                        Change in rhythm? ── Yes ──► to appropriate algorithm
  │                          │
  │                          No
  │                          ▼
  │                        Lidocaine 100 mg IV (or 1 mg/kg)*
  │                          │
  │                          ▼
  │                        Check pulse
  │                          │
  │                          ▼
  │                        Reversion to normal rhythm? ── Yes ──► lidocaine infusion 2 to 4 mg/min*
  │                          │
  │                          No
  │                          ▼
  │                        Cardioversion 20 to 100 joules delivered energy
  │                          │
  │                          ▼
  │                        Check pulse
  │                          │
  │                          ▼
  │                        Reversion to normal rhythm? ── Yes ──► lidocaine infusion 2 to 4 mg/min*
  │                          │
  │                          No
  │                          ▼
  │
  └── No ──► (Precordial thump and immediate countershock if monitored)
              │
              ▼
            CPR
              │
              ▼
            Countershock 200 joules delivered energy—otherwise same as for ventricular fibrillation
```

Algorithm below

Check pulse
↓
Reversion to normal rhythm? —— Yes→lidocaine infusion 2 to 4 mg/min
↓
No
↓
Algorithm below

Recurrent Ventricular Tachycardia
(after maximum lidocaine infusion)

Procainamide 20 mg/min IV—up to 100 mg/5 min until—dysrhythmia suppressed or hypotension ensues or QRS widens by 50% or total of 1 g administered

    or   Bretylium 5 mg/kg IV bolus followed by infusion— 1 to 2 mg/min
↓
Check pulse
↓
Reversion to normal rhythm? —— Yes→continue bretylium infusion 1 to 2 mg/min
↓
No
↓
Bretylium 10 mg/kg IV bolus May repeat if needed
↓
Overdrive pacing

Follow with infusion of procainamide 1 to 4 mg/min
↓
Check pulse

Reversion to normal rhythm? —— Yes→Continue procainamide 1 to 4 mg/min
↓
No
↓
Bretylium
↓
Overdrive pacing

*A second loading dose of 0.5 mg/kg should be given in 5 to 10 minutes.

Bradycardia

Bradycardia (rate <50); or rate <60 plus hypotension (systolic <90) and/or PVCs
↓
Atropine 0.5 mg IV
May be repeated as necessary every five minutes to 2.0 mg
↓
Rate > 60 ——————Yes→ BP obtainable—Yes < 90 → Assess volume status; trial of volume infusion
                                Yes > 90↗   systolic   Dopamine infusion (titrated)
                                                        Norepinephrine infusion (titrated)
↓ No   ↑↓ No
                          Observe
Isoproterenol infusion
2 to 20 μg/min IV   Pulse present ——— Yes → CPR → Trial of volume infusion
                                                       ↓
Rate > 50   Yes   ↓ No   Epinephrine 0.5 to 1.0 mg IV
↓ No   Electromechanical   ↓
                                Dissociation   Sodium bicarbonate 1 mEq/kg IV
*Pacemaker   Algorithm   or according to ABGs
                                                                             ↓
                                                                             Calcium chloride 10% solution 5 ml
                                                                             ↓
                                                                             Dopamine infusion (titrated)
                                                                             ↓
                                                                             Norepinephrine infusion (titrated)

Supraventricular Rhythm with Pulse

(following termination of ventricular
fibrillation or ventricular tachycardia)
↓
IV if not in place
↓
Lidocaine 100 mg IV bolus (1 mg/kg) after termination of ventricular
tachycardia or ventricular fibrillation followed by infusion of
2 to 4 mg/min*
↓
Ventilate as necessary
Intubate if not done and patient unresponsive
↓
Oxygenate 100% O_2
↓
Support circulation as necessary

*If bradycardia requires maintenance of isoproterenol drip, pacemaker should be considered.

*A second loading dose of lidocaine (0.5 mg/kg) should be given in five to ten minutes. If recurrent ventricular tachycardia or ventricular fibrillation is not suppressed by lidocaine, consider procainamide, bretylium, or overdrive pacing. Do not use propranolol to slow sinus tachycardia that occurs in the immediate postresuscitative period. Consider causes of sinus tachycardia (hypovolemia, pump failure, catecholamine excess).

Drugs Used in Cardiac Arrest: How Supplied, Usual Dose (Average Adult)

Drug	Concentration and volume of prefilled syringe	Dose	Infusion rate	Remarks
Atropine sulfate	0.1 mg/ml in 10-ml syringe	0.5–1.0 mg = 5–10 mL	Bolus . . .	Repeat at 5-minute intervals to achieve desired rate. Generally, do *not* exceed 2 mg
Bretylium tosylate	50 mg/ml in 10-ml ampule	5 mg/kg 350–500 mg as initial dose	500 mg in 5% dextrose in water (in 250 ml = 2 mg/ml; in 500 ml = 1 mg/ml) Infusion: 1–2 mg/min	Infusion started after loading dose to control recurrent ventricular tachycardia or ventricular fibrillation
Calcium chloride 10%	100 mg/ml in 10-ml syringe	500 mg = 5 ml	Bolus . . .	May repeat dose every ten minutes as needed
Dopamine	200 mg in 5-ml ampule	. . .	200 mg in 250 ml dextrose in water = 800 µg/ml Infusion: 2–10 µg/kg/min	. . .

Epinephrine 1:10,000	0.1 mg/ml in 10-ml syringe	0.5 mg–1.0 mg = 5–10 ml IV or intratracheal	1 mg in 5% dextrose in water (in 250 ml = 4 μg/ml; in 500 ml = 2 μg/ml) Infusion: 1 μg/min for maintenance of BP	Avoid intracardiac injection. Repeat dose every 5 minutes as needed in cardiac arrest
Isoproterenol	0.2 mg/ml in 5-ml ampule	. . .	1 mg in 5% dextrose in water (in 250 ml = 4 μg/ml; in 500 ml = 2 μg/ml) Infusion: 2–20 μg/min. Titrate	Beware of PVCs
Lidocaine	For IV bolus: 2% (20 mg/ml) in 5 ml = 100 mg For infusion after bolus: 4% (40 mg/ml) in 25 ml = 1 g	75 mg = 3.75 ml	2 g in 500 ml 5% dextrose in water (or 1 g in 250 ml) = 4 mg/ml Infusion: 1–4 mg/min	For breakthrough ventricular ectopy: additional 50 mg bolus every 5 minutes to suppress, or total of 225 mg. Increase drip to 4 mg/min
Sodium bicarbonate	1 mEq/ml in 50 ml = 50 mEq	1 mEq/kg or 75 ml initial dose (average-size adult) or preferably according to pH	. . .	Repeat according to pH. If not available, use ½ initial dose every 10 minutes

APPENDIX 7

American Heart Association Cardiopulmonary Resuscitation and Emergency Cardiac Care Rationale For One Rescuer CPR (Heartsaver)

ELAPSED TIME (Seconds)		ACTIVITY AND TIME (Seconds)	CRITICAL PERFORMANCE	RATIONALE
Min.	Max.			
4	10	Establish unresponsiveness and call out for help. Allow 4–10 sec. if face down and turning is required.	Tap, gently shake and shout—"Are you OK?" Call out—"Help!" Turn if necessary.	Frequently victim will be face down. Effective external chest compression can only be provided with victim flat on back on hard surface.
			Adequate time.	Accurate diagnosis is important. 4 to 10 seconds gives time to do that and to review mentally the sequence of CPR.
7	15	Open airway. Establish breathlessness. (Look, Listen, and Feel) (3–5 sec.)	Kneels properly.	
			Head tilt with one hand on forehead and neck lift or chin lift with other hand.	Airway must be opened to establish breathlessness. Many victims may be making respiratory efforts that are ineffective because of obstruction.
			Ear over mouth, observe chest.	

10		Four ventilations. (3–5 sec.)	Ventilate properly 4 times and observe chest rise.
15	20	Establish pulse and simulate activation of EMS system. (5–10 sec.)	Fingers palpate for carotid pulse on near side (other hand on forehead maintains head tilt).	This activity should take 5 to 10 seconds, because not only does it take time to find the right place, but the pulse may be very slow or very weak and rapid.
	30		Know local EMS number.
			Adequate time.
69		Four cycles of 15 compressions and 2 ventilations. (54–66 sec.)	Proper body position.
			Landmark check each time.
			Position of hands.	Precision in hand placement is essential to avoid serious injury.
			Vertical compression.
			Says mnemonic.	Necessary to establish rhythm.
	96		Proper rate.	Should attempt to accomplish 60 compressions and 8 ventilations per minute.
			Proper ratio.
			No bouncing.
			Ventilates properly.
72	101	Check for return of pulse and spontaneous breathing. (Pupil check optional) (3–5 sec.)	Check pulse and breathing. (Pupil check optional)	Pupil size helps to monitor changes in the patient.

APPENDIX 8

American Heart Association Cardiopulmonary Resuscitation and Emergency Cardiac Care Rationale For One and Two Rescuer CPR

ELAPSED TIME (Seconds) Min. Max.	ACTIVITY AND TIME (Seconds)	CRITICAL PERFORMANCE	RATIONALE
	1st rescuer resumes CPR. 2nd rescuer identifies himself and checks pulse for effective compressions.	Technique for single rescuer. 2nd rescuer says, "I know how to do CPR." Fingers palpate for carotid pulse.	To locate the carotid pulse.
	2nd rescuer calls out "Stop compressions" and checks for spontaneous pulse and breathing. (5 sec.)	Five second pause to check for spontaneous pulse and breathing. 2nd rescuer should inform the 1st rescuer of the status of the victim and the need for either ventilations, compressions or both. Says, "No pulse, continue CPR."	Provides a second assessment of pulse and breathing and the need for CPR.

TWO RESCUERS

2nd rescuer ventilates once.	Ventilates properly and observes chest rise.	
1st rescuer resumes compressions.	Two-rescuer rate and ratio.	2nd rescuer ventilation triggers change of rate and ratio.
Minimum of two cycles of 5 compressions and 1 ventilation. (8–10 sec.) Switch and repeat until examiner is satisfied.	Correct rate of compressions.	
	Says mnemonic.	Necessary to establish rhythm.
	Interposes breath.	
	No pause for ventilation.	
	Calls for switch.	Signal for change must be clear.
	Switches.	
	Switches back.	
	Checks pulse (by ventilator).	
	Technique as above.	

APPENDIX 9

American Heart Association Cardiopulmonary Resuscitation and Emergency Cardiac Care Rationale For Complete Obstruction Conscious Choking Infant

ELAPSED TIME (Seconds)		ACTIVITY AND TIME (Seconds)	CRITICAL PERFORMANCE	RATIONALE
Min.	Max.			
2	3	Rescuer checks for airway obstruction. (2–3 sec.)	Rescuer must identify complete obstruction by looking, listening, and feeling for ventilation and for blueness of the lips.	The presence of complete airway obstruction must be properly diagnosed before proceeding with treatment.
5	8	4 Back blows (3–5 sec.)	The infant is straddled over the rescuer's arm with the head lower than the trunk. The 4 back blows are delivered rapidly and forcefully between the shoulder blades.	Back blows when used alone may relieve the obstruction.

9	13	4 Chest thrusts (4–5 sec.)	The infant is supported between 2 hands, turned onto the back, and the thrusts are delivered in the mid-sternal region in the same manner as external chest compression. The head is lower than the trunk.	The combination of back blows and chest thrusts is superior to one technique when used alone. Abdominal thrusts are not recommended in infants because of the potential injury to the abdominal organs.
		Verbally indicate repeat of above sequence until effective.	Verbalize alternating the above maneuvers in rapid sequence.	Time is of the essence. The two techniques are rapidly repeated alternatively until obstruction is relieved or unconsciousness occurs.

APPENDIX 10

American Heart Association Cardiopulmonary Resuscitation and Emergency Cardiac Care Rationale For Infant Resuscitation

ELAPSED TIME (Seconds)		ACTIVITY AND TIME (Seconds)	CRITICAL PERFORMANCE	RATIONALE
Min.	Max.			
3	5	Establish unresponsiveness and call out for help. (including turning) (3–5 sec.)	Tap, gently shake shoulder, and see if infant responds. Call out—"Help!" Turn if necessary.	Diagnosis must be equally accurate in children and infants. With this emotionally charged situation, time must be taken to establish the diagnosis of cardiac arrest. Horizontal position aids effective circulation.
			Infant horizontal.	
			Adequate time.	

6	10	Open airway. Establish breathlessness. (3–5 sec.) (Look, Listen, Feel)	Tip head back. Do not hyperextend.	Hyperextension can collapse trachea or cause cervical spine injury.
			Put ear over mouth and look toward chest to look, listen, and feel for breathing.	
9	15	Four ventilations. (3–5 sec.)	Use small breaths to ventilate.	Lung capacity of infant smaller than adult. Avoid gastric distention.
14	25	Establish pulse and simulate activation of EMS system. (5–10 sec.)	Fingers palpate for brachial pulse in infant.	Brachial pulse easier to feel in infant than carotid.
			Know local EMS number.	
44	55	10 cycles of 5 compressions and 1 ventilation. Continue uninterrupted. (30 sec.)	Two fingers on mid-sternum in infant for compressions at rate of 100 compressions per minute.	Infants (100/min) need a more rapid cardiac compression rate with breaths interposed every 5 compressions.

APPENDIX 11

American Heart Association Cardiopulmonary Resuscitation and Emergency Cardiac Care Rationale For Infant Obstructed Airway Choking Infant Who Becomes Unconscious Or Is Found Unconscious

ELAPSED TIME (Seconds)		ACTIVITY AND TIME (Seconds)	CRITICAL PERFORMANCE	RATIONALE
Min.	Max.			
4	10	Establish unresponsiveness. Call for help. Turn victim. (4–10 sec.)	Gently shake, tap, call out for help. Turn infant horizontal and supine.	An accurate diagnosis of unresponsiveness must be made before resuscitation begins or continues.
7	15	Open airway. Establish breathlessness. (Look, Listen, Feel) (3–5 sec.)	Tip head back, do not hyperextend. Rescuer looks toward chest with ear over mouth to look, listen and feel for breathing. Utilize head tilt-neck lift or, if needed, head tilt-chin lift.	Hyperextension of the head can collapse the trachea or cause cervical spine injury in the infant. An accurate diagnosis must be made to establish the presence of cardiopulmonary arrest or airway obstruction.

10	20	Attempt to ventilate. (3–5 sec.)	Ventilate—airway remains obstructed.	Complete airway obstruction or a foreign body is assumed.
13	25	Reattempt to ventilate. (3–5 sec.)	Reposition the head. Airway remains obstructed.	Improper head tilt is the most common cause of airway obstruction. Airway obstruction is confirmed.
15	27	Activate EMS system. (2 sec.)	If a second rescuer is present he should activate the EMS. Know local EMS number.	ALS capability will be needed.
19	33	4 Back blows (4–6 sec.)	Same as for conscious infant.	
24	39	4 Chest thrusts (5–6 sec.)	Same as for conscious infant.	
30	47	Tongue-jaw lift (6–8 sec.)	Thumb in victim's mouth over tongue. Lift tongue and jaw forward with fingers wrapped around lower jaw. Remove foreign body if visualized.	Blind finger sweeps are to be avoided in the infant since the foreign body can easily be pushed back and cause further obstruction.
		Verbally indicate repeat of above sequence until effective.	Verbalize alternating the above maneuvers in rapid succession.	Persistent attempts are rapidly made in sequence in order to relieve the obstruction.

V
MULTIPLE-CHOICE QUESTIONS AND ANSWERS

Questions

CHAPTER 1

1. The main functions of the PARR nurse include all the following except:
   a. Recognition and initial treatment of respiratory problems
   b. Measuring temperature
   c. Maintaining accurate records
   d. Monitoring the cardiovascular system
   e. Determining which patients should be admitted to the recovery room

2. During transport of the patient from the operating room to the recovery room:
   a. Adequate monitoring should be maintained
   b. Resuscitative equipment should be readily available
   c. Two people should be in attendance
   d. No more than 5 minutes should elapse
   e. All of the above

3. The initial report from the anesthesiologist to the PARR nurse need not include:
   a. Patient's name
   b. Operation performed
   c. Past medical history
   d. Name of insurance carrier
   e. Physical impairments

4. All of the following are important in the initial respiratory observation of the patient coming to the recovery room except:
   a. Lip and fingernail color
   b. Ability to talk or cry
   c. Respiratory rate
   d. Chest excursion
   e. Adequate arterial blood gases at the beginning of surgery

5. Assessment of recovery from anesthesia may be simply made by:
   a. The Aldrete score

b. Electroencephalographic recording
c. Observation
d. Blood pressure recording
e. All of the above

6. Each of the instructions evaluate the ability to comprehend and perform a motor function except:
   a. "Lift your head"
   b. "Open your eyes"
   c. "Put out your tongue"
   d. "Are you having pain?"
   e. "Can you move your toes?"

7. In using the postanesthetic recovery score, which of the following does not score 1 point?
   a. Ability to move only the lower extremities
   b. Dyspnea
   c. Arousable on calling
   d. Dusky color
   e. Blood pressure 15 percent below preanesthetic level

8. Negative inspiratory pressure:
   a. Cannot be easily measured at the bedside
   b. Should be measured only by the respiratory therapist
   c. Must be at least -40 cm H_2O to allow adequate coughing
   d. Can only be measured if the patient has an endotracheal tube in place
   e. Is of little value

9. Phase 2 neuromuscular blockade:
   a. Develops after prolonged succinylcholine administration
   b. May be a residual effect of pancuronium administration
   c. Is associated with posttetanic facilitation
   d. Is not increased by administration of penicillin
   e. All of the above

10. A flow directed balloon tipped pulmonary artery catheter (Swan-Ganz) is used to measure all of the following except:
    a. Cardiac output
    b. Pulmonary capillary wedge pressure
    c. Central venous pressure
    d. Right ventricular pressure
    e. Left ventricular pressure

CHAPTER 2

1. Pain impulses to the spinal cord are transmitted through:
   a. β fibers

b. φ fibers
   c. Unmyelinated C fibers
   d. Myelinated B fibers
   e. Nodes of Ranvier
2. Which of the following are endogenous peptides exhibiting opioid properties?
   a. Somatostatin
   b. Diamorphine
   c. Beta-lipoprotein
   d. Met-enkaphalin
   e. Alpha-endorphin
3. Opioid receptors are found in which of the following parts of the central nervous system?
   a. Baroreceptor trigger zone
   b. Anterior horn cells
   c. Substantia gelatinosa of the dorsal horn
   d. Basal ganglia
   e. Reticulo-spinal tract
4. Which of the following opioids have agonist effects primarily at μ receptors?
   a. Pentazocine
   b. Heroin
   c. Fentanyl
   d. Nalbuphine
   e. Naloxone
5. Morphine:
   a. Is highly lipophilic
   b. Is a Kappa receptor antagonist
   c. Is an agonist at μ receptors
   d. Antagonizes labyrinthine vomiting
   e. Is highly suitable for epidural analgesia
6. Methadone:
   a. Is a naturally occurring opioid
   b. Has a very long elimination half-life
   c. Is unsuitable for intravenous administration
   d. Has a fast clearance
   e. Is metabolized to a highly active metabolite
7. Bupivacaine:
   a. Is an aminoester local anesthetic
   b. Is poorly lipid soluble
   c. Should never be repeated until the effects of a previous block have worn off
   d. Produces intense motor nerve blockade
   e. Has a longer onset of action than lidocaine

8. Opioids suitable for intravenous infusion analgesia:
   a. Should have a slow hepatic clearance
   b. Are usually partial agonists at μ receptors
   c. Should have a short elimination half-life
   d. Do not cause ventilatory depression
   e. Are not suitable for patient-controlled demand analgesia
9. Narcotic (morphine) overdose:
   a. Is associated with dilatation of the pupil
   b. May be treated with naloxone
   c. Is characterized by rapid shallow breathing
   d. Should be treated with metaclopramide
   e. May be completely reversed by buprenorphine
10. Midthoracic segmental (T4–12) epidural block in the postoperative period:
    a. Cannot be achieved by the use of opioids
    b. Is best achieved by repeated lidocaine injection
    c. Is associated with weakness of leg movements
    d. Can be produced by 15 ml 0.5 percent bupivacaine injected at T8 interspace
    e. Blocks the sympathetic nerve supply to the adrenal gland

CHAPTER 3

1. Postoperatively, the trachea may be extubated safely:
   a. Even if the respiratory pattern is irregular
   b. As long as the patient is kept in a lateral position
   c. When the patient is responsive to commands
   d. Only when the surgeon has given the order
   e. As soon as the temperature reads 35° C
2. All of the following are important in the initial respiratory observation of the patient coming into the recovery room except:
   a. Lip and fingernail color
   b. Patient's ability to talk or cry
   c. Respiratory rate
   d. Chest excursion
   e. Adequate arterial blood gases at the beginning of surgery
3. Respiratory insufficiency is least likely to develop after 1 hour in the recovery room if:
   a. The initial temperature was 30° C
   b. 10 mg morphine is given intravenously
   c. 1.5 liters of normal saline has been infused over 1 hour

d. Trendelenburg position is employed to correct hypotension
e. 12.5 mg meperidine is given intravenously
4. Signs of inadequate ventilation include all of the following except:
   a. Cyanosis
   b. Sternal retraction
   c. Respiratory rate of 38 per minute
   d. PaO_2 of 60 mm Hg with an FiO_2 of 0.35
   e. $PaCO_2$ 32 mm Hg
5. Immediate postoperative hypoxia may be due to all of the following except:
   a. Intraoperative hyperventilation
   b. Intraoperative hypoventilation
   c. 2 liters normal saline intraoperatively
   d. Epidural anesthesia to T-10 level
   e. 150 mg meperidine in the previous hour
6. The alveolar-arterial oxygen tension gradient:
   a. Indicates no pulmonary damage as long as it is < 200 mm Hg
   b. Bears no relationship to the barometric pressure
   c. Is a conveniently calculated number used to assess the ability of pulmonary oxygen transfer
   d. Increases as pulmonary function improves
   e. Has an ideal value of 100 mm Hg
7. Respiratory criteria which should be met before the patient may be safely discharged include all of the following except:
   a. A vital capacity of > 1.5 liters
   b. Respiratory rate stability for 15 minutes
   c. Ability to cough
   d. $PaCO_2$ 35 mm Hg
   e. PaO_2 120 mm Hg at FiO_2 of 0.25
8. The vital capacity is:
   a. The amount of air moved in or out during normal respiration
   b. Measured by a Wright respirometer
   c. Not affected after upper abdominal surgery
   d. An inspiratory measurement
   e. Part of the dead space to tidal volume ratio
9. Negative inspiratory force:
   a. Cannot be suitably measured at the bedside
   b. Should be at least 15 mm Hg if ventilation is to be considered adequate
   c. Must be at least −25 cm H_2O to allow effective gas exchange
   d. Can only be measured if the patient has a tracheostomy tube in place
   e. Is of little value

368   MULTIPLE CHOICE QUESTIONS AND ANSWERS

10. All the following drugs are likely to result in significant ventilatory depression in the recovery period except:
    a. Meperidine 25 mg IV 15 minutes after discontinuing general anesthesia
    b. Diazepam 10 mg orally, given 30 minutes before cystoscopy in an 85-year-old man.
    c. Succinylcholine 550 mg given intraoperatively over a 90-minute period
    d. Curare 3 mg given prior to intubation
    e. Meperidine 25 mg IM after an anesthetic technique which employed 12.5 mg droperidol (5 ml)

CHAPTER 4

1. The treatment of choice for a patient with hypotension complicating sinus bradycardia is:
    a. Methoxamine 2 mg IV
    b. Digoxin 0.25 mg IV
    c. Atropine 0.6 mg IV
    d. Phentolamine
    e. Epinephrine infusion 1 µg/kg per minute
2. A characteristic sign of pulmonary edema arising in the postoperative period is:
    a. Bradypnea
    b. ST segment depression
    c. Basal crepitations
    d. Sinus bradycardia
    e. Prolonged P-R interval
3. Which of the following is a complication of postoperative hypertension?
    a. Pulmonary embolism
    b. Cerebral thrombosis
    c. Atrial fibrillation
    d. Cor pulmonale
    e. Pulmonary edema
4. A high systolic pressure with a wide pulse pressure, but normal diastolic pressure, is compatible with:
    a. Pheochromocytoma
    b. Renovascular hypertension
    c. Coronary artery disease
    d. Coarctation of the aorta
    e. Arteriosclerosis

5. The rate of change of arterial pressure (dP/dT) is a measure of:
   a. Cardiac conduction
   b. Systemic vascular resistance
   c. Stroke volume
   d. Myocardial contractility
   e. Venodilatation
6. Propranolol (1-2 mg) IV is indicated for which of the following circumstances?
   a. Junctional bradycardia
   b. Sinus tachycardia
   c. Möbitz Type II block
   d. First-degree heart block
   e. R on T extrasystoles
7. Lidocaine (1 mg/kg) IV is indicated in which of the following?
   a. R on T phenomenon
   b. Junctional tachycardia
   c. Sinus bradycardia
   d. First-degree heart block
   e. Atrial fibrillation
8. In which of these conditions should postoperative hypertension *not* be treated?
   a. After carotid endarterectomy
   b. In the presence of raised intracranial pressure
   c. When CVP is low
   d. When the urinary bladder is distended
   e. After administration of methylprednisolone
9. Septicemia should be suspected when:
   a. Tachycardia is associated with hypertension
   b. Low cardiac output is associated with raised left atrial pressure
   c. Hypotension is associated with high cardiac output
   d. Paroxysmal tachycardia will not respond to propranolol
   e. Bradycardia will not respond to atropine
10. Subendocardial ischemia is manifest in the ECG as:
    a. Raised, coved ST segments
    b. Widening of the QT interval
    c. Depressed ST segments
    d. Widened QRS complexes in precordial leads
    e. μ waves

CHAPTER 5

1. Who are candidates for platelet transfusion?
   a. Patients who are actively bleeding

b. Patients who are to undergo surgery and have platelet counts under 50,000 per cu mm
   c. Persons with platelet counts less than 20,000 per cu mm
   d. Patients who have had massive transfusions or open heart surgery
   e. All of the above
2. How much colloid would a 70-kg man with 10 percent burn require over 24 hours?
3. In the postoperative patient:
   a. Ringer's lactate should never be used
   b. Salt retention is a dreaded complication
   c. Normal saline is preferable to Ringer's lactate
   d. A certain degree of fluid retention is expected
   e. Dextrose 5 percent water is complete replacement
4. Use of colloid solutions:
   a. Are indicated in the burn patient
   b. Are controversial for resuscitation of patients other than those with burns
   c. May impair organ function
   d. All of the above
   e. None of the above
5. Whole blood:
   a. Should be used instead of packed red cells at every opportunity
   b. Is useful for 3 years if frozen
   c. Is rich in clotting factors
   d. Is useful for acute massive blood loss
   e. Rarely causes allergic reactions
6. Platelet concentrates:
   a. Should be used for patients with an elevated protime
   b. Are useful for bleeding due to a low platelet count
   c. Have a long shelf life (over one year)
   d. Can last at room temperature for 2 to 4 days
   e. Can be obtained immediately from the blood bank
7. Following a TURP, a patient should be observed for:
   a. Water overload
   b. Hyponatremia
   c. Changes in mental function
   d. Congestive heart failure
   e. All of the above
8. Patients receiving chronic diuretic therapy:
   a. Are often salt depleted and have increased fluid requirements
   b. Should be run "dry"
   c. May have increased body stores of potassium

d. Should be maintained with a blood pressure over 150 mm Hg at all times
e. Are usually tachycardic

9. Total body water:
   a. Is the largest single component of body weight
   b. Is least in young, muscular males
   c. Is greatest in elderly obese females
   d. Is made up at least 50 percent by rate of oxidation
   e. Is replenished daily

10. Extracellular fluid:
    a. Is increased during shock
    b. Decreases with resuscitation
    c. Is altered by permeability of cell membranes
    d. Is independent of ion exchange
    e. Averages about 15 percent of normal weight

CHAPTER 6

1. Immediate postoperative hypoxia may be due to all of the following except:
   a. Intraoperative hyperventilation
   b. Intraoperative hypoventilation
   c. 2 liters normal saline intraoperatively
   d. Epidural anesthesia to T-10 level
   e. 300 µg fentanyl in the previous hour

2. Rapid emergence from anesthesia is usually seen following:
   a. Droperidol and fentanyl
   b. Methoxyflurane
   c. Continuous pentothal infusion
   d. Isoflurane 0.5 percent for 4 hours
   e. Fentanyl 25 µg/kg—muscle relaxant technique for 2 hours

3. Therapy of a patient in whom there has only been partial reversal of muscle relaxant action should include all of the following except:
   a. Ventilatory support
   b. Supportive verbal communication
   c. Neostigmine and atropine
   d. Sodium bicarbonate
   e. Naloxone

4. 25 mg demerol in the postoperative period will cause hypoventilation:
   a. In old patients only
   b. In 25 percent of all patients
   c. Especially in a patient who has just had a gastrectomy

d. In 80 percent of patients
e. Only if the surgical dressing is too tight

5. Prolonged effects of muscle relaxants are least likely to occur:
   a. In patients who received 0.4 mg atropine and 2.0 mg neostigmine at the end of the operation
   b. In patients who have an arterial pH of 7.28
   c. In incipient myasthenia gravis
   d. If the patient has received 75 mg curare over 3.5 hours
   e. If a single dose of 200 mg succinylcholine was used for intubation 30 minutes previously

6. A patient who is admitted to the recovery room with a temperature of 31° C:
   a. Must have continuous cardiac monitoring
   b. Must be rewarmed with hot blankets immediately
   c. Can be safely moved for diagnostic X rays within 15 minutes
   d. Should be catheterized to monitor urinary output
   e. Should be given large doses of diazepam to prevent shivering

7. The least common cause of postoperative coma is:
   a. Blood sugar level of 1200 mg%
   b. Regional epidural anesthesia at T-5 level
   c. Intraoperative intracranial aneurysm rupture
   d. Incision and drainage of a fascial abscess of thigh
   e. Temperature of 30° C

8. Respiratory insufficiency exists if:
   a. Respiratory rate is 12 per minute
   b. Tidal volume is 350 ml
   c. Vital capacity is < 1 liter
   d. Oxygen saturation in arterial blood is 98.5 percent
   e. $PaCO_2$ is 37 mm Hg

9. Therapy of postoperative hypoventilation does not include:
   a. Assisted ventilation
   b. Naloxone
   c. Continuous ECG monitoring
   d. Diazepam to decrease confusion
   e. Increased FiO_2

10. Which of the following is not commonly observed in allergic drug response?
    a. Skin wheal
    b. Bronchospasm
    c. PaO_2 65 mm Hg
    d. Blood pressure 80/50
    e. Bradycardia 50 per minute

CHAPTER 7

1. According to JCAH, a patient may be discharged from PACU by:
   a. The PACU nurse manager or staff nurse
   b. The patient's surgeon or anesthesiologist
   c. The hospital administrator or OR supervisor
   d. The patient or family
   e. Any physician in the unit
2. Written discharge criteria should include:
   a. The physiologic parameters of the patient to be evaluated
   b. The length of time a patient may remain in PACU
   c. The time a patient is discharged from PACU
   d. The destination of the patient
   e. All of the above
3. A postanesthesia scoring system provides:
   a. Long-term evaluation of the patient's recovery
   b. More paperwork for the PAN
   c. An objective measurement of the patient's recovery from anesthesia
   d. A standard for discharge criteria
   e. An essential part of the patient's record
4. Which of the following classifications of patients *do not* require specific discharge criteria?
   a. Pediatric patients
   b. Ambulatory surgery patients
   c. Critical care patients
   d. Abdominal surgery patients
   e. Postcraniotomy patients
5. Established discharge criteria provide:
   a. A tool for evaluating discharge eligibility
   b. Professional accountability for the PAN
   c. A means to comply with JCAH guidelines
   d. Improved patient care
   e. All of the above
6. Standards identified for written discharge criteria should include all of the following except:
   a. A definition of acceptable temperature range
   b. A definition of stability for vital signs
   c. The patient's ability to drive himself home
   d. Documentation requirements
   e. Discharge to the care of a responsible adult
7. The Aldrete postanesthetic recovery score is most similar in concept to the:
   a. Glasgow coma scale

b. Carignan scoring system
c. Apgar score
d. Graphic score
e. None—it is a new concept

8. An anesthesiologist's discharge signature is required:
   a. In 32 states and 6 countries
   b. By JCAH
   c. When that is the policy in a particular institution
   d. When the patient is ready to leave the PACU
   e. Throughout the United States

9. The pediatric patient in PACU, upon discharge, should be able to:
   a. Cry or talk
   b. Retain fluids
   c. Focus his eyes
   d. Maintain stable vital signs
   e. All of the above

10. A verbal report from the PACU nurse to the next nurse who will be caring for the patient is important for all of the following reasons except:
    a. Alerts the nurse to the patient's imminent arrival
    b. Provides continuity in the patient's care
    c. Enables the PACU nurse to use nursing assistants for transport
    d. Assists the next nurse to plan for the patient's continuing care needs
    e. Expands the role of the recovery room nurse to the wards

CHAPTER 8

1. The estimated blood volume of a 3 kg neonate is:
   a. 90 ml
   b. 120 ml
   c. 195 ml
   d. 240 ml
   e. 300 ml

2. The minimum systolic blood pressure (mm Hg) considered normal in a healthy 6-hour-old full-term infant is:
   a. 70
   b. 60
   c. 50
   d. 40
   e. 30

3. Heat loss in the newborn infant is enhanced by each of the following except:
   a. Large surface area to body weight ratio

b. Environmental temperature of 21°C (70°F)
   c. Presence of only small amounts of subcutaneous tissue
   d. Heat loss from brown fat deposits
   e. Radiation to surrounding surfaces (e.g., incubator walls)
4. True statements about the infant airway include all the following except:
   a. The larynx is more cephalad than in the adult
   b. The widest part is just below the cords
   c. Edema following intubation may critically compromise the airway
   d. An appropriately sized endotracheal tube allows a leak
   e. Humidified oxygen is appropriate therapy to treat early edema
5. A 2-year-old 15-kg child, after an uneventful endotracheal general anesthetic becomes restless in the recovery room, with a "croupy" cough, mild retractions and a respiratory rate of 45 per minute. Appropriate initial therapy is:
   a. Epinephrine, 0.2 mg subcutaneously
   b. Endotracheal intubation
   c. Nebulized racemic epinephrine and cool mist
   d. Dexamethasone, 15 mg intravenously
6. In addition to 5 percent dextrose in 0.2 percent normal saline solution, a 3-day-old infant undergoing surgery for bowel resection should be given:
   a. An electrolyte containing solution at a rate of 4 to 6 ml/kg per hour
   b. Five percent dextrose in water at a rate of 4 to 6 ml/kg per hour
   c. No additional fluids
   d. Whole blood as replacement for third space loss
   e. Plasmanate 5 ml/kg per hour
7. One hour after tonsillectomy, a 4-year-old 20-kg child vomits approximately 300 ml of fresh blood. He is restless, blood pressure is 60/40 mm Hg, and the pulse is 160 per minute. The best approach is to:
   a. Draw blood for hemoglobin and hematocrit determination
   b. Administer lactated Ringer's solution
   c. Await fully cross-matched blood before operative intervention
   d. Alert the surgeon immediately and administer partially cross-matched blood
8. Appropriate doses of agents used in pediatric cardiopulmonary resuscitation include all the following except:
   a. Atropine, 0.02 mg/kg
   b. Epinephrine, 1:10,000 solution, 0.01 ml/kg
   c. Calcium chloride, 10 mg/kg
   d. Sodium bicarbonate, 2 mEq/kg
   e. 100 percent O_2

9. When using an inflatable cuff to measure blood pressure:
   a. The width of the cuff should equal two-thirds the length of the upper arm
   b. Use of a narrower cuff leads to pressure measurements lower than actual pressures
   c. The width of the cuff should be related to age
   d. Pressures are measured in the arm
   e. All of the above
10. Drugs and techniques to relieve postoperative pain include all the following except:
    a. Narcotics
    b. Regional analgesia
    c. Acetaminophen
    d. Diazepam
    e. Parental visit

CHAPTER 9

1. The normal intracranial pressure is:
   a. 22 mm Hg
   b. 10 mm Hg
   c. 32 mm Hg
   d. 40 mm Hg
   e. 5 cm H_2O
2. The following physiological variable will increase ICP:
   a. Hypocarbia
   b. Hypercarbia
   c. Hypothermia
   d. Hypotension
   e. Hypoxia to 70 mm Hg PaO_2
3. The factor that will decrease the ICP is:
   a. Tachycardia
   b. Hypertension
   c. Nitroprusside
   d. Mannitol
   e. Nitroglycerin
4. Persistent poor neurological function in the recovery room may be due to all of the following except:
   a. Intracranial bleeding
   b. Spasm of cerebral vessels

c. Pneumocephalus
d. Shivering
e. Hypoxia

5. The ideal position for a patient following craniotomy is:
   a. Head low
   b. Feet up
   c. Head turned to the left
   d. Head up
   e. Flat

6. Patients following cervical cord injury are liable to manifest all of the following except:
   a. Pulmonary edema
   b. Hypotension
   c. Respiratory disease
   d. Increased ICP
   e. Hallucinations

7. Increasing intracranial pressure is detected by:
   a. Monitoring ICP
   b. Diuresis
   c. Low arterial $PaCO_2$
   d. Hypothermia
   e. Falling blood pressure

8. Clinical deterioration in the neurological function can be detected by all except:
   a. Pupillary reaction to light
   b. Unequal size of pupils
   c. Shivering (nonconvulsive)
   d. Deteriorating mental status
   e. Decreasing handshake

9. All of the following are true features in direct intraventricular ICP monitoring except:
   a. Early detection of neurological deterioration
   b. Withdrawal of CSF to decrease ICP
   c. Sterile heparinized saline in a highly pressurized system is used
   d. Intracranial hemorrhage and infection can result
   e. Requires making a burr hole

10. Glasgow coma scale uses all of the following parameters except:
    a. Motor response
    b. Verbal response
    c. Eye opening ability
    d. Pupillary reaction to light
    e. Response to commands

CHAPTER 10

1. Which of the following patients is most likely to have a local anesthetic reaction when he arrives in the recovery room?
   a. A man who had a spinal anesthetic an hour ago for hernia repair
   b. A patient who had multiple intercostal blocks 20 minutes ago and was brought to the recovery room prior to surgery
   c. A patient who had a digital nerve block with 5 cc of 1 percent xylocaine 10 minutes ago
   d. Any patient who received bupivacaine 0.25 percent
   e. Any case in which epinephrine was added to the solution

2. Which of the following procedures is least likely to result in a pneumothorax?
   a. Supraclavicular brachial plexus block
   b. Multiple intercostal block for gall bladder surgery
   c. Lumbar epidural for varicose vein surgery
   d. Subclavian placement of CVP catheter
   e. Internal jugular placement of a Swan-Ganz catheter

3. A T6-level spinal anesthetic may result in all except which of the following?
   a. Make most vascular beds below the waist vasodilate
   b. Block all nerve supply to the bladder
   c. Generally increase the blood pressure
   d. Relax the lower abdominal muscles
   e. Cause a decrease in blood pressure

4. Which of the following is not appropriate treatment for significant hypotension from spinal anesthesia?
   a. Place patient in head up position to keep spinal from going higher
   b. Give 5 1/m nasal oxygen
   c. Infuse 200 ml of Ringer's lactate solution quickly
   d. Place patient in head down position
   e. Give ephedrine 12.5 mg

5. The adverse reaction to spinal anesthesia most likely to be seen in the recovery room is:
   a. Pneumothorax
   b. Local anesthetic toxicity
   c. Sympathetic nerve block causing hypotension
   d. Headache
   e. Backache

6. Possible adverse reactions after topical anesthesia for bronchoscopy include all the following except:
   a. Seizures
   b. Hypotension

c. Aspiration
   d. Pneumothorax
   e. Tachycardia
7. Which statement about epidural morphine is not true?
   a. It has been used for surgical anesthesia
   b. It is used most for postoperative pain relief
   c. Since small doses are used, it is safer than morphine administered intramuscularly
   d. It may cause itching
   e. Its use is still controversial
8. Which statement about the respiratory effects of spinal anesthesia is true?
   a. Spinal anesthesia rarely paralyzes the diaphragm
   b. Hypotension from a spinal anesthesia may cause respiratory arrest
   c. Spinal anesthesia can have a significant effect on respiration
   d. Narcotics given to supplement spinal anesthesia may cause respiratory depression
   e. All of the above
9. Which statement about spinal headaches is not true?
   a. There is evidence that lying flat after a spinal anesthetic does not help prevent a headache
   b. It is unlikely that a patient would get a headache after epidural anesthesia
   c. If a patient is going to get a spinal headache, it will be starting in the recovery room period
   d. Increasing fluid administration helps to prevent and treat spinal headache
   e. Severity of headache is related to the gauge of the spinal needle
10. Heat loss in the recovery room is:
    a. More of a problem with a high spinal
    b. More of a problem after general anesthesia
    c. No different after spinal or general anesthesia for similar operations
    d. Increased by shivering
    e. Decreased by narcotic administration

CHAPTER 11

1. The most useful indicator of renal function is:
   a. Urine output
   b. Serum creatinine
   c. Urine specific gravity

    d. U/P creatinine
    e. Blood urea nitrogen
2. Which of the following statements about the patient with chronic renal disease is true?
    a. Congestive heart failure is rare
    b. Should never receive Na^+-containing solutions because Na^+ cannot be excreted
    c. Alteration of dosages of all drugs is required
    d. Anemia is caused by decreased red blood cell synthesis
    e. None of the above
3. All of the following are ECG signs of hyperkalemia except:
    a. Presence of U waves
    b. Tall, peaked T waves
    c. Loss of P waves
    d. Wide QRS complexes
    e. ST segment changes
4. The anephric adult at rest requires:
    a. ~1200 ml H_2O per day to replace insensible loss
    b. ~ 500 ml H_2O per day to replace insensible loss
    c. ~2500 ml H_2O and electrolytes per day to replace gastrointestinal and respiratory loss
    d. ~ 500 ml H_2O and electrolytes per day to replace gastrointestinal and respiratory loss
    e. ~1000 ml colloid daily
5. Which of the following parameters will give the least information about the patient with chronic renal disease during the perioperative period?
    a. ECG
    b. Urine specific gravity
    c. Central venous pressure
    d. Blood pressure
    e. Serum electrolytes
6. All of the following statements about acute renal failure are true except:
    a. Acute renal failure may be the result of administration of aminoglycoside antibiotics
    b. Perioperative acute renal failure carries a poor prognosis
    c. Acute renal failure may occur 2° to sepsis
    d. Perioperative oliguria is always an indication of acute renal failure
    e. None of the above
7. The correct treatment of established acute renal failure includes all of the following except:
    a. "Flushing" the kidneys to remove pigments

b. Hemodialysis
   c. Fluid restriction
   d. Peritoneal dialysis
   e. Precise fluid balance charting
8. Hyperkalemia may be treated by administration of all of the following except:
   a. Sodium bicarbonate
   b. Diuretics
   c. Insulin and glucose
   d. Exchange resins
   e. Normal saline infusion
9. Each of the following tests may be useful in distinguishing prerenal from renal oliguria except:
   a. Urine specific gravity
   b. Fractional excretion of Na^+
   c. U/P potassium
   d. U/P creatinine
   e. None of the above
10. Which of the following statements about the patient with chronic renal failure is true:
    a. Insensible loss is greater than in the patient with normal renal function
    b. Urine output, when present, should be replaced with infusion of 0.5 or 0.33 normal saline
    c. Colloid solutions should never be administered
    d. Perioperative Na^+ requirements are less than in the patient with normal renal function
    e. Low hemoglobin concentrations are poorly tolerated

CHAPTER 12

1. The greatest decrease in vital capacity following thoracic surgery occurs:
   a. Within 24 hours of surgery
   b. On the second postoperative day
   c. On the third postoperative day
   d. On the fourth postoperative day
   e. Immediately
2. In order to tolerate extubation and maintain adequate ventilation, a patient should have a vital capacity of at least:
   a. 3 ml/kg
   b. 30 ml/kg

c. 15 ml/kg
d. 7 ml/kg
e. 50 ml/kg

3. A patient who is intubated has been evaluated and is considered ready for extubation. He is awake with stable vital signs and good arterial blood gas values. His inspiratory force has been measured and found to be:
   a. -30 cm H_2O
   b. -15 cm H_2O
   c. -10 cm H_2O
   d. -8 cm H_2O
   e. -5 cm H_2O

4. Tension pneumothorax can develop in the postoperative thoracic patient when: (1) air leak is present from the lung; or (2) the patient's chest tube is kinked.
   a. (1) only occurs
   b. (2) only occurs
   c. Either (1) or (2) occur separately
   d. Both (1) and (2) occur simultaneously
   e. Unrelated to (1) or (2)

5. The suction control chamber is filled to 20 cm depth and the suction is applied:
   a. No bubbles in this chamber means that the suction is too great.
   b. If bubbles appear in this chamber, increasing the suction will increase the suction applied to the patient's pleural space.
   c. If bubbles appear in the chamber, increasing the suction will only increase the amount of bubbling, and the suction being applied to the patient will remain at -10 cm.
   d. If bubbles appear in the chamber, increasing the suction will only increase the amount of bubbling, and the suction being applied to the patient will remain at -20 cm.
   e. There should be no bubbles in the system.

6. The function of the water seal chamber is: (1) to allow air to pass from a leak in the lung with little resistance; or (2) to prevent air from entering the pleural space through the chest tube.
   a. (1) only
   b. (2) only
   c. (1) and (2)
   d. Neither (1) or (2)
   e. Partial effect from both (1) and (2)

7. The postoperative thoracic patient requires analgesia:
   a. To keep the noise level low in the recovery room
   b. To be able to breathe

c. To be able to cough effectively and clear secretions
d. To be able to sleep in the recovery room
e. Because anesthesia intraoperatively was inadequate

8. The myasthenic patient can develop difficulty breathing because of: (1) weakness of respiratory muscles; or (2) difficulty swallowing.
   a. (1) only
   b. (2) only
   c. Only with (1) and (2) simultaneously
   d. Either (1) or (2)
   e. Neither (1) or (2)

9. Pulsus paradoxus is:
   a. A paradoxical slowing of the pulse during inspiration
   b. A paradoxical increase of the pulse during inspiration
   c. A paradoxical increase of the blood pressure during inspiration
   d. A greater than normal decrease of blood pressure during inspiration
   e. Associated with heart failure

10. The patient who has had a pneumonectomy is different from the patient who has had a lobectomy in that he is more likely to develop:
    a. Congestive heart failure and arrhythmias
    b. Tension pneumothorax
    c. Hemorrhage
    d. Cardiac tamponade
    e. More pain

CHAPTER 13

1. The advantages of using the recovery room as a special procedures unit include all the following except:
   a. Proximity to the operating room
   b. Improvement in recovery room efficiency
   c. Accessibility of sterile precautions
   d. Ready availability of an anesthesiologist
   e. No need to wear operating room garb

2. Special procedures which may conveniently be performed in the operating room include all of the following except:
   a. Electroconvulsive therapy
   b. Celiac plexus block
   c. Swan-Ganz catheter insertion
   d. Administration of last rites
   e. Blood patch for spinal headache

3. The nursing role in special procedures in the recovery room includes all of the following except:
   a. Verification of signed consent forms
   b. Careful monitoring of vital signs
   c. Application of the current during cardioversion
   d. Emotional support
   e. Completion of the customary preanesthetic checklist if anesthesia is to be administered
4. Cardiovascular complications after electroconvulsive therapy:
   a. Are mainly due to excess vagal tone
   b. Usually resolve in 10 to 15 minutes
   c. Are exaggerated if there is preexistent vascular disease
   d. Are characterized by hypertension and tachycardia after 5 minutes
   e. All of the above
5. In considering cardioversion, which of the following is not true?
   a. It is an effective means of converting cardiac arrhythmias to sinus rhythm
   b. It is indicated mainly for atrial flutter and atrial fibrillation
   c. Fairly deep general anesthesia is required because of burn pain
   d. On rare occasions, pulmonary edema may be a severe complication
   e. It is less likely to be successful if the patient is receiving large doses of propranolol
6. Epidural anesthesia:
   a. Provides patchy pain relief
   b. Has a sympatholytic effect
   c. Does not increase blood supply to the legs
   d. Is performed through a 22- or 25-gauge needle
   e. None of the above
7. A brachial plexus block:
   a. Takes about 20 to 30 minutes for total blockade
   b. Involves placement of a small-gauge needle close to the brachial plexus sheath
   c. Requires 5–10 ml local anesthetic solution
   d. Can only be completely successful if a supraclavicular route is used
   e. Is the first line of treatment for angina pectoris
8. The most common severe complication of nerve block is:
   a. Allergic response
   b. Peripheral rash
   c. Cardiovascular collapse
   d. Tachycardia
   e. Hemiplegia
9. Following hemolytic transfusion reaction, all of the following steps should be taken except:
   a. Blood administration should be immediately discontinued

b. The patient's blood and urine should be checked for free hemoglobin
c. No diuretics should be given as the patient is already hypovolemic
d. Steroids should be given to modify the antigen-antibody reaction
e. Step-by-step documentation on the hospital record is essential
10. The least common complication of blood transfusion is:
   a. Hemolytic transfusion reaction
   b. Shivering due to hypothermia
   c. Septicemia due to pyrogens
   d. Transmission of serum hepatitis
   e. Congestive cardiac failure if the blood is given over 2 hours

CHAPTER 14

1. Endotracheal intubation:
   a. Should always be performed as a first step in CPR
   b. Should be preceded by oxygenation of the lungs by other methods of ventilation
   c. Allows adequate lung inflation but also causes gastric distention
   d. Makes it difficult to use a chest compression rate of 80 per minute
   e. Is best done through the nose
2. Aspiration of gastric contents:
   a. May follow removal of an esophageal airway
   b. Is potentially lethal
   c. May follow removal of an endotrachael tube
   d. Is particularly hazardous if the pH of the aspirate is less than 5
   e. All of the above
3. Lidocaine:
   a. Can cause seizures
   b. Is usually given as a 10 ml bolus of 2 percent solution
   c. Is given as 2 mg/kg bolus
   d. Increases ventricular automaticity
   e. Is not used any more as a first-line drug
4. Calcium chloride:
   a. Is never dangerous in digitalized patients
   b. Does not enhance myocardial contractility
   c. May be given by IV push 5-7 mg/kg
   d. Is not a first-line drug
   e. Is the same as calcium gluconate
5. Basic life support does not include:
   a. Establishment of the airway
   b. Maintenance of alveolar ventilation
   c. Cannulation of a vein

386 MULTIPLE CHOICE QUESTIONS AND ANSWERS

   d. Cardiac compression rate of 60 per minute
   e. Protective measures against corneal abrasions
6. Atropine sulfate:
   a. Is of no value in ventricular tachycardia
   b. Is always required if the heart rate is less than 60 beats per minute
   c. Is usually given in 2-mg boluses up to a total of 10 mg
   d. Is not indicated in high-degree atrioventricular block
   e. Should not be given to children because it causes fever
7. Verapamil:
   a. Is given in an initial bolus of 0.075–0.15 mg/kg over 1 minute
   b. May be repeated at 5-minute intervals
   c. May be given safely to a total dose of 30 mg in 30 minutes
   d. Is not indicated for AV nodal reentrant tachydysrhythmias
   e. Is highly successful in terminating many dysrhythmias
8. Ventricular tachycardia:
   a. Is defined as five or more sequential ventricular complexes occurring at a rate greater than 100 per minute
   b. Causes an irregular rate
   c. Always generates a pulse
   d. Occurs in the absence of normal sinoatrial node activity
   e. Is best treated initially by intravenous lidocaine 1 ml/kg
9. Hazards associated with the rapid administration of sodium bicarbonate include:
   a. Dysrhythmia secondary to ion shifts across cell membrane
   b. Metabolic acidosis
   c. Shift in the hemoglobin dissociation curve to the right
   d. Hyperkalemia
   e. None of the above
10. An intraaortic balloon:
    a. Requires preheparinization
    b. Must be inserted surgically
    c. Is useful in the treatment of cardiogenic shock refractory to fluid and pharmacologic therapy
    d. Includes a sensor to read the ECG
    e. All of the above

CHAPTER 15

1. A fatally injured head trauma patient is transferred to the recovery room for kidney donation. His blood pressure suddenly falls from 90/60 mm Hg to 40/0 mm Hg. The appropriate response is:
   a. To monitor vital signs every 3 minutes

b. To inform kidney transplant team of hypotension when they arrive
   c. To call physician if urine output falls below 30 ml per hour
   d. To increase infusion rate of vasopressor
   e. To commence immediate CPR
2. Patients with brain death are characterized by coma:
   a. Which is transient
   b. Which is accompanied always by loss of all reflexes
   c. With inappropriate verbalization
   d. With intact spinal reflexes
   e. With pharyngeal reflexes
3. Brain death implies:
   a. Death of all cells in the brain
   b. Cessation of nail growth
   c. Cessation of skin growth
   d. Nonviable cornea
   e. Non-functioning brainstem
4. The following are true statements about the value of EEG in brain death diagnosis except:
   a. It is the most frequently employed test in USA
   b. It is of limited value due to artifact
   c. It requires specialized training for interpretation
   d. Its recording time of electrosilence is five minutes
   e. It requires a minimum of eight scalp electrodes
5. In comas due to known etiology the following criteria are acceptable except:
   a. Low barbiturate blood levels
   b. Rectal temperature lower than 34°C
   c. Patient not in shock
   d. Patient not hypoxic
   e. Age-dependent criteria
6. Reversible brain damage is possible with all the following conditions except:
   a. Drug intoxication
   b. High velocity bullet injury
   c. Metabolic disorders
   d. Hypothermia
   e. Endocrine disorders
7. Patients with drug overdose coma:
   a. Will not show signs of brain death
   b. May be tested for brain death after 12 hours
   c. Must have minimal levels of drugs before brain death testing
   d. Are considered as brain dead after 48 hours
   e. Can never be declared as brain dead

8. The absence of brainstem function is suspected if:
   a. Patient breathes with $PaCO_2$ of 75 mm Hg (normal = 40 mm Hg)
   b. Patient is apneic but has occasional seizures
   c. Patient has flacid limbs and is apneic
   d. Patient is comatose with negative "doll's eye"
   e. Patient following general anesthesia is unresponsive on arrival in recovery room
9. Functions of the brainstem include all except
   a. Initiation of spontaneous respiratory activity
   b. Acts as a two-way relay station to allow cortical function and maintain consciousness
   c. Maintains systemic blood pressure
   d. Contains speech centers
   e. Holds the nuclei of the cranial nerves
10. Brain death is definite if
    a. The heart stops
    b. Respiration has ceased
    c. No flow is demonstrated on four vessel angiography
    d. There are no spinal reflexes
    e. Coma has persisted for 72 hours

CHAPTER 16

1. The structural configuration of the recovery room unit which is capable of accommodating a large bed capacity (over 15 beds) is the:
   a. Rectangle
   b. Circle
   c. Square
   d. Semicircle
   e. Oval
2. Dividing walls between individual patient units in the recovery room provide:
   a. Complete visual surveillance of all patients
   b. Patient privacy
   c. Cost-efficient staff requirements
   d. Complete auditory observation of the patient
   e. Structural improvement
3. The intubation cart or tray (adult and pediatric) provides:
   a. All necessary emergency medications
   b. ECG monitoring capabilities
   c. All equipment necessary to manage a respiratory emergency

d. Cardiac pacing equipment
   e. Defibrillator
4. The ambient temperature in the recovery room should be maintained at:
   a. 18.5°C (70°F)
   b. 24.0°C (80°F)
   c. 20.75°C (75°F)
   d. 26.25°C (85°F)
   e. Temperature is not important if humidity is high enough
5. The relative humidity in the recovery room should be maintained at:
   a. 50–60 percent
   b. 60–70 percent
   c. 40–50 percent
   d. 80–90 percent
   e. Depends on temperature
6. To reduce sensory stimulation in the recovery room:
   a. Lighting should be bright and direct
   b. Colors of walls, wallpaper, and draperies should be pastels or beige
   c. Ceiling tiles should be of an intricate design involving twisting shapes and patterns
   d. Discussion should occur at the patient's bedside
   e. Auditory signal on the ECG should be turned off
7. For every OR surgical suite there should be at least the following number of available patient care units in the recovery room:
   a. 0.5–1
   b. 1.5–2
   c. 2.5–3
   d. 3.5–4
   e. Varies from day to day
8. An alternative location if a recovery room isolation room is not available for recovering a patient who is on strict or respiratory isolation is:
   a. The patient's private room
   b. A semiprivate room on the patient's unit
   c. An open design recovery room unit
   d. An open design SICU
   e. The OR until recovered
9. Fire extinguishers (regardless of type) must be located in the recovery room every:
   a. 300 square meters (3300 square feet)
   b. 200 square meters (2200 square feet)
   c. 100 square meters (1100 square feet)
   d. 400 square meters (4400 square feet)
   e. 50 square meters (500 square feet)

390   MULTIPLE CHOICE QUESTIONS AND ANSWERS

10. It is highly recommended that these mandatory items, sphygmomanometer, oxygen therapy, suction, ECG monitor, be:
    a. Ceiling-suspended
    b. Wall-mounted
    c. Portable
    d. Retrieved from a central location within the RR
    e. Easily and quickly borrowed from the Department of Anesthesiology

CHAPTER 17

1. Elements of the nursing process include:
   a. Assessment
   b. Plan
   c. Intervention
   d. Evaluation
   e. All of the above
2. Assessment skills include all the following except:
   a. Observation
   b. Evaluation
   c. Percussion
   d. Auscultation
   e. Palpation
3. Criteria to be considered when designing a classification system would not include:
   a. Size of patient
   b. Admission score
   c. Length of stay
   d. Degree of nursing intervention required
   e. Monitoring requirements
4. When determining staffing patterns, the following statistics are vital:
   a. Census
   b. Hours of operation
   c. Peak activity levels
   d. Acuity levels
   e. All of the above
5. The use of flowsheets and checklists is advisable in the recovery room setting for all the following except:
   a. Time element
   b. Ease of documentation
   c. Eliminates need for direct observation
   d. Data retrieval
   e. Objective vs. subjective

MULTIPLE CHOICE QUESTIONS AND ANSWERS   391

6. Prior to writing nursing care standards, it is essential to have pre-established:
   a. Policies
   b. Procedures
   c. Standing orders
   d. Role delineations
   e. All of the above
7. Components of a good quality assurance program would not include:
   a. Established criteria
   b. Method of monitoring
   c. Unlimited time elements
   d. Problem-solving techniques
   e. Isolating problems
8. Resources to be used when establishing standards of care include all the following except:
   a. Accreditation manual for hospitals
   b. State guidelines for care
   c. ASPAN guidelines
   d. ASA guidelines
   e. AORN standards
9. Responsibilities that can be delegated to ancillary personnel include all the following except:
   a. Transportation
   b. Stocking
   c. Charting
   d. Requisitions
   e. Maintenance of equipment
10. The role of the LPN in the recovery room is limited to all but which of the following?
    a. Monitoring
    b. Direct patient care
    c. Assessment
    d. Reporting to RN
    e. Charting

CHAPTER 18

1. One of the major premises of adult learning principles is that the adult learner wants to learn.
   True/False
2. Programmed instruction is the least time-consuming and, therefore, has become the most widely used teaching method.
   True/False

3. No matter what method of evaluation is used, the greater the frequency of feedback, the greater the possibility of performance consistent with a standard.
   True/False
4. How long should a typical recovery room orientation program be for a new nurse?
   a. 1 day
   b. 1 week
   c. 6 weeks
   d. 8 to 12 weeks
   e. More than 3 months
5. Which method do orientees prefer when learning a recovery room skill?
   a. Dynamic lecture
   b. Hands on experience
   c. Reading policy and procedure manuals
   d. Involvement in paper work and charting
   e. Acting as ward liaison
6. Nursing personnel policies should be written by:
   a. Head nurse
   b. Assistant director
   c. Director of the unit
   d. Staff nurses
   e. All of the above
7. The recovery room nurse should have training in:
   a. Anesthetic drugs
   b. Cardiopulmonary resuscitation
   c. ECG interpretation
   d. Basic anesthetic techniques
   e. All of the above
8. Planning for staff development include:
   a. Assessment
   b. Planning
   c. Implementation
   d. Evaluation
   e. All of the above
9. A preceptor should be:
   a. The head nurse
   b. The clinical instructor
   c. The senior staff nurse
   d. A collaboration of all three
   e. Separate from the day-to-day recovery room nurse

10. Orientation to any new work environment is a time of adjustment and stress.
    True/False

CHAPTER 19

1. Health may be defined as:
   a. Absence of disease
   b. Balance of equilibrium
   c. Complete state of well-being
   d. Maintenance of homeostasis
   e. All of the above
2. A holistic concept of human beings includes:
   a. Endogenous and exogenous environment
   b. Physiologic, psychologic, socioeconomic processes
   c. Metaphysical/spiritual process
   d. Homeostatis of all systems
   e. All of the above
3. The preoperative visit:
   a. Contributes to client apprehension and fear
   b. Has a definite effect on length of stay
   c. May cause tension between surgeon and patient
   d. Is a methodology in a holistic approach for increased communication and patient teaching
   e. Is not necessary
4. Recommended preparation for preoperative teaching should include the following:
   a. Discussion with surgeon regarding patient
   b. Discussion with unit RN, review of chart, identification of previous surgery and type
   c. Discussion with surgeon and unit RN
   d. Review of chart and identification of previous surgery and type
   e. Knowledge of patient's value systems and life experience
5. Recommended teaching aids are structured:
   a. According to patient's age and financial status
   b. To include staff participation
   c. To accommodate consumer and staff schedules
   d. According to availability of institutional financial resources and staffing patterns
   e. For adaptation in certain surgical specialties only
6. Interviewing techniques may be classified as:
   a. Direct, nondirect, communicative

    b. Non-direct, communicative, transactional analysis (child, parent, mature adult)
    c. Direct, Rogerian, transactional analysis (child, parent, mature adult)
    d. Direct, assertive, Rogerian
    e. Direct, assertive, transactional analysis (child, parent, mature adult)
7. The nursing process applied to the perioperative role of the recovery room nurse involves:
    a. Preoperative interviews and patient teaching
    b. Identification of patient problems and potential problems
    c. Individualized nursing care plan
    d. Evaluation of postanesthetic care
    e. All of the above
8. The pediatric patient:
    a. Requires no special preoperative preparation or treatment
    b. Should never be spoken to directly
    c. Cannot be identified by an individual teaching care plan
    d. Is assessed depending on developmental level and determination of language and comprehensive skills
    e. Is difficult to handle when the parents are present
9. Recommendations regarding pediatric patients:
    a. Preoperative teaching need not include both child and parents
    b. Medical equipment for handling is not significant (show and tell)
    c. Preoperative class or tour is not meaningful to children or parents
    d. Presence of parents in the holding area and recovery room alleviates the child's fear of separation (from parents)
    e. All of the above
10. Ambulatory patients:
    a. Do not require preoperative teaching since length of stay is short
    b. Require no reenforcement of instructions
    c. Cannot be included in preoperative classes, tours, or interviews
    d. Should not be communicated with via phone, pre- and postoperatively
    e. Should have specific preoperative instructions as well as discharge instructions

CHAPTER 20

1. Medical malpractice:
    a. Is a form of negligence
    b. Involves imprudent acts

c. Shows a lack of conformance with the standards of the medical community
   d. Is not a criminal act
   e. All of the above
2. A plaintiff is:
   a. The person who institutes the lawsuit
   b. The person to be defended in a lawsuit
   c. Often the godparents, in the case of an infant
   d. Often a spouse, in the case of a paralyzed adult
   e. The lawyer's friend
3. The standard of care:
   a. Cannot be explained in a courtroom
   b. Is presented by expert witnesses
   c. Is an imaginary concept which holds no weight in a lawsuit
   d. Is determined by what a reasonably prudent nonmedical person would do
   e. All of the above
4. The statute of limitations:
   a. Varies from state to state
   b. Is the period during which a lawsuit may be instituted
   c. Sometimes begins when the patient discovers the injury
   d. Is of extreme importance when a lawsuit is initiated
   e. All of the above
5. The doctor's order is for 5.0 mg digoxin. You believe this is an excessive dose. You:
   a. Give the medication because you trust and respect the doctor
   b. Question the anesthesia resident on call for the recovery room
   c. Contact the physician who wrote the order to clarify it
   d. Do not give it and forget about it
   e. None of the above
6. A medication you are unfamiliar with is ordered by the physician. You:
   a. Ask other staff members about it
   b. Look it up in the *Physician's Desk Reference*
   c. Give it because you trust and respect the doctor
   d. Give it, and hope for the best
   e. Give something you know and believe the patient needs
7. The physician calls and gives a telephone order. You:
   a. Have another staff nurse verify the order
   b. Write it as it is being said
   c. Repeat what you have written back to the doctor
   d. All of the above
   e. None of the above

8. Your patient's condition suddenly starts to deteriorate. You:
   a. Page the doctor stat
   b. Take the necessary nursing actions
   c. Document everything that is done while awaiting the doctor
   d. Continue to call for help until there is a response
   e. All of the above

9. Your patient suffers complications in the recovery room and needs to be brought back to surgery. You:
   a. Call the risk management department to report the complication
   b. Refuse to sign your nursing note because you do not want to be implicated
   c. Tell the patient's family that they should sue
   d. Do not follow up on the patient's condition
   e. All of the above

10. Exposure on a case can be minimized by:
    a. Reporting fewer cases to the risk management department
    b. Extremely careful record keeping
    c. Signing your note illegibly
    d. Refusing to care for more than one patient
    e. All of the above

Answers

CHAPTER 1

1. e
2. e
3. d
4. e
5. a
6. d
7. e
8. c
9. e
10. e

CHAPTER 2

1. c
2. d
3. c
4. c
5. c
6. b
7. e
8. c
9. b
10. e

CHAPTER 3

1. c
2. e
3. e
4. e
5. d
6. c
7. e
8. b
9. c
10. d

CHAPTER 4

1. c
2. c
3. e
4. e
5. d
6. b
7. a
8. b
9. c
10. c

CHAPTER 5

1. e
2. 350 ml
3. d
4. d
5. d
6. b
7. e
8. a
9. a
10. c

CHAPTER 6

1. d
2. d
3. e
4. d
5. a
6. a
7. b
8. c
9. d
10. e

CHAPTER 7

1. b
2. e
3. c
4. d
5. e
6. c
7. c
8. c
9. e
10. c

CHAPTER 8

1. d
2. b
3. d
4. b
5. c
6. a
7. d
8. b
9. a
10. d

CHAPTER 9

1. b
2. b
3. d
4. d
5. d
6. d
7. a
8. c
9. c
10. d

CHAPTER 10

1. b
2. c
3. c
4. a
5. c
6. d
7. c
8. e
9. c
10. a

CHAPTER 11

1. b
2. d
3. a
4. b
5. b
6. d
7. a
8. b
9. c
10. b

CHAPTER 12

1. a
2. c
3. a
4. d
5. d
6. c
7. c
8. d
9. d
10. a

CHAPTER 13

1. e
2. d
3. c
4. e
5. c
6. b
7. a
8. b
9. c
10. e

CHAPTER 14

1. b
2. e
3. a
4. c
5. e
6. a
7. a
8. e
9. a
10. e

CHAPTER 15

1. d
2. d
3. e
4. d
5. b
6. b
7. c
8. c
9. d
10. c

CHAPTER 16

1. a
2. b
3. c
4. c
5. a
6. b
7. b
8. b
9. b
10. b

CHAPTER 17

1. e
2. b
3. a
4. e
5. c
6. e
7. c
8. e
9. c
10. c

CHAPTER 18

1. True
2. False
3. True
4. d
5. b
6. e
7. d
8. e
9. d
10. True

CHAPTER 19

1. e
2. e
3. d
4. b
5. d
6. c
7. e
8. d
9. d
10. d and e

CHAPTER 20

1. e
2. a
3. b
4. d
5. c
6. b
7. d
8. d
9. a
10. b

INDEX

Index

f = figure; *t* = table

Abdominal surgery, pain, 34
Abbreviations, standard, 333-335
Acetaminophen (Tylenol), 258
 pediatric dosage, 142
Acetylsalicylic acid (Aspirin), 142, 258
Acid-base balance *See also* Acidosis;
  Alkalosis
 disorders, 339-340
 and neuromuscular paralysis, 89
Acidosis, 34
 AHA assessment rules, 230
 effect on neuromuscular blockade, 8
 metabolic, 131, 187, 229-230
 respiratory, 49, 339
 treatment, 231
ACLS *See also* Advanced cardiac life support
Activity, postanesthetic scoring, 5, 108
Acute renal failure
 diagnosis, 192-194
 etiology, 191-192*t*
 risk and perioperative situations, 182
Acute respiratory failure, in children, 131-132
Acute tubular necrosis (ATN)
 diagnosis, 192-193
 etiology, 191-192
 prevention, 194-195
 treatment, 195-196
ADH (Antidiuretic hormone), secretion abnormalities, 97-98*t*, 186
Admission to recovery room
 assessment, 4-5
 checklist, 277*f*
Adults, anatomic differences from children, 121-122
Advanced cardiac life support (ACLS), 239
 defibrillators, 234-236
 drug therapy, 229, 231*t*, 353-354

 dysrythmia, 231-234, 235*t*
 algorithms, 342-352
 intravenous fluids, 229
Aerosol therapy, high humidity mask, 37, 39*f*
Affective learning, 297
Age
 and baseline fluid requirements, 76*t*
 and brain death criteria, 246-247
 pain perception and, 134
Agitation, in children postoperatively, 134-135
Air, intracranial, 100
Airway(s)
 of children, 121-122
 maintenance, 225-226
 obstruction, 29
  in children, 127-128
  treatment of infant, 364-365
 problems in burn patients, 145
 and superior laryngeal blocks, 170
Albert Einstein College of Medicine, brain death protocol, 245
Albumin, resuscitation, 66, 80, 190
Albuterol (Solbutamol; Ventolin), 45*t*
Alcohol
 plasma half-life, 243
 intoxication
  delayed awakening, 89
  morphine and, 92
Aldomet (Methyldopa), 91, 188
Aldrete scoring, 5, 9
Alfentanil, 16, 21
Alkalosis
 metabolic, 73-74, 340
 respiratory, 91, 340
Allergic reaction(s)
 to blood transfusion, 223

Allergic reaction(s) (*Continued*)
   to drugs, 98, 99t
Alupent (Metaproterenol), 45t
Alveolar-arterial oxygen tension gradient (P(A-a) O, 2, 32
Alveolar-capillary block, 30
AMBU bag, 227
Ambulatory surgery, 211
   equipment requirements, 212
   patients
      discharge criteria, 113, 115f, 116f
      education, 301
      instructions, 212, 213t
      pediatric, 146-148
      postsurgical instructions, 116f
   types, 212
American Heart Association (AHA)
   ACLS, 229-231t, 235t, 342-354
      defibrillators, 234-236
      drug therapy, 229-231t, 353-354
      and dysrhythmia, 231-234, 235t, 342-352
   BLS, 225-229, 239
   golden rules to assess acidosis, 230t
American Medical Association (AMA), brain death protocol, 245
American Society of Anesthesiologists (ASA), discharge criteria, 104
American Society of Postanesthesia Nurses (ASPAN), discharge criteria, 104-105
Aminoglycosides, toxicity, 188
Aminophylline, 258
Amitriptyline, 91
Analgesia
   caudal, 25
   patient-demand, 21-22
   postlobectomy, 203
Analgesic(s). *See also* specific analgesic
   classification, 15, 17t
   pediatric dosages, 142
Anaphylaxis tray, chemonucleolysis, 260-261
Anectine *See* Succinylcholine
Anemia, of renal insufficiency, 186-187
Anesthesia
   decreased SVR and, 65
   postoperative somnolence, 87
   services, proximity to RR, 265
Anesthesiologist(s)
   admission assessment information, 4
   discharge by, 109, 111f
Anesthetic(s) *See also* specific anesthetic(s)
   effect on neuromuscular blockade, 8
   and fluid and electrolyte changes, 79
   interacting drugs, 90t
   general, and postoperative opioids, 91
   and junctional tachycardia, 64
   local

   pharmacology, 18-19
   supplementation for pain relief, 25-27
   myocardial depression and, 59
   prolonged effect, 87-90t
   residual effect, 33-34
   and respiratory insufficiency, 94
   techniques
      and discharge criteria, 114
      and postoperative pain, 134
Aneurysm, intracranial rupture, 100
Anion gap, 74
Antibiotic(s)
   and chronic renal disease, 188
   drug interactions, 91
   effect on neuromuscular blockade, 8
   observation period, 111
Anticholinergics, 135
Antidiuretic hormone secretion (ADH)
   secretion abnormalities, 97-98t, 186
Antiemetic(s), 24-25
   observation period, 111
Antihistamine(s), 99t
Antihypertensive(s), 188-189, 200
Antilirium (Physostigmine), 135, 258
Antishock garment, 228
Anuria, 192
Apgar scoring, 5, 9, 105
Apnea, in premature infants, 132
Apresoline. *See* Hydralazine
Aquamephyton, 258
Arrhythmias, 95. *See also* Dysrhythmia
   cardioversion, 216-217, 218t
   and electrocardiogram change, 163-164
   and thermoregulatory dysfunction, 96
Arterial pressure
   high, caused by increased CO, 66-68
   low
      causes and treatment, 59-62f
      and decreased CO, 59-65
      and decreased SVR, 65-66
   monitoring, 53-54
      automatic nonivasive, 55
      direct intraarterial, 54-55f, 56f
      intermittent manual, 56
      systolic, in calculation of RPP, 67-68
Arteriosclerosis, 66
Aspiration. *See* Pulmonary aspiration
Aspiration pneumonia, 35
Aspirin (Acetylsalicylic acid), 142, 258
Assessment, nursing, 280f
Association of Nurse Anesthetists, 112
Asystole, 69
   algorithm, 345-346
Atelectasis, 35, 204-205
ATN. *See* Acute tubular necrosis
Atracurium, 33
Atrial fibrillation, 65, 68
Atropine, 258
   bradycardia treatment, 62

Atropine (*Continued*)
  counteraction of muscle relaxant, 34, 99*t*
  and ECT, 215
  as first-line drug, 231, 233, 235*t*, 353
  inhalation, 45*t*
  pediatric dosage, 143
  and effectiveness of neostigmine, 90
Audit, 281, 282*f*
Autonomic nervous system, of children, 124
Autonomic hyperreflexia, 167*t*
Autoregulation, 161–162*f*
Awakening, delayed
  causes, 87
  and prolonged anesthetic effect, 87–90*t*
Axillary block, 79

Babinski sign, 99*t*
Barbiturate(s), 215
  allergic or atypical response, 99*t*
  biotransformation, 89
  drug interaction, 92
  hypnotic effect, 88
  pediatric dosage, 142
  postoperative agitation, 135
Basic life support (BLS), 239
  airway management, 225–226
  breathing, 226–227
  circulation, 227–229
Bed(s), patient care unit, 263
Benadryl (Diphenylhydramine), 258
Benzodiazepine(s), drug interaction, 92
Beta-adrenergic blocker(s), 188, 200
Beta-endorphins, 14, 15*t*
Bicarbonate, 75*t*, 184. *See also* Sodium bicarbonate
Bigeminy, 69
Bile, 74
Blanket(s), fire, 268
Blindness, infantile, 203
Block-aid monitor, 99*t*
Blood
  component guidelines, 315–317
  loss and hypotension, 61–62
  transfusions, 221–223*t*
    in children, 140–141
Blood bank, proximity to RR, 265
Blood-brain barrier, 141
Blood gas(es)
  analysis, 338–339
  arterial, normal values, 200*t*, 338
  monitoring, 31–32
Blood patches, 221
Blood pressure, 7. *See also* Arterial pressure; Hypotension; Hypertension
  normal range, 8*t*, 337
Blood urea nitrogen (BUN), 184
Body composition, normal, 71–72

Body surface area rule, 142
Body temperature regulation, 96
  in children, 125, 135–138
  in burn patients, 146
Body weight, and hydration status, 82
Brachial plexus block, 218
Bradycardia
  algorithm, 351
  junctional, 62, 63*f*
  sinus, 62
  and sympathetic block, 174, 176
  treatment, 62–63
  with hypertension, 68
Brain death
  circumstances of care, 241
  clinical tests, 243–244
  definition, 241–242
  legal and international status, 247
  protocols, 244–247
  special tests, 244
Brain stem
  death, 243–244
  functions, 242
  nuclei, 243*t*
Breathing, basic life support, 226–227
Bretylium tosylate (Bretylol), 258
  as first-line drug, 231, 234, 235*t*, 353
Bronchiolitis, 131
Bronchoconstriction, 166
Bronchodilator(s), 45*t*
Bronchoscopy, 207
Bronkosol (Isoetharine), 45*t*
BUN (Blood urea nitrogen), 184
Bupivicaine (Marcaine), 171*t*
  caudal analgesia, 25
  lumbar epidural blockade, 26
  pharmacology, 18, 19
  thoracic epidural blockade, 26–27
Buprenorphine
  classification, 16, 17
  epidural, 23*t*
Burn injuries
  cardioversion complication, 218*t*
  in children, 144–146
  fluid and electrolyte changes, 79–80
Butorphanol, 16, 17*t*, 17–18
Butyrophenone(s), 91

Calcium, increased serum levels, 137
Calcium channel blocker(s), 200
Calcium chloride, 258
  as first-line drug, 231, 235*t*, 353
  and junctional bradycardia, 62
  pediatric dosage, 143
Calcium gluconate, 187, 258
Cannula(s), nasal, 36–37*f*
Carbocaine (Mepivicaine), 18, 171*t*

404 INDEX

Carbon dioxide, failure, 30–32
Cardiac arrest, 69, *See also* Cardiopulmonary arrest
  cardioversion complication, 218t
  drugs, 353–354
Cardiac compression, 227–228, 233
Cardiac glycosides, 65
Cardiac index, 8t, 60f
Cardiac output (CO)
  decreased, 35, 59–60f
  increased, 66–68
  normal range, 8t
Cardiac resuscitation, 228
Cardiac standstill, 233
Cardiac surgery, 208
Cardiac tamponade, 62, 206, 228
Cardiogenic shock, 59–60f, 228
Cardiopulmonary arrest, 69
  cardioversion complication, 218t
  drug therapy, 229–231
  equipment, 238–239
  guidelines for CPR, 225
  intravenous fluids, 229
  postresuscitation management, 237–238t
Cardiopulmonary resuscitation (CPR), 69, 233
  of choking infant, 360–361
  one rescuer, 356–357
  one and two rescuer, 358
Cardiovascular drug(s). *See also* specific drugs
  drug interactions, 91
Cardiovascular system
  of children, 122
  complications, postoperative, 166–167t
  instability, 95, 161–164
  local anesthetic toxicity and, 170t
  management of disturbances, 59–69
  monitoring, 7–8, 53–59f
  symptomatology in chronic renal disease, 185–186
Cardioversion, 216–217, 218t
  synchronized, 236
Carfentanil, 16
Carignan scoring system, 9, 105, 106f
Carotid endarterectomy, 67, 101
Catheter(s)
  cardiac, preoperative placement, 223–224
  pulmonary artery balloon-tipped, 57
  urinary, 67
Caudal analgesia, 25, 134
CBC (complete blood count), 184
CDAP (continuous distending airway pressure), 48
CEDP (continuous expiratory distending pressure), 48
Celiac plexus block, 219
Central nervous system
  of children, 124

complications, postoperative, 166
dysfunction, 131
effect of cardiopulmonary arrest, 237–238
local anesthetic toxicity and, 170t
Central venous pressure (CVP), 57
  and cardiac failure, 192–193
  and hemorrhage, 62
  normal range, 8t
Cephaloridine, 8, 91
Cephradine, 8, 91
Cerebral blood flow, 160f, 161, 162f
Cerebral edema, 159, 163t
Cerebral function, postoperative evaluation, 9–10
Cerebral hemorrhage, 67
Cerebral perfusion pressure (CPP), 152, 237
Cerebral vessels, spasm, 163t
Cerebrospinal fluid (CSF), normal values, 336
Chair(s), recovery room, 256
Chemonucleolysis anaphylaxis tray, 260–261
Chest tube(s), 201–203f
Cheyne-Stokes respiration, 6
Children. *See also* Infants
  acute respiratory failure, 131–132
  agitation, postoperative, 134–135
  ambulatory surgery, 212
  autonomic nervous system, 124
  blood replacement, 140–141
  burns, 144–146
  caudal analgesia, 25
  central nervous system, 124
  differences from adults
    anatomic, 121–122
    physiologic, 122–125
    psychological, 125
  discharge criteria, 114
  drug dosages, 141–143
  fluid replacement, 138–140
  intubation tray contents, 259–260
  kidneys, 123
  outpatient surgery, 146–148
  pain, postoperative, 133–134
  plastic surgery, 143–144
  postintubation croup, 128–129
  preoperative preparation, 300, 301t
  respiratory support, 132–133
  respiratory system, 122–123t
  temperature regulation, 135–138
Chloride, 75t
Chloroprocaine (Nesacaine), 18, 171t
Chlorpromazine, 91
Chlorpropamide, 97
Cimetidine, 92, 238
Circular configuration, of recovery room, 252–253f

Circulation
  basic life support, 227–229
  postanesthesia scoring, 108–109
  postanesthetic assessment scoring, 5
Circulatory system, failure, 131
Choking, infant
  conscious, 360–361
  unconscious, 364–365
Clark formula, 142
Classification system, patient, 274, 275t
Cleft lip and palate, 143–144
Clindamycin, 91
Clinical instructor, 285–286
Clonidine, 68, 188
Cocaine, 171t
Codeine, 15, 258
  pediatric dosage, 142
Cognitive learning, 297
Colistin, 91
Colloid(s), 190
  in fluid resuscitation, 80
  treatment of septicemia, 66
Color of patient, postanesthetic scoring, 5, 109
Coma, 95, 96, 238
  cerebral function evaluation, 9–10
  hyperosmolar nonketotic, 97
  hypoglycemic, 97
  intraoperative factors, 100t
Communication, in holistic approach, 295–296, 297f
Compazine (Prochlorperazine), 25, 258
Complete blood count (CBC), 184
Compression dressing, 34
Congenital anomalies, surgical correction, 143–144
Congestive heart failure, 131
Consciousness
  monitoring of levels, 9–10
  postanesthesia scoring, 5, 109
Continuous distending airway pressure (CDAP), 48
Continuous expiratory distending pressure, (CEDP), 48
Continuous positive airway pressure (CPAP), 130
  minimizing cardiac depression, 49
  terminology, 48
Continuous positive pressure mask(s), 41
Convalescence, fluid and electrolyte requirement, 80–81
Conversion factor(s), 337–338
Corticosteroid(s), 189
Countershock(s), 233
CPAP. See Continuous positive airway pressure
Cranium, content(s), 151
Crash cart, 238–239
  equipment and medications, 258–259

Creatinine
  clearance, 184
  serum levels, 183
  U/P ratio, 193
Critical care patients, discharge criteria, 114
Croup
  postintubation, 128–129
  tents, 42, 44f
Crystalloid solution(s), vs. colloids, 80
Curare. See d-Tubocurarine
Cushing's reflex, 163
CVP. See Central venous pressure (CVP)
Cyanosis, 29, 30
Cyclazocine, 17t
Cyclopropane, drug interactions, 91

Dantrolene, 96
DC countershock, 65
1-Deamino-8-D-arginine vasopressin (DDAVP), 98, 164
Death
  of brain, 241–242
  of brainstem, 242–244
  definition, 242
  pediatric, 130
Defendant, 304
Defibrillation, 233, 233–234
  pediatric dosage, 143
  steps, 235–236
Defibrillator(s), 234–236
Dehydration, 75
Demerol. See Meperidine
Desipramine, 91
Dexamethasone (Decadron), 129, 258
  treatment of septicemia, 66
Dextrose, 78, 258
Diabetes insipidus, 98t
Diabetes mellitus, 96–97
Diabetic Ketoacidosis, 74
Diacetyl morphine. See Heroin
Dialysis, 190–191
Diamorphine, epidural, 23t
Diazepam (Valium), 172, 258
  drug interaction, 92, 99t
  pediatric dosage, 142
Diazoxide, 258
Diffusion hypoxia, 35
Digitalis
  drug interactions, 91
  and renal insufficiency, 189
  toxicity, 64–65
Digoxin, 258
  atrial fibrillation treatment, 65
  treatment of cardiogenic shock, 60
Dimenhydrinate (Dramamine), 147
Diphenylhydramine (Benadryl), 258

Discharge
  checklist, 278f
  criteria, 117
    ASA, 104
    JCAH, 103-104
    special, 113-115f
    University Hospitals, Cleveland Ohio, 112
    written, 113
  following spinal and epidural anesthesia, 178
Disease, definition, 293
Disseminated intravascular coagulopathy (DIC), 222, 241
Diuretic(s), 96, 200, 222
  ATN prophylaxis, 195
  chronic administration, 91
  and renal insufficiency, 189
  therapy, 75, 78
  treatment of pulmonary edema, 60
  water overload therapy, 186
Dobutamine (Dobutrex), 238t, 258
Documentation, general measures, 309
Doll's eyes maneuver, 244
Donor(s), kidney, 196-197f
Door(s), recovery room, 268
Dopamine, 59, 61, 258
  for cardiac arrest, 353
  infusion, pediatric dosage, 143
  as second-line, 238t
Doxapram (Dopram), 24, 258
Doxepine, 91
Dramamine (Dimenhydrinate), 147
Droperidol (Inapsine), 91, 258
  allergic or atypical response, 99t
  antiemetic effect, 24
  drug interaction, 92
  pediatric dosage, 142
Drug interaction(s). See also specific drugs
  allergic, 98, 99t
  and delayed awakening, 90-92t
  and postoperative neuromuscular paralysis, 89
Dynamap, 55, 56
Dynorphins, 14-15t
Dysrhythmia. See also Arrhythmias; specific dysrhythmia
  AHA algorithms, 342-352
  and arterial pressure, 53, 55, 56f
  identification and treatment, 231-234
  synchronized cardioversion, 236
  without hypotension or hypertension, 68-69f

Edrophonium (Tensilon), 8, 90, 208, 258
Education of patient
  ambulatory, 301
  pediatric, 300-301t
  role of nurse, 296-297
  teaching aids, 298-299
EFD (estimated fluid deficit), 138, 139
EFR (estimated fluid requirement), 138, 139
Elderly, fluid and electrolyte balance, 76t, 96, 97
Electrical safety, recovery room, 261
Electrocardiogram (ECG), 7
  and arrhythmias, 163-164
    ventricular fibrillation, 233
    ventricular tachycardia, 232
  CM5 lead placement, 58f
  heart block patterns, 64f
  monitoring of dysrythmias, 56-57
  postresuscitation management, 237
  subendocardial ischemia, 61f
  transmural ischemia, 61f
Electroconvulsive therapy (ECT), 214-216t
Electroencephalogram (EEG), 9-10
  and brain death, 244, 246
Electrolyte(s)
  changes in injury, 76-80
  evaluation of patient, 81-83
  gastrointestinal tract loss, 74-75
  imbalance, 7, 96-98
    in neurological patient, 164
  metabolism in children, 124-125t
  monitoring, 10
  normal, 72, 73, 184
  requirements during convalescence, 80-81
  serum concentrations, 73-74, 184
  urinary, 9
Electromechanical dissociation (EMD), 213, 233
  algorithm, 347
Elevator(s), recovery room, 266
Emergency Cardiac Care (ECC), 225
Emergency equipment, 258-261
Emphysema, 203-204
Encephalitis, 131
Endobronchial intubation, 204-205
Endotoxin shock, 65-66
Endotracheal intubation
  benefits, 46
  in children, 132-133
  complications, 46-47
Enflurane, 88, 135
Enkephalins, 14, 15t
EPAP (expiratory positive airway pressure), 48
Ephedrine, 188, 258
  treatment of decreased SVR, 65
Epidural administration, 22-23
Epidural anesthesia, 176-180t
  decreased SVR, 65
  vs. spinal anesthesia, 179, 180t
Epidural blockade, 26-27, 218

Epidural hematoma, 181
Epidural monitoring, of ICP, 154, 156f
Epinephrine, 99t, 258
  as first-line drug, 231, 233, 234, 235t, 354
  pediatric dosage, 143
  pharmacology, 18-19
  racemic, 128
  toxic effects, 170t, 172-173
Erythromycin, 91
Escherichia coli, 66
Esophageal gastric tube airway (EGTA), 226
Esophageal obturator airway (EOA), 226
Estimated fluid deficit (EFD), 138, 139
Estimated fluid requirement (EFR), 138, 139
Ether, 88, 91
Etidocaine, 18, 171t
Executor, 304
Expert witness, 304
Expiratory positive airway pressure (EPAP), 48
Extracellular fluid (ECF), 72, 77, 78t
Extrasystole(s), ventricular, 69f
Extubation, 50
  safe, criteria for, 204t
  technique, 201-203f
Eyes, pupillary reflex monitoring, 10

Face tent(s), 37, 39f
FE/Na, 194
Fentanyl, 15
  epidural, 23t
  intravenous infusion, 21
  pharmacology, 17
  and postoperative somnolence, 89
Fever. *See* Hyperthermia
Fibrillation
  atrial, 68
  ventricular, 69
Fire extinguishers, 268
Fire regulations and codes, 267-269
Fluid(s)
  imbalance, 96-98
  in injury, 76-80
  in neurological patient, 164
  intravenous, 229
  metabolism in children, 124-125t
  monitoring, 10
  overload and respiratory insufficiency, 94
  requirements
    and body weight, 82
    evaluation, 81-83
    during convalescence, 80-81
    factors that modify, 82
    and increased metabolism, 83

  replacement therapy, 99t
    baseline requirements, 75, 76t
    in burn patients, 145
    in children, 138-141
    in chronic renal disease, 189-190
    formula for burn patients, 79-80
  restriction, 78
Functional residual capacity (FRC), 48
Furosemide (Lasix), 9, 222, 258
  ATN prophylaxis, 195
  pediatric dosage, 143
  for pulmonary congestion, 60
  and renal insufficiency, 189
  SIADH treatment, 98

Gallamine, 91
Gastric juice, 74, 75t
Gastrointestinal tract, water and electrolyte losses, 74-75t
Gate control theory of pain, 14
Gentamycin, 66, 91, 188
Glasgow coma scale (GCS), 9
  as discharge criteria, 109, 110f
  monitoring of neurologic patients, 152, 155t
Glomerular filtration rate (GFR), 191
Glomerulonephritis, 189
Glucose
  bedside determination, 97
  monitoring, 10
  with insulin, 187
Glycolysis, anaerobic, 136
Glycosides, cardiac, 65
Graft(s), arterial, 67
Guanethidine, 188
Guardian, 304
Guidelines for Recovery Room Care, 112

Hallucinations, 99t
Halothane
  awakening, 88
  drug interactions, 91
  myocardial depression, 54f
  postoperative agitation, 135
Harvard criteria of brain death, 244-245
Headache(s)
  spinal, 177-178, 179
  treatment by blood patches, 221
Health, definition, 293
Heart. *See also* Myocardial entries
  blocks, 63, 64f
  congenital disease, 144
  decreased stroke volume, 59-65f
  impaired filling, 61-62
  rate, and calculation of RPP, 67-68
  sounds, 7
  surgery, 208

Hematocrit, 184
Hematology, symptoms of renal disease, 186-187
Hematoma
  epidural, 181
  intracranial, 152, 163t
Hemodilution, 66
Hemoglobin, 184
Hemorrhage
  cerebral, 67
  and CVP, 57
Hemorrhagic shock, 76-77
Hemothorax, and intrapulmonary shunting, 205
Heroin (diacetyl morphine), 15, 22
Holistic concept, 293, 294f
Holistic medicine, 293, 294f
  approach, 295
  interrelatedness of approach, 297f
Homeostasis, maintenance, 295f
Hope bag, 227
Humidification system(s), 42-46
Hydralazine (Apresoline), 258
  and decreased SVR, 65
  hypertensive therapy, 67, 163
  and tachycardia, 68
Hydrochlorothiazide, 189
Hydrocortisone, 189, 258
Hydrocortisone hemisuccinate, 66
Hydromorphine (Dilaudid), 258
Hydroxyzine, drug interaction, 92
Hyperactivity, 135
Hypercapnia, 131, 163t, 203-204
Hypercarbia, 135
Hyperglycemia, 97t
Hyperkalemia, of renal disease, 187-188
Hypermagnesemia, 8
Hypernatremia, 98, 186, 231
Hyperosmolality, 231
Hypertension
  arterial pressure wave form, 54f
  causes, 162-163
  and chronic renal disease, 188-189
  definition, 66
  treatment, 163
Hyperthermia
  in children, 136-137
  malignant, in children, 137-138
  postoperative, 96
Hyperthyroidism, 83
Hyperventilation, 91, 96
  prolonged intraoperative, 34-35
  provoked by pain, 34
  and respiratory insufficiency, 94
  water loss, 82
Hypocalcemia, 9, 136
Hypocarbia, 30
Hypoglycemia, 97t, 136

Hypokalemia, 231
Hyponatremia, 79, 186
Hypoproteinemia, 74
Hypotension
  causes, 99t
  cardiovascular instability, 161, 162
  cardioversion, 218t
  hemothorax, 205
  local anesthesia, 172, 174, 176, 178
  and coma, 95
  orthostatic, 174
  variability from sympathetic block, 176
Hypothermia, 9
  in children, 135-136
  effect on neuromuscular blockade, 8
  and postoperative paralysis, 89
Hypoventilation, 29, 30, 99t
Hypovolemia
  arterial pressure wave form, 54f, 55
  and impaired cardiac filling, 61
  treatment, 62
Hypoxia (Hypoxemia)
  anion gap, 74
  of burn patients, 145-146
  causes, 29-30
  in lobectomy, 204-205
  chronic, 203-204
  correction, 229-230
  and compression dressing, 34
  diffusion, 35
  and hypothermia, 136
  increased ICP, 163t
  following intraoperative hyperventilation, 34-35
  management, 161
  physiologic criteria, 131
  and ventilation/perfusion mismatch, 35-36

IAV (intermittent assisted ventilation), 48
IDV (intermittent demand ventilation), 48
Imipramine, 91
IMV (intermittent mandatory ventilation), 48
Infant(s)
  acute respiratory failure, 131-132
  cardiovascular system, 122
  drug dosages, 141-143
  fluid compartments, 124t
  postintubation croup, 128-129
  premature
    and oxygen concentration, 203
    complications, 132
  respiratory support, 132-133
  respiratory system, 122-123t
  temperature regulation, 135-138

Infection(s)
 of burn patients, 146
 control guidelines, 266-267
Inhalation agent(s), 92. *See also*
 Anesthetic(s); specific agents
Inspiratory force, 7
Insulin, 96, 97, 258
Intercostal block, 25-26, 218
Intermittent assisted ventilation (IAV), 48
Intermittent demand ventilation (IDV), 48
Intermittent mandatory ventilation (IMV), 48
Intermittent positive pressure breathing (IPPB), 45t, 47
Intermittent positive pressure ventilation (IPPV), 45t, 47
International status, of brain death, 247
Intraaortic balloon, 228
Intracellular fluid (ICF), 72, 77
Intracranial content(s), 151f
Intracranial lesion, 100-101
Intracranial pressure (ICP), 151-152, 237
 classification, 155
 increased, 163t
  and bradycardia, 68
  causes, 153f
  effects of, 158, 159f
  management, 159
  monitoring, 152, 154f
  types of waves, 157-158f
  volume curve, 156-157f
Intraoperative complication(s)
 catastrophic, 98-99, 100t
 and respiratory insufficiency, 94-95
Intrathoracic surgery. *See also* specific types of surgery
 preoperative evaluation, 199-201t
Intravenous administration, 20-21
Intraventricular monitoring, of ICP, 154, 156f
Intubation tray(s), contents, 259-260
Invasive monitoring systems, preoperative placement, 223-224
IPPB. *See* Intermittent positive pressure breathing (IPPB)
IPPV. *See* Intermittent positive pressure breathing (IPPB)
Isocarboxazid, 91
Isoetharine (Bronkosol), 45t
Isoflurane, 8
 awakening, 88
 drug interactions, 91, 92
Isolation rooms, 266-267
Isoproterenol (Isuprel), 233, 234, 258
 for cardiac arrest, 354
 infusion, pediatric dosage, 143
 inhalation, 45t
 as second-line, 238t

 treatment
  of heart block, 63
  of junctional bradycardia, 62-63
  of myocardial depression, 59
Isordil, 200
Isosorbide dinitrate, 60
Isuprel. *See* Isoproterenol

Jaw thrust, 226
Joint Commission on Accreditation of Hospitals (JCAH), 276
 discharge criteria, 103-104
 quality assurance standards, 281
 requirements for nurses, 272

Kanamycin, 91, 188
Kayexalate, 187, 196
Ketamine
 allergic or atypical response, 99t
 drug interaction, 92
 postoperative agitation, 135
Keto acid(s), 74
Ketosis, treatment, 97
Kidney(s)
 of children, 123
 disease
  clinical symptomatology, 185-188
  prevention, 194-195
  sodium wasting, 73
 failure, 74
  with previously normal function, 191-192
  fractional excretion of sodium (FE/Na), 194
 function
  laboratory evaluation, 183-184
  monitoring, 9
 transplants, 196-197f
Korotkoff sounds, 56, 206
Kussmaul's sign, 206

Laboratory(ies), clinical
 evaluation of renal disease, 183-184
 proximity to RR, 265
Lactic acid, 74
Landry-Guillain-Barre syndrome, 67
Laryngeal spasm, 127-128
Laryngoscope, use on children, 133
Laryngospasm, after extubation, 50
Larynx, of children, 121-122
Learning, types of, 297
Legal aspect(s), 224
 of brain death, 247
 of malpractice, 303-305
 and nursing liabilities, 305-309

Legal aspect(s) (*Continued*)
  and persons involved in lawsuit, 306
  of standard of care, 304–305
  of statute of limitations, 305
Licensed practical nurse(s) (LPN), 273
Lidocaine (Xylocaine), 258
  and ECT, 215
  effect on neuromuscular blockade, 91
  as first-line drug, 231, 233, 235t, 353
  and multifocal ventricular extrasystoles, 69
  pediatric dosage, 143
  pharmacology, 18–19, 171t
  for ventricular tachycardia, 232
Lincomycin, 91
Lip, cleft, 143–144
Lissauer's tract, 14
Lithium, 91
Lobectomy
  care of chest tubes, 201–203f
  causes of hypoxemia, 204–205
  criteria for safe extubation, 204t
  pain relief, 203
Local anesthetic(s), toxicity, 170–173
Lofentanil, 16
Lumbar spine, epidural blockade, 26
Lung(s). *See also* Pulmonary edema
  disease, 131
  embolism, 35
  problems in burn patients, 145–146

Maintenance medications, drug interactions, 90t, 91
Malignant hyperthermia, 260
Malpractice, 303–305
Mannitol, 159, 195, 222
Marcaine *See* Bupivacaine
Mask(s), oxygen
  continuous positive pressure, 41
  nonrebreathing, 37, 40, 42f
  partial rebreathing, 37, 41f
  simple, 37, 38f, 39f
  venturi, 40–41, 43f
MAST (Military antishock trousers), 228
Mediastinoscopy, 207
Membrane potential (MV), 78t
Meperidine (Demerol), 15, 258
  pediatric dosage, 142
  epidural, 23t
  intravenous infusion, 21
  pharmacology, 16–17
  postoperative IM administration, 20
Mephentermine (Wyamine), 258
Mepivicaine (Carbocaine), 18, 171t
Metabolic acidosis, 131, 187, 229–230, 340
Metabolic alkalosis, 73–74, 340
Metabolism, increased, 83

Metaproterenol (Alupent), 45t
Metaraminol, 238t
Methadone, 16, 17
Methoxamine, 65
Methoxyflurane, 88
Methyldopa (Aldomet), 91, 188
Methylphenidate (Ritalin), 95, 99t
Methylprednisolone, 66
Metoclopramide, 24–25
Metocurine, 8, 9
Metoprolol, 68, 188
Metronidazole, 66
Military antishock trousers (MAST), 228
Minnesota criteria of brain death, 245
Mobitz type heart block(s), 63, 64f
Monitoring, 5
  of cardiovascular system, 7–8
  of children, 126
  of chronic renal disease, 190
  of fluid and electrolyte balance, 10
  of neurological patients, 150, 152, 155t
  of neuromuscular transmission, 8–9
  nursing failure in, 306
  of renal function, 9
  of respiratory system, 6–7t
  of temperature, 9
Monoamine oxidase inhibitors, 91
Morphine, 66, 231, 258
  drug interactions, 91
  epidural, 23t, 181
  epidural injection, 22
  as first-line drug, 235t
  intrathecal, 23t
  intravenous administration, 21
  intravenous infusion, 21
  pediatric dosage, 142
  pharmacology, 16, 17t
  plasma half-life, 243
  postoperative IM administration, 20
  receptors, 15
  respiratory depression, 92
  subcutaneous administration, 20
Muscle relaxant(s)
  allergic or atypical response, 99t
  and brain death, 243
  nondepolarizing, 33, 92, 190
  polarizing, 33–34
  postoperative neuromuscular paralysis and, 89
  prolonged action, 88
Muscle spasm, 13, 166
Myasthenia gravis, and removal of thymus, 207–208
Myocardial depression, 54f
Myocardial infarction, 68, 99
Myocardial ischemia
  forms, 60–61f
  secondary to hypertension, 67

Myocardial ischemia (*Continued*)
  subendocardial, 68
  transmural, 68
  treatment, 60-61

Nalbuphine, 16, 17t, 18
Nalorphine, 17t
Naloxone (Narcan), 17t, 23, 99t, 181, 258
  counteraction of narcotics, 99t, 181
  observation period, 111
  pediatric dosage, 143
  pharmacology, 17t, 23
  reversal of respiratory depression, 24, 129
  reversal of analgesia, 89
Narcosis, residual, 30
Narcotic antagonist(s), 33
Narcotic(s), 258
  allergic or atypical response, 99t
  analgesic effect, 33, 34
    in children, 134
  drug interactions, 92
  epidural, 181
  observation period, 111
  overdose, 23-24
  pediatric dosage, 142
  postoperative somnolence, 89
  prolonged action, 88
Nasal cannulas, 36-37f
Nausea, treatment, 24-25
Nebulizer(s), 43-44, 45t
Nembutal. *See* Pentobarbital
Neomycine, 91
Neonate(s). *See* Infants
Neostigmine (Prostigmine), 99t, 258
  and bradycardia, 62, 68, 91
  and neuromuscular transmission, 8, 34
Nerve block(s)
  diagnostic, 217-221t
  intercostal, 25-26
  and local anesthetic toxicity, 170, 172
  and pneumothorax, 173
Nerve fiber(s), differential block, 177
Nesacaine (Chloroprocaine), 18, 171t
Neurological patient(s)
  fluid and electrolytes, 164
  pathophysiology, 151-152
  postoperative complications, 149
  restlessness and pain, 164-165
  temperature, 164
  transportation, 150
Neuromuscular blockade
  and metabolic acidosis, 187
  prolonged, 91
Neuromuscular drug(s), and antibiotics, 91
Neuromuscular paralysis, residual, 29, 34
Neuromuscular transmission, 8-9

Neurosurgical patient(s), 149, 150. *See also* Neurological patient(s)
Nipride. *See* Sodium nitroprusside
Nitroglycerin, 60
Nitroglycerine, 200, 258
  as second-line, 238t
Nitroprusside, 163, 238t
Nondepolarizing block, residual tests, 8
Nonrebreathing mask, 37, 40, 42f
Norepinephrine, 188, 234, 238t
Numerical scoring system(s), 105-109f, 110f
Nurse(s)
  failure
    to adequately monitor patient, 306
    to administer medications, 306-307
    to follow physicians's orders, 307-308
    to report significant changes, 308-309
    to take correct telephone orders, 308
  head, responsibilities of, 271-272
  licensed practical (LPN), 293
  postanesthetic discharge guidelines, 104-105
  position requirements, 272-273
  and preoperative teaching, 296-297
  PACU, verbal discharge report, 117
Nurses station, location, 255-256, 257f
Nursing
  assessment, 280f
  chain of command, 272f
  holistic, 293-296f
  liabilities, 305-309
  process steps, 273f
  requirements of head nurse, 271-272
  staff, position requirements, 272-274
  standards of care, 278, 280t, 321-323
Nutritional depletion, 77

Obesity
  and prolonged anesthetic effect, 33, 88
  and pulmonary embolism, 35
  and total body water, 71
Observation period(s), length, 111
Oliguria, 75, 192, 193
Open-chest massage, 228
Operating room (OR)
  patient transfer, 3, 4
    children, 125-126
  proximity to RR, 264-265
Operation site
  and pain, 134
  and respiratory insufficiency, 94
Opioid(s)
  pharmacology, 16-18
  route of administration, 19-23
  treatment of side effects, 23-25
  types and receptors, 14-16

Opioid receptor(s), 15, 16t
Orientation checklist, 325-331
 clinical instructor, 285-286
 preceptor selection and training, 286-287
 weekly outline, 287-291
Orthostatic hypotension, 174
Osmolality
 gastrointestinal secretions, 74
 serum, 184
 urine, 9
Outpatient surgery. See Ambulatory surgery
Overdose, drug, 89, 131, 243
Oxygen
 consumption with rebound shivering, 9
 discontinuance of therapy, 111
 failure, 29-30
 as first-line drug, 235t
 low inspired, 32
 tension, arterial, 48
 tents, 42, 44f
 therapy, 36-46f
 toxicity, 32
Oxytocin (Pitocin), 258

PACU. See Postanesthesia care unit
Pain
 from burns, 146
 consequences of, 13
 impulse origin and transmission, 14
 postoperative
  in children, 133-134
  in neurological patients, 164-165
 relief
  in lobectomy, 203
  practical aspects, 19-23
  regional and local anesthetics, 25-27
 respiratory dysfunction from, 34
 from spinal column surgery, 165
 types, 14
Palate, cleft, 143-144
Pancreatic juice, 74
Pancuronium bromide (Pavulon), 8, 9, 258
 and body temperature, 89
 excretion, 190
 and metabolic acidosis, 187
 residual effects, 33-34
 reversal time, 91
Paralysis, neuromuscular postoperative, 89
Pargyline hydrochloride, 91
Parkland formula, 79-80, 145
PARR. See Postanesthetic recovery room (PARR)
Partial rebreathing mask, 37, 41f
Party to the suit, 304
Patient care units, individual, 263-264
Pediatric patient(s). See Children

PEEP. See Positive-end expiratory pressure
Penicillin, 99t
Penicillin G, 8, 91
Pentazocine, 16, 17t
Pentobarbital (Nembutal), 91, 142
Pentothal, 216t
Peptide(s), endogenous, 14-16t
Pericardial window, 206-207
Perphenazine, 25, 91
Phenelzine sulfate, 91
Phenergan (Promethazine), 91, 258
Phenobarbital, 243, 258
Phenothiazine(s), drug interactions, 91
Phenylephrine (Neo-synephrine), 92, 258
Phenytoin (Dilantin), 258
Phrenic nerve damage, 166
Physician's orders, failure to follow, 307-308
Physostigmine (Antilirium), 135, 258
Pierre Robin's syndrome, 144
Pitressin, 164
Plaintiff, 304
Plastic surgery, in children, 143-144
Pleur-evac unit, 201-203f
Plumbing, of recovery room, 261
Pneumocephalus, 163t
Pneumonectomy, 205-206
Pneumonia
 aspiration, 35
 viral, 131
Pneumothorax, 173-174, 205
Polymyxin, 91
Pontocaine (Tetracaine), 18, 171t
Positioning of patient, in spinal column surgery, 165
Positive-end expiratory pressure (PEEP), 48, 49
Postanesthesia care record, 115-117
Postanesthesia care unit. See also Recovery room
Postanesthesia care unit (PACU)
 discharge, 115-117f
  by anesthesiologist, 109, 111f
  and Glasgow coma scale, 110f
 discharge criteria, 111-115f
  ASA, 104
  ASPAN, 104-105
  JCAH, 103-104
  use of numerical scoring systems, 105-109f
 discharge or transfer, 115-117f
 written discharge criteria, 111-113
Postanesthetic recovery room nurse, main functions of, 3-4
Postanesthetic recovery score (PARS), 5, 105, 108-109f
Postextubation croup, 128-129
Posttetanic potentiation, 8

Potassium
  content of gastrointestinal secretions, 75t
  daily intake, 73
  exchangeable, 72
  excretion in chronic renal disease, 187–188
  exogenous, 190
  normal serum level, 184
  serum concentrations, 73
  treatment of ATN, 196
  supplementation, 98
Preceptorship program
  clinical instructor, 285–286
  preceptor selection and training, 286–287
  weekly orientation outline, 287–291
Preoperative medication, 88t, 200
Preoperative state, 101
Pressure unit conversions, 338
Procainamide (Pronestyl), 231, 235t, 258
Procaine (Novocaine), 96, 171t
  effect on neuromuscular blockade, 91
  pharmacology, 18
Prochlorperazine (Compazine), 25, 258
Promethazine, 91
Promtehazine (Phenergan), 258
Propranolol (Inderal), 258
  and chronic renal disease, 188
  drug interactions, 91
  pediatric dosage, 143
  as second-line, 238t
  treatment
    of hypertension, 66–67, 163
    of tachycardia, 65, 68
    of Wolff-Parkinson-White syndrome, 65
Protamine sulfate, 258
Protein, 74, 88
Pruritus, 23
Pseudocholinesterase, atypical, 90
Pseudomonas, 44
Psychological factor(s)
  and pain perception, 134
  causing problems in burn patients, 145
Psychomotor learning, 297
Psychotropic drug(s), drug interactions, 91
Puerperium, 89, 90
Pulmonary artery
  balloon-tipped catheters, 57
  pressure, normal range, 8t
Pulmonary artery wedge pressure, 60f
Pulmonary aspiration
  in children, 129–131
  and respiratory insufficiency, 95
Pulmonary capillary pressure, 8t
Pulmonary capillary wedge pressure (PCWP), 192–193
Pulmonary compliance, 48
Pulmonary edema, 67, 75
  and cardiogenic shock, 59–60f
  cardioversion complication, 218t
  interstitial, 80
  and postoperative hypoxia, 35
  treatment, 60
Pulmonary embolism, 35
Pulmonary function test(s), 199, 200t
Pulse, 7, 8t, 337
Pulse monitor(s), 57, 59
Pulsus paradoxus, 206
Pupils, reflexes, 10
Pyridostigmine, 8
Pyrogens, 222

Quality assurance programs, 281, 282f
Quinidine, 216–217
  effect on neuromuscular blockade, 91

Racepinephrine, 45t
Rate-pressure product (RPP), 67–68
Record(s)
  postanesthesia care, 115–117
  recovery room, 274, 276–279f
Recovery room. *See also* Postanesthesia care unit
  central nurses' station, 255–256
  considerations after spinal and epidural anesthesia, 181t
  dividing walls, 256
  documentation, 274, 276–278f, 279f
  educational programs
    preceptor selection and training, 286–287
    role of clinical instructor, 285–286
    weekly outline, 287–291
  electrical safety, 261
  elevators, 266
  entrances and exits, 266
  equipment and supplies
    location, 256–262f
    in patient care unit, 263–264
  fire regulations and codes, 267–269
  fundamental purpose, 251
  individual patient care units, 263–264
  liabilities
    malpractice, 303–305
    nursing staff, 305–309
  monitoring of children, 126
  patient observation, 254–255
  personnel
    requirements, 271–274
    staffing pattern, 276f
    staffing patterns, 274
  physical structure
    general considerations, 252–256f
    configuration, 252–245f

Recovery room (*Continued*)
  physical support structures, 255
  plumbing, 261
  proximity of support services, 264-266
  quality assurance programs, 281, 282f
  and sensory bombardment, 262
  and sensory deprivation, 262
  as special procedures unit, 211
  standing orders and protocols, 277-278
  supply cabinets, 261
  transfer, 125-126
Recovery Room Nurses Association, 112
Recovery room orders, routine, 6f
Regional anesthesia, general considerations after, 169-170
Renal disease, chronic. *See also* Kidney(s)
  clinical symptomatology, 185-188
  dialysis, 190-191
  fluid therapy, 189-190
  laboratory evaluation, 183-184
  medications, 188-189
  monitoring, 190
Renal failure, and neuromuscular blockade, 9
Renal transplant, 196-197f
Reserpine, 91, 188
Respiratory acidosis, 34, 49, 339
Respiratory alkalosis, 91, 340
Respiratory system
  adequacy in lobectomy, 203-204
  assistance, 46-50
  of children, 122, 123t
  complications
    in children, 126-132
  depression
    in children, 129
    from epidural morphine, 181
    narcotic-induced, 92, 134
  distress, from spinal column surgery, 166-167
  dysfunction, 32-36t
  effects of spinal and epidural anesthesia, 178
  failure, 29-32
  postanesthesia scoring, 5, 108
  infection, 166
  insufficiency
    causes, 93t
    diagnostic criteria, 92, 93t
    in neurological patients, 160-161
    monitoring, 6-7t
  support, for children, 132-133
Restlessness, postoperative, 164-165
Retrolental fibroplasia, 203
Reye's syndrome, 131
Right atrial pressure, normal range, 8t
Right ventricular pressure, normal range, 8t

Ritalin (Methylphenidate), 95, 99t
Rule of nines, 144-145

Salicylate intoxication, 74
Saline, 22. *See also* Sodium
  balanced, 80
  postoperative administration, 76
  treatment of hyponatremia, 79
Saliva, 74, 75t
Salt tolerance, postoperative, 76
Secobarbital (Seconal), pediatric dosage, 142
Sedative(s), pediatric dosages, 142
Seizure(s), 164
Semicircle configuration, of recovery room, 253f
Sensory bombardment, 262
Sensory deprivation, 262
Septicemia, 65-66
Shivering, 200
  effect on oxygen consumption, 35-36
  following spinal and epidural anesthesia, 178
  postoperative, 95
Shock
  anion gap and, 74
  cardiogenic, 59-60f, 228
  decrease of cardiac output, 35
  endotoxin, 65-66
  hemorrhagic, 76-77
Shunting
  intrapulmonary or intracardiac, 29
  and ventilation/perfusion mismatch, 35
SIADH (syndrome of inappropriate antiduretic secretion), 97-98t, 186
SIMV (synchronous intermittent mandatory ventilation), 48
Skin reactions, allergic, 99t
Society of Anesthesiologists, 112
Sodium, 71
  content of gastrointestinal secretions, 75t
  exchangeable, 72
  intake
    in chronic renal disease, 185
    daily intake, 73
  loss, and dehydration, 75
  normal serum level, 184
  postoperative administration, 76
  renal fraction excretion (FE/Na), 194
  resorption indices, 194
  serum concentrations, 73
Sodium bicarbonate, 231, 233 *See also* Bicarbonate
  acidosis treatment, 187
  as first-line drug, 235t, 354
  pediatric dosage, 143

Sodium heparine, 258
Sodium nitroprusside (Nipride), 65, 259
    arterial pressure waveform, 54f
    contraindication, 189
    control of arterial pressure, 68
    and hypertensive emergency, 67
Sodium thiopental, 33, 88
Solbutamol (Albuterol), 45t
Somnolence, postanesthetic, 87
Special procedures unit, recovery room as, 211, 213-214
Specific gravity, urinary, 9, 184
Spinal anesthesia
    background physiology, 176-177
    continuous techniques, 181
    of different nerves, 177
    discharge criteria, 179
    vs. epidural anesthesia, 179, 180t
    headache, 177-178
    recovery room considerations, 181t
    respiratory effects, 178
    shivering, 178-179
Spinal column surgery, 165-167t
Spinal headache, 179
Sprinkler system(s), 269
Square configuration, of recovery room, 253-254f
Standard of care, 304-305
Standards and Guidelines for Cardiopulmonary Resuscitation (CPR), 225
Status asthmaticus, 131
Statute of limitation(s), 305
Stellate ganglion block, 219
Steroid(s), 96
Streptomycin, 91
Stretcher(s), patient care unit, 263
Subarachnoid block, 79, 218
Subarachnoid bolt, 145
Subglottic stenosis, 144
Succinylcholine (Anectine), 8, 258
    abnormal responses, 33-34
    ECT dosage, 216t
    laryngeal spasm treatment, 128
    for laryngospasm, 50
    postoperative paralysis and, 89-90
Sufentanil, 16
Supraventricular rhythm, with pulse, 352
Surgical intensive care unit (SICU), proximity to RR, 265-266
SVR (systemic vascular resistance), decreased, 65-66
Sweating, 82
Sympathetic nervous system blockage, 174, 175f
Synchronous intermittent mandatory ventilation (SIMV), 48

Tachycardia, 99t
    and arterial hypotension, 61-62
    and decreased SVR, 65-66
    junctional, 63f, 64-65
    sinus, 63-64
    ventricular, 69
    with hypertension, 67-68
Tachypnea, 205
Teaching aids, patient, 298-299
Technetium 99 pryophosphate infarct scintigram, 99
Telephone orders, failure in taking, 308
Temperature
    body, 96
        of children, 125, 135-138
        effect on muscle relaxants, 89
        and neurological patient, 164
        regulation of burn patient, 146
    conversion factors, 337
    of recovery room, 262
Tensilon (Edrophonium), 8, 90, 208, 258
Tent(s)
    face, 37, 39f
    oxygen or croup, 42, 44f
Tetanus, 67
Tetracaine (Pontocaine), 18, 171t
Tetracycline, 91, 188
Thermoregulatory dysfunction, 96
Thiocyanate, 189
Thoracic spine, epidural blockade, 26-27
Thymectomy, 207-208
Thyrotoxicosis, 67
Tidal volume, 6, 7t
Tigan (Trimethobenzamide), 258
Tobramycin, 91
Total body water (TBW), 71-72
Toxicity, of local anesthetics, 170-173
Trachea, of children, 121-122
Tracheostomym masks, 37, 40f
Train-of-four response, 8, 90
Tranquilizer(s), prolonged action, 88
Transfer of patient, 3-4
Transportation of patient(s), neurological, 150
Trans-urethral resection of prostrate (TURP), 79
Tranylcypromine, 91
Treacher Collin's syndrome, 144
Tricyclic antidepressant(s), 91
Trimethaphan, 65, 92
Trimethobenzamide (Tigan), 258
d-Tubocurarine (Curare), 8, 187, 258
    effect of temperature on, 89
    excretion, 190
    lithium and, 91
Tylenol (Acetaminophen), pediatric dosage, 142

Urea. *See also* Blood urea nitrogen (BUN)
 U/P ratio, 193
Urine
 decreased output, 75
 excretion in chronic renal disease, 186
 osmolality, 193
 production, 184
 specific gravity, 184, 193
 volume measurement, 9

Vaponefrine (Racepinephrine), 45t
Vascular resistance, systemic (SVR),
  decreased, 65-66
Vasodilator(s), 60, 65, 200
Vasopressin tannate, 98
Ventilation. *See also* Respiration
 arrest, from narcotics overdose, 23-24
 assistance, 47-48
 essentials of monitoring, 31t
 frequency, 22-23
 intraoperative, 99
 MV and ECF changes following, 78t
 support, 99t
Ventolin (Albuterol), 45t
Ventricular asystole, 233
Ventricular failure, acute left, 67
Ventricular fibrillation (VF), 232-233
 algorithm. 342-344
Ventricular tachycardia (VT), 232
 algorithm, 348-350
Venturi mask(s), 40-41, 43f
Verapamil, 231, 235t
 treatment of junctional tachycardia, 65
 treatment for Wolff-Parkinson-White
   syndrome, 65
Vital capacity measurement, 7
Vital sign(s), normal, 337
Vitamin K, 258
V/Q abnormality, 32

Wall(s), recovery room, 256, 268
Water
 endogenous, 81
 factors modifying requirements, 82
 loss, 74-75
 normal daily balance, 72-73
 overload, 186
 resorption indicies, 193
 total body (TBW), 71-72
Weight gain, due to fluids, 77
Wenkebach heart block, 63, 64f
Witness, expert, 304
Wolff-Parkinson-White syndrome, 65
Wyamine (Mephentermine), 258